Electrocardiographic Interpretation

A SELF-STUDY APPROACH
TO CLINICAL ELECTROCARDIOGRAPHY

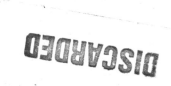

Electrocardiographic Interpretation

A SELF-STUDY APPROACH
TO CLINICAL ELECTROCARDIOGRAPHY

EMANUEL STEIN, M.D., M.P.H., F.A.C.P., F.A.C.C., F.C.C.P.
Director, Eastern Virginia Graduate School of Medicine and
    Associate Dean, Eastern Virginia Medical School
Professor of Internal Medicine and
Professor of Family and Community Medicine
    Eastern Virginia Medical School
    Norfolk, Virginia
Medical Director, United States Public Health Service, Ret.
Diplomate, American Board of Internal Medicine and
    Subspecialty Board of Cardiovascular Disease

Illustrations by THOMAS XENAKIS, M.A., A.M.I.

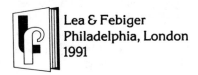 Lea & Febiger
Philadelphia, London
1991

Lea & Febiger
200 Chester Field Parkway
Malvern, Pennsylvania   19355
U.S.A.
(215)251-2230
1-800-638-0672

An audio cassette series consisting of 10 tapes geared to the didactic material in this manual is available from Lea & Febiger.
Call toll free 1-800-638-0672 for more information.

Library of Congress Cataloging-in-Publication Data
Stein, Emanuel
   Electrocardiographic interpretation: a self-study approach to clinical electrocardiography / Emanuel Stein; illustrations by Thomas Xenakis.
      p.   cm.
   Includes index.
   ISBN 0-8121-1378-0. — ISBN 0-8121-1380-2 (tapes). — ISBN (invalid) 0-8121-1379-0 (package)
   1. Electrocardiography—Programmed instruction. I. Title. [DNLM: 1. Electrocardiography—programmed instruction. WG 18 S819e]
RC683.5.E5S74   1991
616.1'207547—dc20
DNLM/DLC
for Library of Congress   90-13671
                                                                                          CIP

Reprints of chapters may be purchased from Lea & Febiger in quantities of 100 or more.

PRINTED IN THE UNITED STATES OF AMERICA

Print number: 5   4   3   2   1

TO THE MEMBERS OF THE
HEALTH PROFESSIONS

who will benefit from this effort
and from whom I continue to learn

FOREWORD

I am pleased to have the opportunity to write this short foreword to Dr. Stein's obviously first-class syllabus.

Two or three decades ago, electrocardiography was pronounced dead. Shortsighted as this pronouncement was, it had numerous adherents. But a number of bystanders have breathed new life into the supposed corpse, so that today, electrocardiography is not only alive and well but flourishes as never before. The electrocardiogram today is still the most often ordered cardiologic test, it is the most cost effective, the most often diagnostic and, alas, probably the most often misinterpreted.

During the past 25 years, electrocardiography has acquired numerous refinements, including the recognition of fascicular blocks, the early suspicions of myocardial infarction, the masking of infarction, and the numerous subvariants of AV block—to mention a few.

Moreover, the role of electrocardiography has been greatly expanded. It is, of course, the chief arbiter in exercise tests and Holter monitoring; it plays the part of indispensable referee for the timing of echocardiographic and nuclear studies; but most important is the way its stature has been enhanced by extrapolation from intracardiac recordings in the electrophysiologic laboratory—in much the same way that phonocardiography and attendant pulse tracings have enhanced and refined the bedside examination. Owing to this mutually beneficial partnership, it has been possible to confirm the validity of many of the morphologic clues for identifying the wide-QRS arrhythmias; and the type of narrow-QRS tachycardias often now can be identified in the clinical tracing thanks to correlation with electrophysiologic findings.

Dr. Stein's excellent course should contribute materially to diminishing the frequency of misinterpretation and to sustaining the diagnostic importance of electrocardiography.

Henry J.L. Marriott, M.D.
Director of Clinical Research
    Rogers Heart Foundation, Inc., St. Petersburg, Florida
Clinical Professor of Medicine (Cardiology)
    Emory University, Atlanta, Georgia
Clinical Professor of Pediatrics (Cardiology)
    University of Florida, Gainesville, Florida

P R E F A C E

The program of electrocardiographic interpretation consists of this manual, the cardiac vector analysis model, and 10 audio cassette tapes and is a complete fundamental course for the full understanding and proper interpretation of the clinical electrocardiogram. It is well balanced for a diverse group, including medical students, house officers, family physicians, noncardiologist internists, nurses, allied health personnel, and members of all other medical and surgical specialties.* The spatial vector approach of Grant† is emphasized. Various criteria, measurements, and "normal values" are given that may change as future knowledge accumulates. The vector concept, however, remains valid. During my training years my mentors were Dr. Ira L. Rubin, Dr. John B. Schwedel, and Dr. Sidney P. Schwartz. Dr. Schwartz had been interested in electrocardiography from his early interning days and made available to me, with characteristic grace, his dearly cherished and carefully preserved collection of electrocardiograms dating back more than a half century. Some of these are included in this work. The three world-renowned cardiologists who have influenced my teaching of electrocardiography are Dr. Robert P. Grant, Dr. Henry J.L. Marriott, and Dr. Leo Schamroth. I am honored to be able to impart some of their scholarship in this fundamental course.

The requirements for the mastery of this subject include diligence, application, patience, and perseverance. This is one area of knowledge where you will learn by doing. Many, both physicians and nonphysicians, have become proficient electrocardiographers. Paramount are your interest and determination.

I am grateful to my distinguished colleague and friend, Dr. Henry J.L. Marriott, for reviewing the course and writing the Foreword, and to Dr. William Fox,‡ Dr. David B. Propert, Dr. Robert D. Patton, Dr. Stephen P. Swersie, Dr. Arnold B. Barr, Mr. Mark A. Belcher, Mr. Charles R. Portner, Mr. John Moscoffian, Ms. Pamela Moscoffian Blake, Dr. Stephen L. Daniel, Ms. Elaine Halverson, and the talented artist, Mr. Thomas Xenakis, for their contributions, which have enriched this work. Special thanks to Mr. R. Kenneth Bussy, Mr. Samuel Rondinelli, Mrs. Tanya Lazar, and Mrs. Holly C. Lukens of Lea & Febiger for their help in making this edition possible.

Norfolk, Virginia   Emanuel Stein, M.D.

---

*This program is the outgrowth of teaching clinical electrocardiography for many years and was recorded earlier for W.B. Saunders, Philadelphia, and the Health Sciences Consortium, Chapel Hill, NC.
†Beckwith, J.R.: Grant's Clinical Electrocardiography, 2nd Ed. New York, McGraw-Hill, 1970.
‡Fox, W., and Stein, E.: Cardiac Rhythm Disturbances, a Step-by-Step Approach. Philadelphia, Lea & Febiger, 1983.

HOW TO USE THIS BOOK
AND THE CORRESPONDING
CASSETTE TAPES

Each of the eight chapters starts with objectives and a pretest. The pretest will help determine how much you already know about specific areas in clinical electrocardiography. Each chapter also has a post-test or tests for self-evaluation. In addition, the first chapter, covering basic concepts and the normal electrocardiogram, has review questions with specific instructions provided. After answering each set of review questions, you should check your responses immediately on the pages indicated. Illustrations relevant to the pretests, post-tests, and review questions are presented in their appropriate sections as well as in the text. For additional self-assessment, a course post-test is included. At the end of the chapters, notes and references have been added. Solutions to the pretests, post-tests, and course post-test are indicated in the manual and/or are presented on the tapes.

Important features are stressed by repeated emphasis. The manual can be used as an introduction, a review, or a study guide. The cassette tapes should be used in concert with the manual, as the illustrations are examined in a formal sequence.

This combination of the manual/workbook, cassette tapes, and vector analysis model is as close as possible to my actual course in electrocardiographic interpretation. Every effort was made to preserve the flavor of the seminars. A few times during the many hours of instruction, I stood too close to the microphone; at other times, a little too far away. It may be necessary, therefore, to adjust the volume of the tape accordingly. To fit the actual tape time within an 8-hour time frame, repetitive material was removed from the original tapes. Occasionally, a few sentences have been added for clarity. PLEASE NOTE: After you have completed side 1 of each tape, DO NOT ADVANCE THE TAPE, but turn to side 2 immediately. Side 2 has been set to begin where side 1 ends.

C O N T E N T S

1

BASIC CONCEPTS AND
THE NORMAL ELECTROCARDIOGRAM

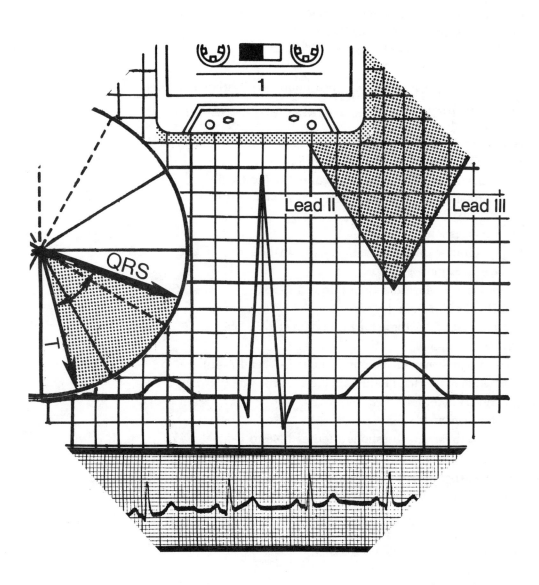

CHAPTER 1

INTRODUCTION

This chapter is the first in the eight-part program. Topics discussed are the formation of the electrocardiographic leads, depolarization, repolarization and the conduction system of the heart, the cardiac vectors in the frontal and horizontal planes, determination of the heart rate, and analysis of electrocardiograms. Numerous electrocardiograms have been included for review and practice. In the remaining chapters you will study right ventricular hypertrophy including right and left atrial enlargement, left ventricular hypertrophy, repolarization (S-T segment and T wave) alterations, myocardial infarction, ventricular conduction disturbances, arrhythmias, and digitalis.

O B J E C T I V E S

Upon completion of this chapter, you should be able to:

1. State the extremities and the polarities which comprise the electrocardiographic leads.

2. Draw the Einthoven triangle and label its components.

3. State the summations of the leads in the frontal plane (I, II, III, aVR, aVL, aVF).

4. Label a diagram of the hexaxial system with the appropriate leads and degrees.

5. Label a diagram with electrocardiographic waves, intervals, and segments.

6. Determine the mean QRS vector in the frontal plane.

7. Determine the normal range for the mean QRS vector.

8. State what is meant by abnormal left axis deviation (LAD).

9. State what is meant by abnormal right axis deviation (RAD).

10. Determine the mean T vector in the frontal plane.

11. Determine the QRS-T angle in the frontal plane.

12. Determine the mean P vector in the frontal plane.

13. Determine the heart rate from the electrocardiogram.

14. State the definition of sinus rhythm.

15. Determine the mean spatial QRS vector in three dimensions.

16. Analyze the normal electrocardiogram.

P R E T E S T

DIRECTIONS. This pretest consists of ten questions. Answer each in the space provided.

1. Draw and fully label the Einthoven triangle.

2. State the summation of leads I, II, and III.

3. State the summation of leads aVR, aVL, and aVF.

4. Place the appropriate leads and degrees on the following diagram.

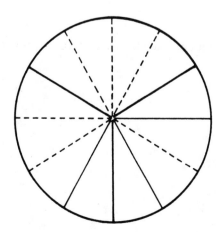

5. Label the electrocardiographic waves, intervals, and segments on the diagram below.

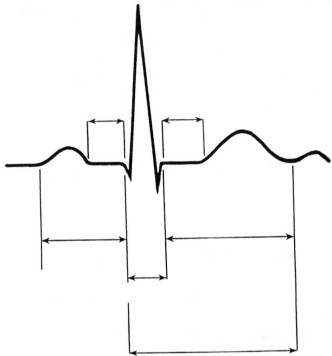

6. What is meant by abnormal left axis deviation (LAD) of the mean QRS vector?

7. What is meant by abnormal right axis deviation (RAD) of the mean QRS vector?

8. Determine the mean P vector of the following electrocardiogram.

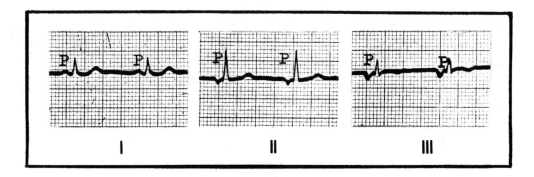

FIGURE 1-44.

9. Determine the QRS-T angle (frontal plane) of the following electrocardiogram.

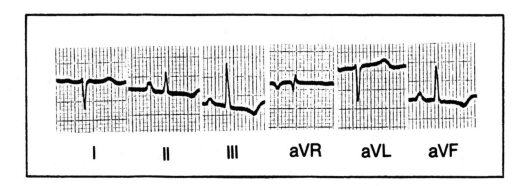

FIGURE 1-49.

10. Analyze the following electrocardiogram.

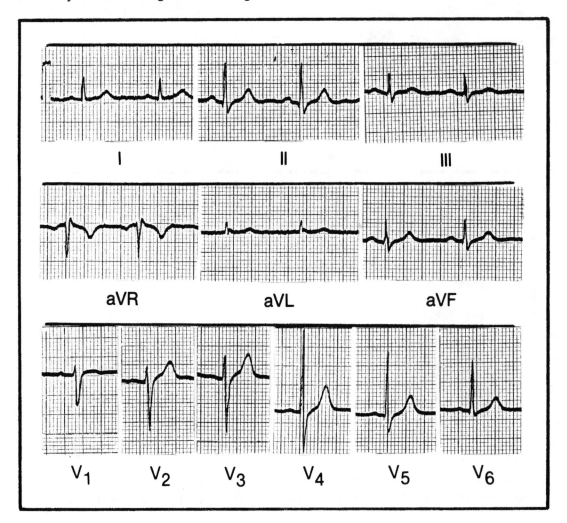

FIGURE 1-78.

Analysis:

> The answers to the pretest will be found on pages 114 to 116.

> When you have completed the pretest, start Cassette Side 1 and continue on the next page.

CASSETTE SIDE 1
Running Time: 27 minutes

100   50   0

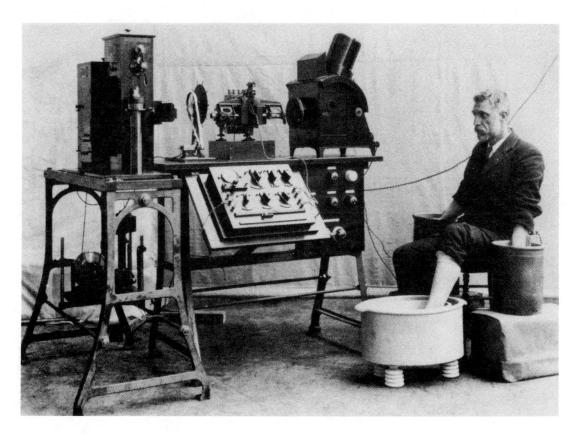

FIGURE 1-1.   Original Cambridge electrocardiograph (1912), built for Sir Thomas Lewis. Produced under agreement with Prof. Willem Einthoven, the father of electrocardiography. It wasn't always easy to take electro-cardiograms. The gentleman whose electrocardiogram is being recorded had both arms and left leg in containers of conducting solution. The electrodes were not directly attached to the patient. (Courtesy of Cambridge Instrument Company, New York.)

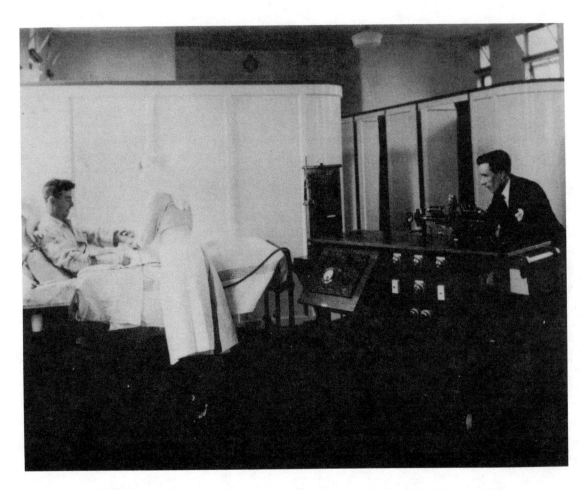

FIGURE 1-2.   *Early electrocardiographic equipment. This machine, of a later date, was still far removed from the streamlined models in use today. Here, however, the electrodes are attached to the patient, avoiding the necessity of containers of conducting solution. (Courtesy of Cambridge Instrument Company, New York.)*

FORMATION OF THE ELECTROCARDIOGRAPHIC LEADS

William Einthoven, who had worked with the string galvanometer, is known as the father of electrocardiography. The galvanometer, which is basic to all electrocardiographs, consists of a movable writing element within a magnetic field. A wire is connected to each end—one the positive electrode and the other the negative electrode. The difference in potential between the two poles can be measured by use of this instrument. When the two electrodes are placed on different positions on the body, the positive electrode on one extremity and the negative on another, they form what is known as a lead. The deflection which is recorded for each lead is a manifestation, at the body surface, of the electrical activity of the heart seen from the vantage point of that particular lead. In this section, the development of the Einthoven triangle, the triaxial and hexaxial systems, and the electrical truths of electrocardiography are discussed.

A. The Einthoven Triangle

Einthoven found that by connecting the right arm to the negative electrode and the left arm to the positive electrode, and inducing a current to flow, a certain deflection was recorded by the galvanometer; this is called lead I (Figure 1-3).

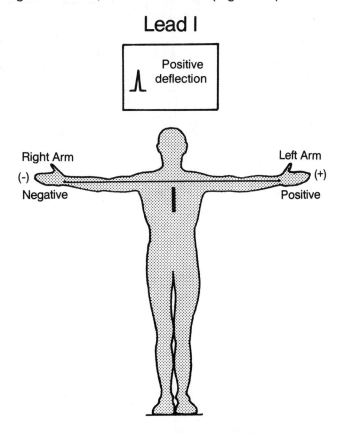

FIGURE 1-3.   Formation of lead I.

By connecting the left arm with the left leg, the left arm to the negative electrode and the left leg to the positive electrode, Einthoven recorded another positive deflection with the galvanometer; this is known as lead III (Figure 1-4).

Lead III

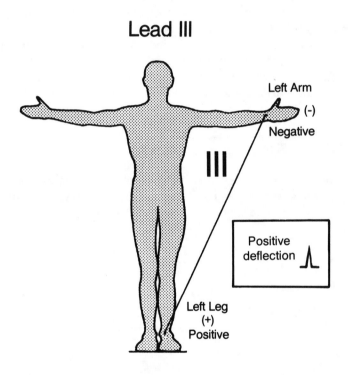

FIGURE 1-4.   Formation of lead III.

In Figure 1-5 we see the original lead II. The information presented in Figures 1-5 and 1-6 is *not* correct today. It is included for the basic understanding of lead development.

By connecting the right arm and the left leg, the right arm to the positive electrode and the left leg to the negative electrode, Einthoven recorded a large negative deflection (Figure 1-5).

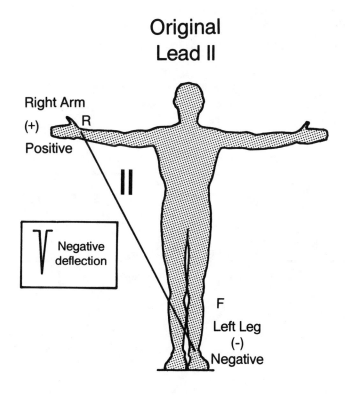

FIGURE 1-5.   Formation of the original lead II. This was to be corrected
later; see Figure 1-7.

In Figure 1-6A, Figures 1-3, 1-4 and 1-5 are brought together into a triangle, the *original* Einthoven triangle. Inspection of the triangle reveals a positive (+) charge and a negative (−) charge at each of the angles. The summation of the deflections also becomes apparent. If the triangle were to remain as indicated it should be noted that since:

   a. the deflection in lead I =   5 mm.
   b. the deflection in lead III =   5 mm.
   c. the deflection in lead II = − 10 mm.
       the summation would be 0

and, therefore, leads I + III + II would equal 0.

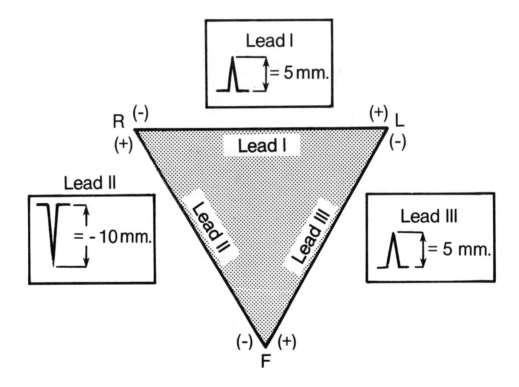

FIGURE 1-6A.   The original *Einthoven triangle.*

In measuring the potentials, Einthoven originally started at the right arm, measuring first lead I, then lead III, then lead II, returning to the right arm (Figure 1-6B). The vectorial sum of these potentials measured consecutively and returning to the point of origin equals 0. It would be as if you had traveled around the entire world and returned to your point of origin. You would have traveled much but without any displacement. Einthoven, however, made a major change; he reversed the polarity of lead II (Figure 1-7). According to Grant, it may be that he was not happy with a large negative deflection in lead II. By reversing the polarity of lead II—by making the right arm *negative* and the left leg *positive*—a positive deflection, of the same magnitude, resulted in lead II.

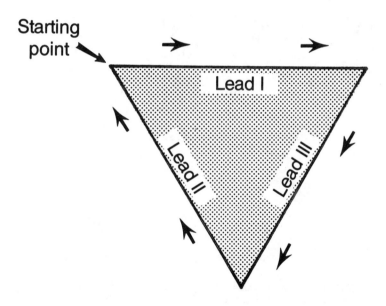

FIGURE 1-6B.   *Summation of the leads in the* original *Einthoven triangle.*

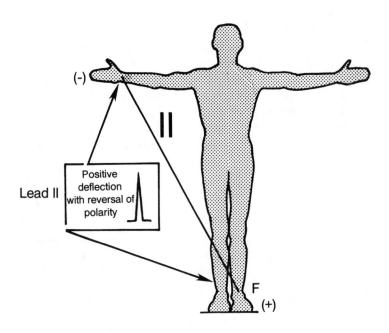

*FIGURE 1-7.   Lead II as known today. The positive is at the left leg
and the negative is at the right arm, following reversal of polarity.*

By reversing the polarity of lead II, a new relationship was established. We no longer
have the equation: leads I + III + II = 0. Note that since:

    a.   the deflection in lead I   =   5 mm.,
    b.   the deflection in lead III =   5 mm., and
    c.   the deflection in lead II   = 10 mm.

the summation is as follows:

lead I + lead III = lead II

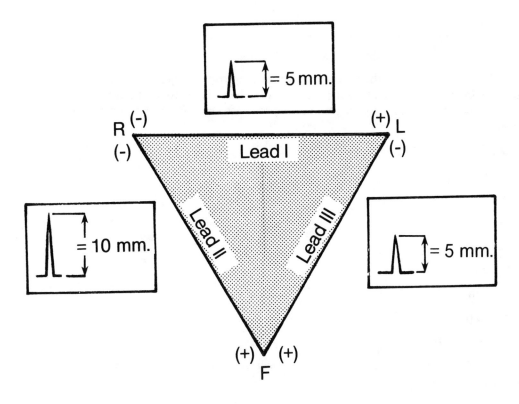

FIGURE 1-8.   The Einthoven triangle as known today.

This is an electrical truth (lead I + lead III = lead II) which always holds for the *areas* encompassed by each and every electrocardiographic deflection. We have used the heights and depths of the deflections as a good approximation.

Several assumptions are made in using the Einthoven triangle which are not strictly true. Note that:

  a.   The heart is not within a uniform volume conductor.
  b.   The leads do not form a true equilateral triangle.
  c.   The heart is not in the center of the triangle.

These, however, do not detract from the value of the Einthoven triangle in helping us to understand clinical electrocardiography.

> After you have reviewed the material you have just studied, stop the tape, and answer the following review questions.

Review Questions

DIRECTIONS. For each of the following bipolar, electrocardiographic leads, write the extremity in the space provided, and indicate whether it is positive (+) or negative (−) according to current usage by placing the appropriate sign after the name of the extremity.

1. Lead I

    a. extremity:

    b. extremity:

2. Lead II

    a. extremity:

    b. extremity:

3. Lead III

    a. extremity:

    b. extremity:

DIRECTIONS. Draw the Einthoven triangle, as it is known today, label its leads, and indicate their polarities.

4.

Check your responses to these review questions on page 117 and continue reading in this guide and listening to the tape.

B. Conversion of the Einthoven Triangle to a Triaxial System

In order to assign degrees, as presently used in electrocardiography, the Einthoven triangle (Figure 1-9A) may be converted into a triaxial system (Figure 1-9B) by bringing the sides of the triangle to the common center. The solid lines represent the positive half of each lead while the broken lines represent the negative half.

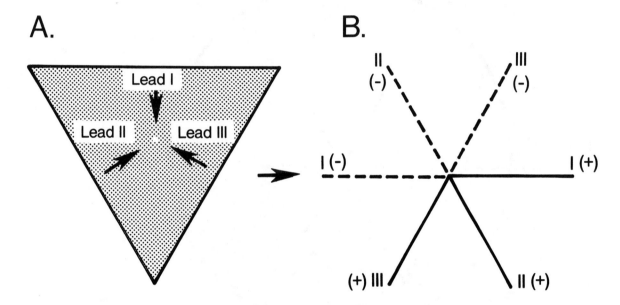

FIGURE 1-9.   The Einthoven triangle (A) converted into a triaxial system (B).

In assigning degrees to the triaxial reference system the axes are 60° apart (Figure 1-10). The positions of the positives and negatives remain as in the Einthoven triangle (Figure 1-8).

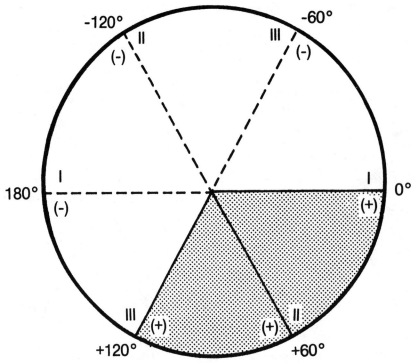

FIGURE 1-10. *Assignment degrees. The solid line represents the positive half of each lead; the broken line represents the negative half.*

In Figure 1-11 we have a further elaboration of the positive, negative, and transitional zones of leads I, II, and III. In Figure 1-11A positive lead I is indicated by the solid line at 0° and negative lead I by the broken line at 180°. Perpendicular to this line is the *transitional* zone of lead I. Lead I is most positive at the extreme left and most negative at the extreme right. As you approach the center from the positive and from the negative, there is decreasing positivity and negativity, respectively. At the center of the circle, forming an angle of 90° with lead I, is the transitional zone, as noted previously, the zone of null, which is neither positive nor negative (arrows). It divides the circle into two parts, one half positive and one half negative. The positive, negative, and transitional zones of leads II and III are seen in Figure 1-11B and C, respectively.

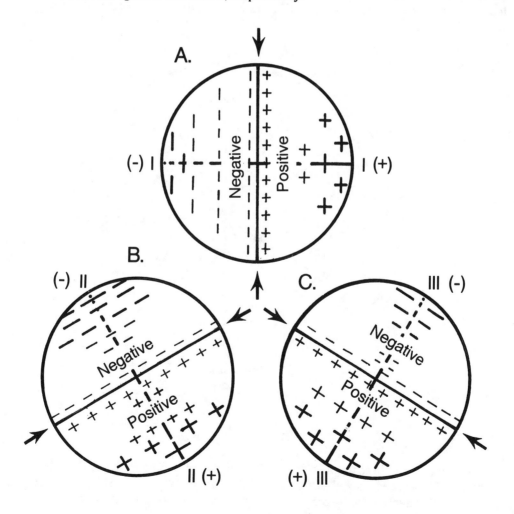

FIGURE 1-11.   *Positive, negative, and transitional zones of leads I, II, and III. The transitional zones are indicated by the arrows. Note the decreasing positivity and negativity as the transitional zone is approached.*

C. *Formation of the Hexaxial System*

Up to now we have been studying three leads, I, II, and III. These are the *bipolar* extremity leads; each lead makes use of *two* extremities, both arms for lead I, the right arm and left leg for lead II, and the left arm and left leg for lead III. For many years these were the principal leads used in electrocardiography. In time other leads were added and became generally accepted. Among these were the *unipolar* extremity leads; only one pole, the *positive,* is attached to the right arm, left arm, and left leg. The negative pole is attached to a central terminal. The letter V refers to these unipolar leads as well as to the precordial unipolar leads to be studied later. The extremity unipolar leads were known as VR (right arm), VL (left arm), and VF (left leg). Following augmentation to produce larger deflections they are now known, respectively, as *aVR, aVL,* and *aVF.* By adding these leads to the triaxial system (Figure 1-10), a hexaxial system is formed. This is summarized in Figure 1-12.

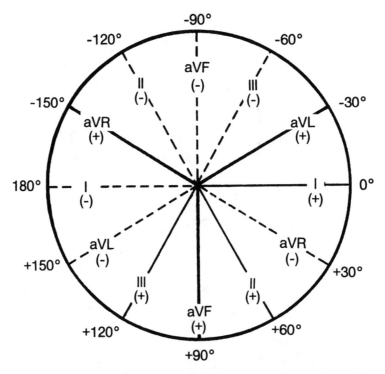

FIGURE 1-12. Formation of the hexaxial system.

The addition of the three unipolar leads, aVR, aVL, and aVF, to the triaxial system (see Figure 1-10) forms a hexaxial system containing six leads. The solid line represents the positive half of each lead; the broken line represents the negative half. The part of the circle most frequently dealt with in clinical electrocardiography contains:

positive aVL	−30°
positive I	0°
negative aVR	+30°
positive II	+60°
positive aVF	+90°
positive III	+120°

Note that negative aVR at +30° is used. Positive aVR is at −150°, not in the part of the circle that is normally used.

We have seen that leads I + III = lead II. The rule for leads aVR, aVL, and aVF is as follows: leads aVR + aVL + aVF = 0. There was no reversal of polarity, as occurred in lead II.

Each of the leads, *with the exception of aVR,* has its positive pole in the part of the circle from −30° to +120°. The positive pole of lead aVR is at −150°, which is outside the part of the circle normally utilized. Negative aVR at +30° is, therefore, frequently used in electrocardiographic evaluation.

In Figure 1-8 the summation for the bipolar extremity leads was shown to be

$$lead\,I + lead\,III = lead\,II$$

The summation for the unipolar extremity leads is as follows:

$$leads\,aVR + aVL + aVF = 0$$

Refer back to the discussion on the reversal of polarity in lead II. There was no such reversal of polarity for the unipolar extremity leads.

These relationships are of importance in the evaluation of every electrocardiogram and will be described in Figures 1-13 to 1-20.

D. Practice Electrocardiograms

Figures 1-13 through 1-20 are provided in order to illustrate the electrical truths:

$$\text{leads I + III = lead II}$$
$$\text{leads aVR + aVL + aVF = 0}$$

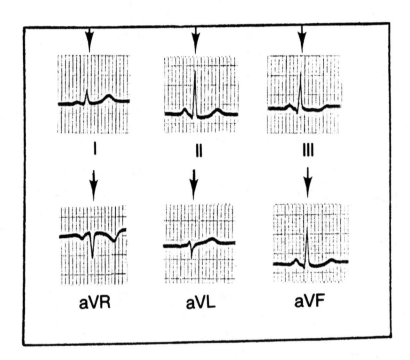

FIGURE 1-13.   The deflection in lead I (arrow) is approximately 3 mm. tall and the deflection in lead III is 9 mm. tall.

Using the rule that

$$\text{leads I + III = lead II}$$

the lead II deflection must be 12 mm. tall. Any time you have two leads, you should be able to solve for the third. The deflection in lead aVR is 6 mm. deep and the deflection in lead aVL is 4 mm. deep. Using the rule that

$$\text{leads aVR + aVL + aVF = 0}$$

the lead aVF deflection must be approximately 10 mm. tall.

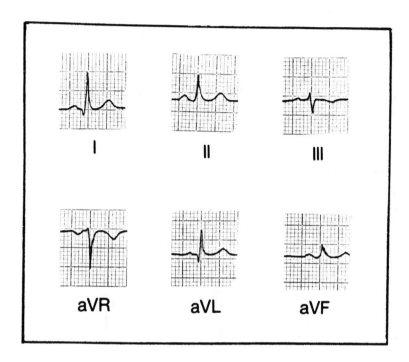

FIGURE 1-14.   *Lead I is taller than lead II; therefore lead III must be negative. Lead aVR is deeper than aVL is tall; therefore, aVF must be small but positive.*

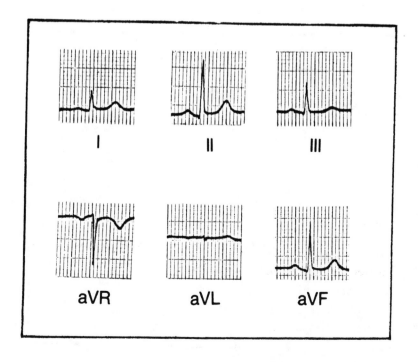

FIGURE 1-15.   *Leads I + III = lead II. Lead aVR is as deep as aVF is tall; therefore aVL must summate to 0, since leads aVR + aVL + aVF = 0.*

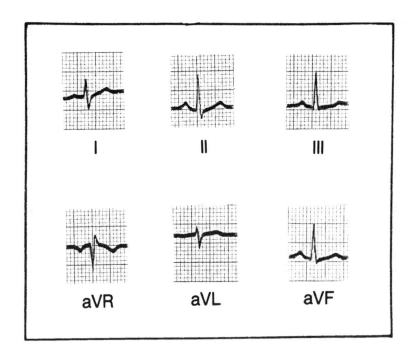

FIGURE 1-16. *Lead II is approximately equal to lead III; therefore, lead I must summate to approximately 0. Lead aVF is slightly taller than aVR is deep; therefore, aVL is slightly more negative than positive.*

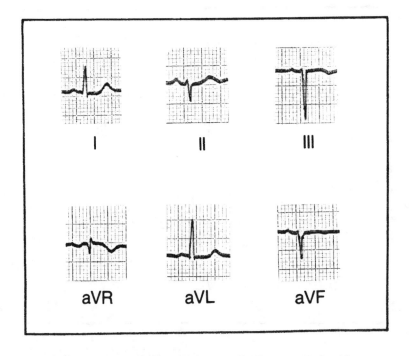

FIGURE 1-17. *Lead I is less positive than lead III is negative. Lead II must then be negative. The negative aVR plus the negative aVF plus the positive aVL equal 0.*

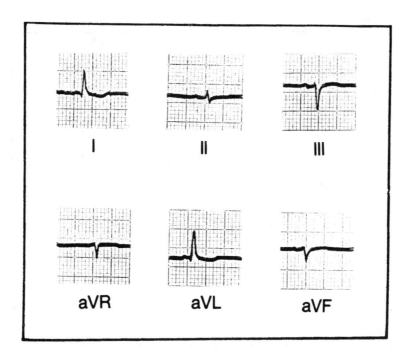

FIGURE 1-18.   *Lead II is small and equiphasic; lead I is then as positive as lead III is negative. Lead aVL is as positive as aVR plus aVF are negative.*

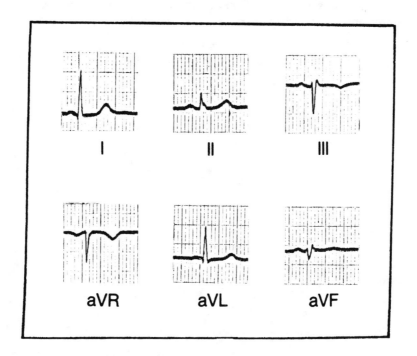

FIGURE 1-19.   *Lead III is less negative than lead I is positive. Lead II must then be smaller than lead I, but positive. The negative aVR plus the negative aVF plus the positive aVL equal 0.*

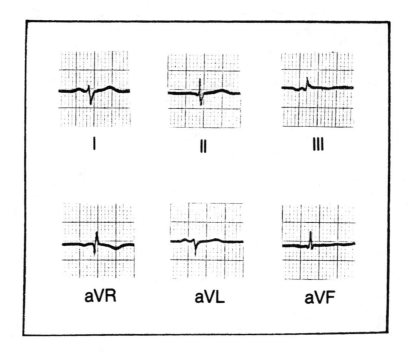

FIGURE 1-20.

To reemphasize, for convenience we have been using the height and depth of the deflections for summation; this gives a good approximation. Actually, for more accurate summation, the area encompassed by the deflections may be used. The rules again:

$$\text{Leads I + III = lead II}$$
$$\text{Leads aVR + aVL + aVF = 0}$$

> After you have reviewed the material you have just studied, stop the tape and answer the review questions on the next page.

Review Questions

DIRECTIONS. Provide the information requested in each of the following:

1. Place the appropriate leads and degrees on the following diagram.

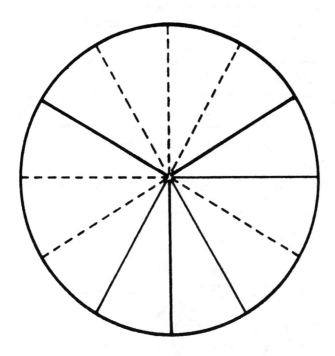

2. State the summation of leads I, II, and III.

3. State the summation of leads aVR, aVL, and aVF.

> Check your responses to these review questions on page 118, and continue reading in this guide and listening to the tape.

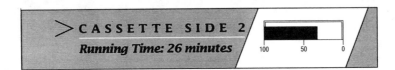

> CASSETTE SIDE 2
> *Running Time: 26 minutes*
> 100   50   0

DEPOLARIZATION, REPOLARIZA-TION, AND THE CONDUCTION SYSTEM OF THE HEART

Positive and negative ions line up on opposite sides of the semipermeable membrane which is found in all excitable tissue, including of course, the heart. If a change occurs in the state of the semipermeable membrane, the ions then may cross. The state when the ions are lined up on their respective sides is the *polarized* state. *Depolarization* refers to the state when the ions have crossed the semipermeable membrane. The process of restoring them to the proper side of the semipermeable membrane is the process of *repolarization.*

The normal site of impulse formation in the heart is the sinoatrial (S-A) node (Figure 1-21). The atria are then depolarized, resulting in the P wave on the electrocardiogram. There is much ongoing research in the area of the specialized conduction system of the atria. The impulse then spreads through the atrioventricular (A-V) node and bundle of His to the left and right bundle branches and then to the ventricular muscle through the Purkinje network. Ventricular depolarization results in the inscription of the QRS complex on the electrocardiogram.

The S-T segment and T wave represent the repolarization of the ventricles (Figure 1-22). Repolarization of the atria is usually obscured on the electrocardiogram by the small size of the waves and by the proximity of the QRS complex.

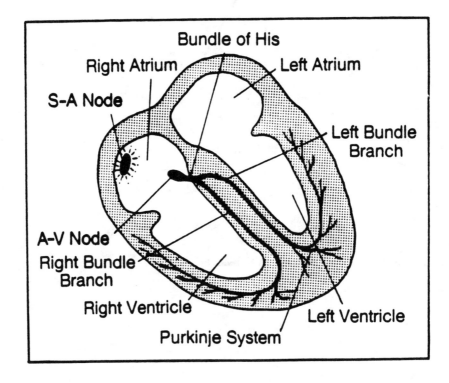

FIGURE 1-21.   Conduction system of the heart.

TABLE 1-1.   Electrocardiographic Waves, Intervals, and Segments
(Refer to Figure 1-22)

P Wave	Produced by the depolarization of the atria
QRS Complex	Produced by the depolarization of the ventricles
Q Wave	The initial negative deflection of the QRS complex preceding the R wave
R Wave	The initial positive deflection of the QRS complex
S Wave	A negative deflection following the R wave and usually the terminal portion of the QRS complex; a second positive deflection (following the S wave) is called an R′ wave, which in turn may be followed by a negative S′ wave
QS Complex	QS complex means that there is no R wave; the entire ventricular complex is negative
T Wave	Produced by the repolarization of the ventricles
U Wave	Follows the T wave; its clinical significance will be illustrated in Chapter 4
P-R Interval	From the beginning of the P wave to the beginning of the QRS complex; when a Q wave is present, the interval may be called a P-Q interval
P-R Segment	From the end of the P wave to the beginning of the QRS complex
QRS Interval	From the beginning of the Q wave to the end of the S wave
S-T Segment	From the end of the S wave to the beginning of the T wave representing the early phase of ventricular repolarization
S-T Interval	From the end of the S wave to the end of the T wave representing the repolarization of the ventricles
Q-T Interval	From the beginning of the QRS complex to the end of the T wave

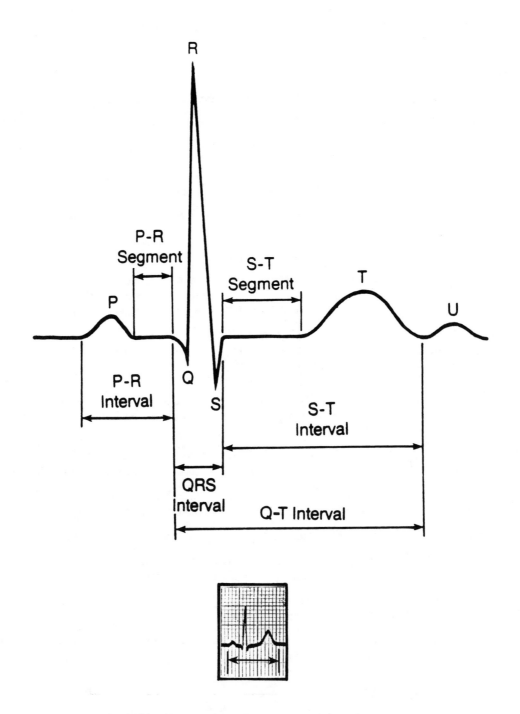

FIGURE 1-22. Electrocardiographic waves, intervals, and segments.

> Examples of types of ventricular complexes are presented on page 122.

> After you have reviewed the material you have just studied, stop the tape and answer the review questions on the next page.

Review Questions

DIRECTIONS. Label the electrocardiographic waves, intervals, and segments.

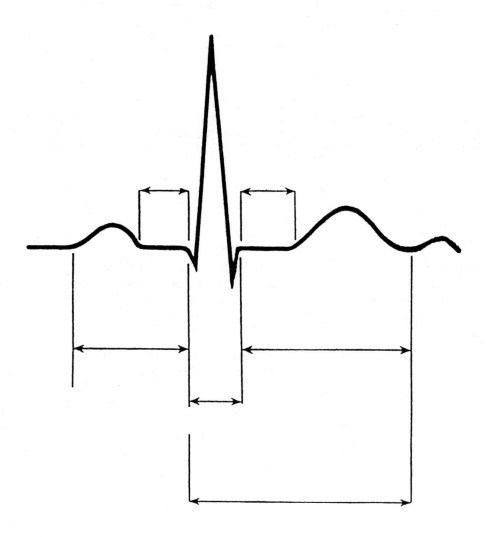

> Check your responses to these review questions on page 32 or 119, and continue
> reading in this guide and listening to the tape.

THE CARDIAC
VECTORS

Electrical forces can be considered vector quantities. (The properties of a vector are magnitude, direction, and sense or polarity. By convention the arrow of the vector is in the positive field.) A vector is represented by an arrow where both size and orientation are easily demonstrated. Let us relate this to the inscription of a single normal QRS complex on the electrocardiogram (Figure 1-23A) within a period of 0.08 sec. (The normal QRS interval, from the beginning of the Q wave to the end of the S wave, does not exceed 0.10 sec.) Figure 1-23B illustrates the sequential instantaneous vectors generated during this single QRS cycle. The greater the muscle mass, the bigger will be the arrow. The magnitude and orientation of the vector will be determined from the position of the heart and the muscle mass and the electrical and conductive properties of the heart. When we connect the arrows, which were drawn as if they arose from the same point of origin, we have what is known as the QRS loop (Figure 1-23C). The *mean QRS vector* is the vectorial sum of all the instantaneous vectors within a single QRS cycle (Figure 1-23D). We will often refer to the mean QRS vector, mean T vector, and mean P vector in our study of electrocardiography. You may hear, because of common usage, the term "mean electrical axis" of the QRS, T, and P when referring to the mean QRS, T, and P vectors, respectively.

A. Determination of the Mean QRS
Vector in the Frontal Plane

The mean QRS vector is a major determinant of the normality or abnormality of the electrocardiogram. In the following series of electrocardiograms we will determine the mean QRS vector in the *frontal plane*. (Leads I, II, III, aVR, aVL, and aVF represent electrical activity in the frontal plane. The boundaries of the frontal plane are illustrated in Figure 1-54.)

Prior to starting, this would be a good place to review the Einthoven triangle, the positive, negative, and transitional zones of the leads, and the "lineup" of the leads around the circle (Figures 1-8 and 1-10 to 1-12).

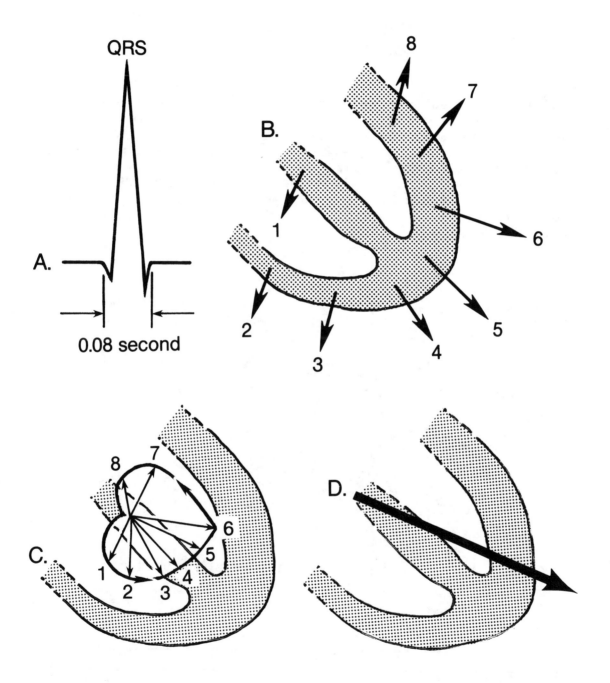

FIGURE 1-23.   A, Inscription of a single normal QRS complex (0.08 sec.). B, Sequential instantaneous vectors generated during this single QRS cycle. C, QRS loop results when we connect the arrows which were drawn as if they arose from the same point of origin. D, Mean QRS vector which is the vectorial sum of all the instantaneous vectors within a single QRS cycle.

In Figure 1-24 let us examine the electrocardiogram as to the positivity and negativity of each QRS complex. In lead I the QRS is positive and is so indicated on the circle next to lead I at 0°. Lead II is also positive, as is lead III. *Negative* aVR is also positive. When lining up the leads remember that *negative* aVR is at +30°; lead aVR must then be inverted before being placed on the circle. Lead aVL is neither predominantly positive nor predominantly negative; it is a transitional lead. Lead aVF is positive. The transition is through lead aVL. The *mean QRS vector* is at right angles to the transitional zone on the positive side. In this electrocardiogram the *transitional* zone is at −30° and the *mean QRS vector* is at 60°.

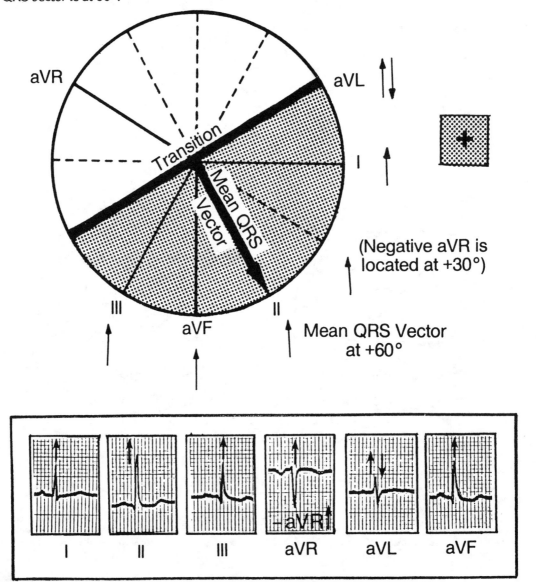

FIGURE 1-24.   *Determination of the transitional zone and mean QRS vector.*

In Figure 1-25 lead I is positive, II and III are negative, while *negative* aVR and aVL are positive. Lead aVF is negative. The transitional zone is somewhere between 30 and 60°, with the mean QRS vector at right angles to the transition, on the positive side, beyond −30°. All the positive QRS complexes are in the positive half of the circle and all the negative QRS complexes are in the negative half of the circle. The positive half is the upper part of the circle; hence the mean QRS vector is within this half.

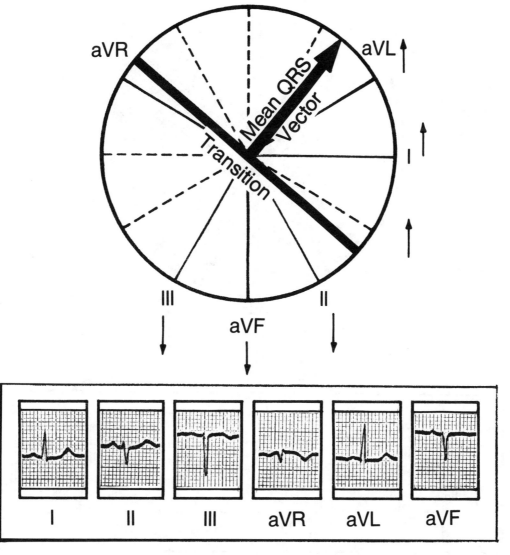

FIGURE 1-25. Mean QRS vector beyond −30°.

In Figure 1-26 all the QRS complexes are positive. The transitional zone must then bypass all six leads so that all the leads fall within the positive half of the circle. The mean QRS vector, at right angles to the transition, on the positive side, is approximately 45°.

The use of the positivity and negativity of the QRS complexes is a good approximation. The exact measurement of the *area* under each deflection would not be practical in a clinical setting.

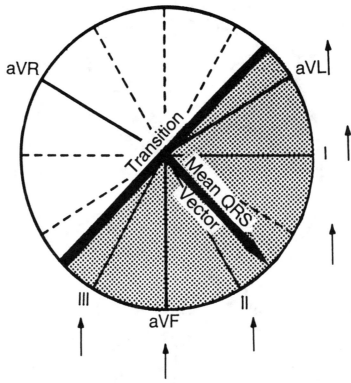

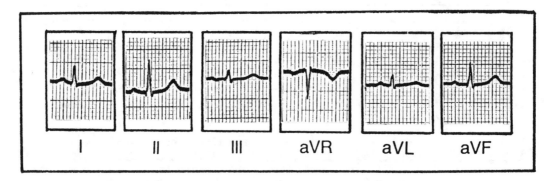

FIGURE 1-26.   Mean QRS vector at approximately 45°.

To determine the mean QRS vector in the frontal plane, the following should be done sequentially.

1. Line up all six leads on the circle from −30 to +120°. Lead aVR must be inverted at +30°.

2. Draw the transition, dividing the circle into positive and negative halves.

3. The mean QRS vector is at right angles to the transition on the positive side.

> At this point stop the tape. The mean QRS vector was studied in three electrocardiograms (Figures 1-24 to 1-26), and the steps used in this determination were outlined. The following electrocardiograms (Figures 1-27 to 1-35) are presented for your evaluation. Determine the mean QRS vector in each electrocardiogram. Do not forget to invert lead aVR since we are dealing with negative aVR at +30°.

Review Questions

DIRECTIONS. Below are nine electrocardiograms. Determine for each the mean QRS vector in the frontal plane.

1.

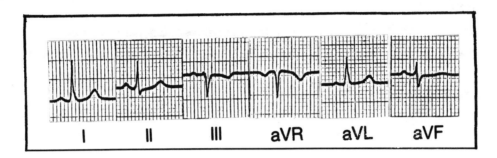

FIGURE 1-27.

Mean QRS vector:

2.

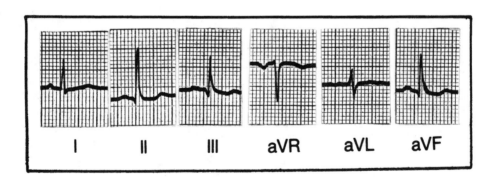

FIGURE 1-28.

Mean QRS vector:

3.

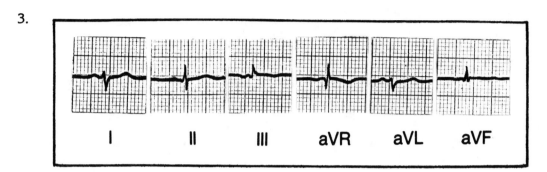

FIGURE 1-29.

Mean QRS vector:

4.

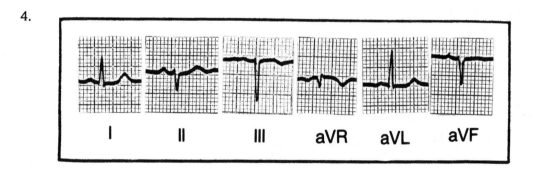

FIGURE 1-30.

Mean QRS vector:

5.

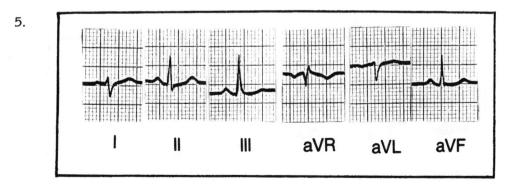

FIGURE 1-31.

Mean QRS vector:

6.

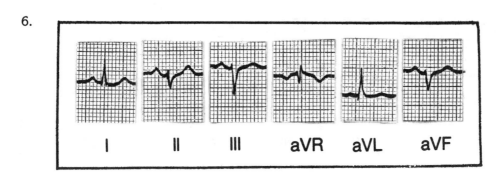

FIGURE 1-32.

Mean QRS vector:

7.

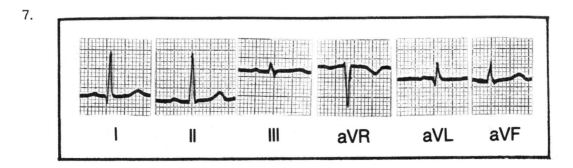

FIGURE 1-33.

Mean QRS vector:

8.

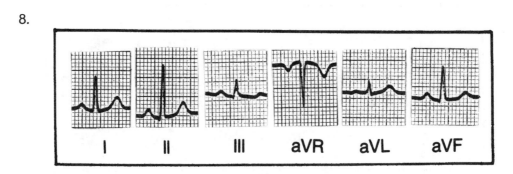

FIGURE 1-34.

Mean QRS vector:

9.

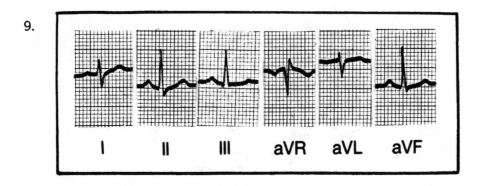

FIGURE 1-35.

Mean QRS vector:

After determining the mean QRS vector in Figures 1-27 through 1-35, restart the tape and listen to the solutions. The analyses are presented in this guide on the following pages. The answers may also be found on page 120.

Solutions to Review Questions
(Figures 1-27 to 1-35)

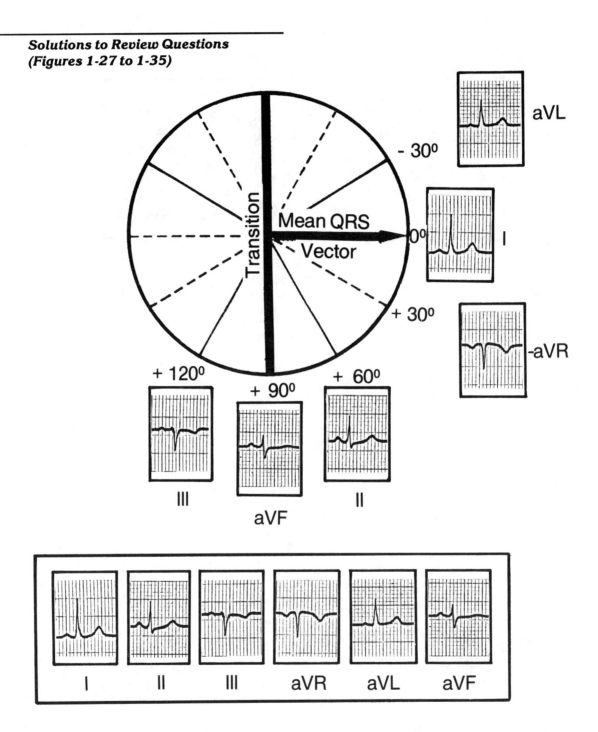

FIGURE 1-27.

Leads aVL, I, − aVR, and II are positive and lead III is negative. Lead aVF is transitional. We draw the transition at aVF, and the mean QRS vector is perpendicular to the transition, on the positive side (lead I at 0°).

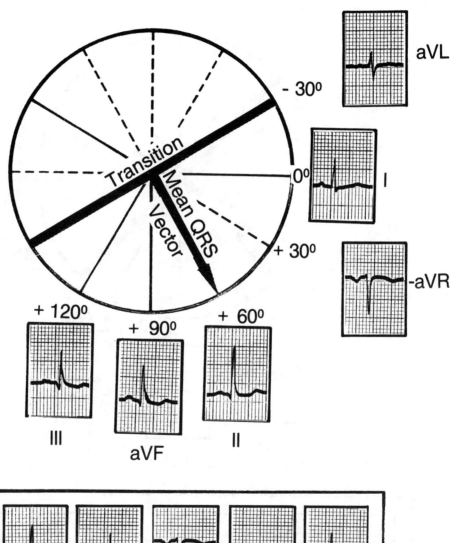

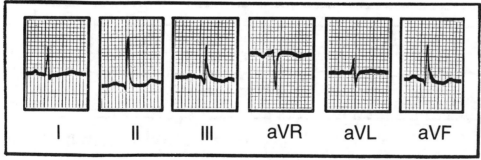

FIGURE 1-28.

Leads I, II, III, negative aVR, and aVF are positive. Lead aVL is transitional. We therefore draw the transition through the axis of aVL. The mean QRS vector is perpendicular to this transition, toward the positive (lead II at 60°).

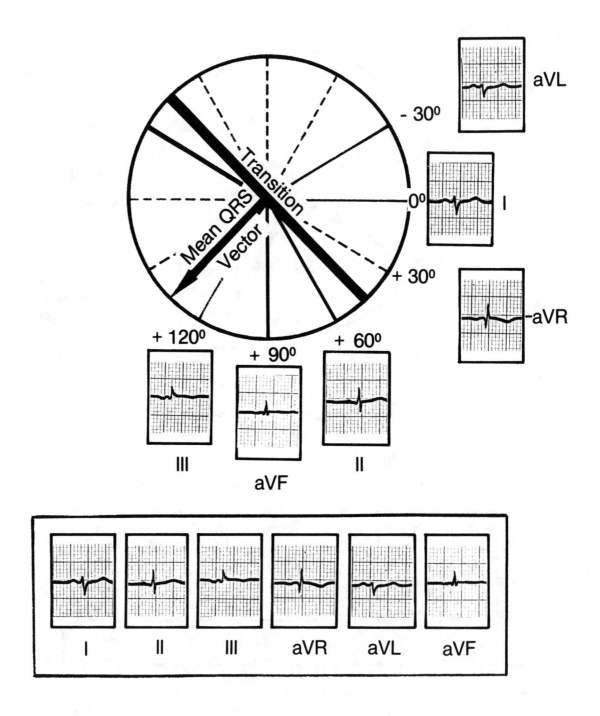

FIGURE 1-29.

Leads I and aVL are negative, while leads III and aVF are positive. Lead II is slightly more positive, while negative aVR is slightly more negative. The transition, therefore, falls between leads −aVR and II, with the mean QRS vector beyond lead III (beyond 120°).

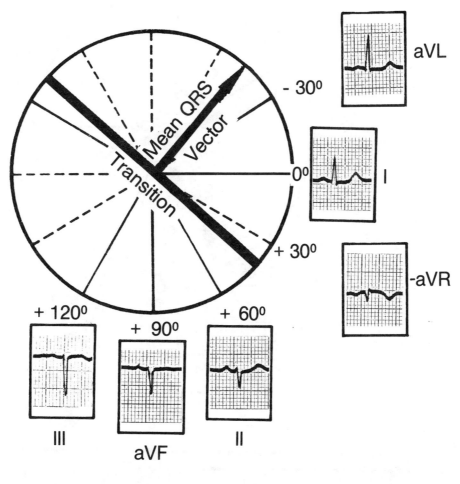

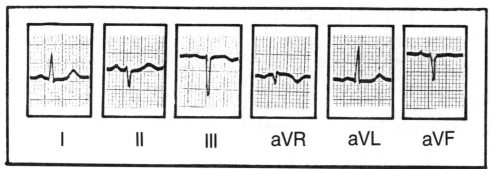

FIGURE 1-30.

Leads aVL, I, and −aVR are positive, and leads II, aVF, and III are negative. The transition is between leads −aVR and II, with the mean QRS vector beyond −30°.

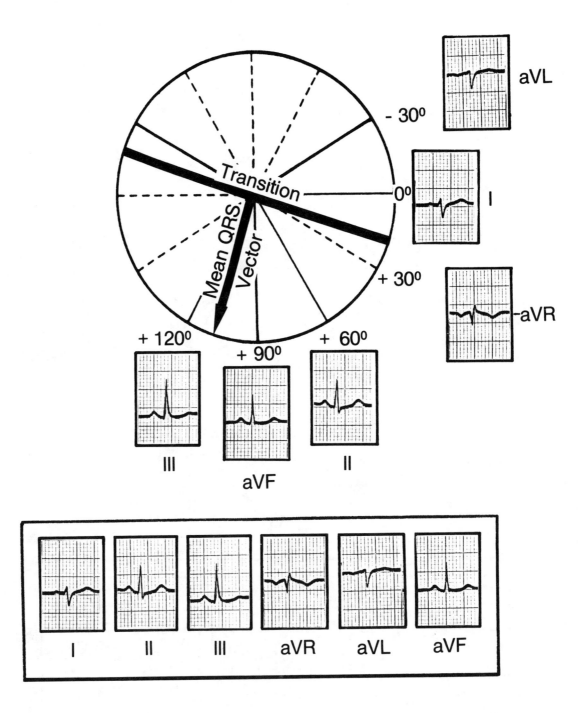

FIGURE 1-31.

Leads aVL and I are negative, and leads −aVR, II, aVF, and III are positive. The transition is between leads I and −aVR, and the mean QRS vector is between leads aVF and III but closer to lead III. Note that the QRS complex is more positive in lead III than in lead aVF. The mean QRS vector is, therefore, at approximately 110°.

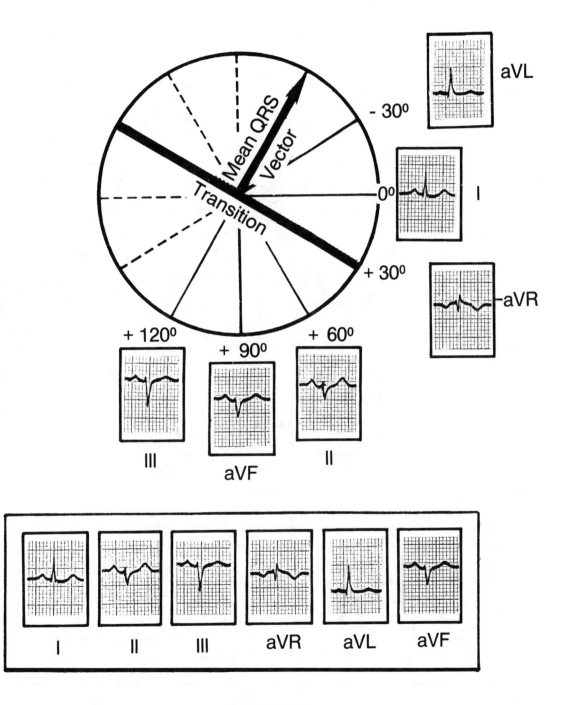

FIGURE 1-32.

Leads aVL and I are positive, while leads II, aVF, and III are negative. The transition is at lead aVR. The mean QRS vector, perpendicular to the transition toward the positive, is beyond −30° (at −60°).

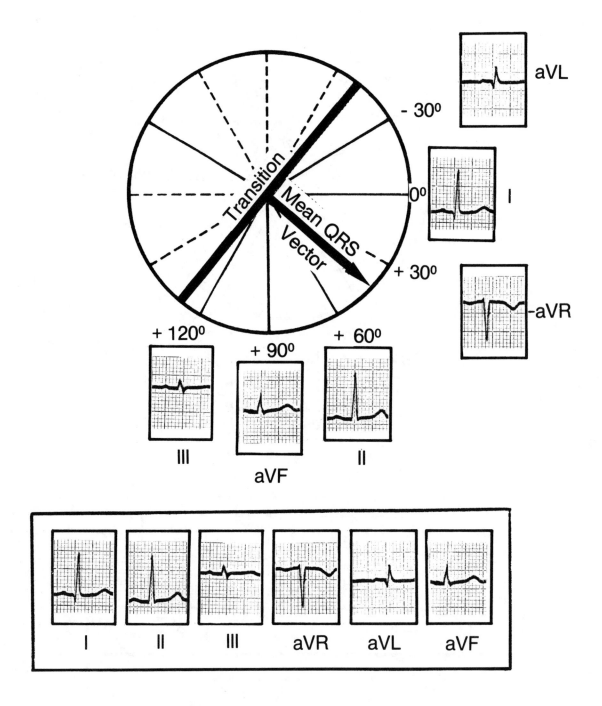

FIGURE 1-33.

All six leads are positive (remember to invert aVR). The transition, therefore, bypasses all the leads, and the mean QRS vector falls between +30 and +60°.

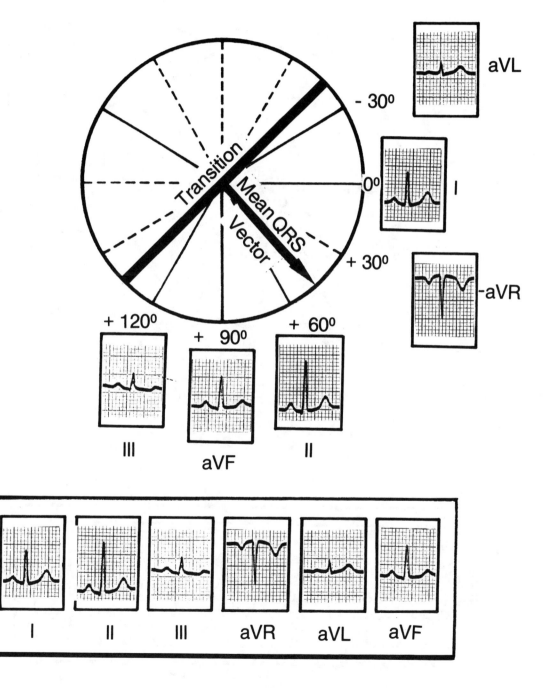

FIGURE 1-34.

This figure is similar to Figure 1-33. All the leads are positive so that the transition bypasses all the leads. The mean QRS vector is between +30 and +60°.

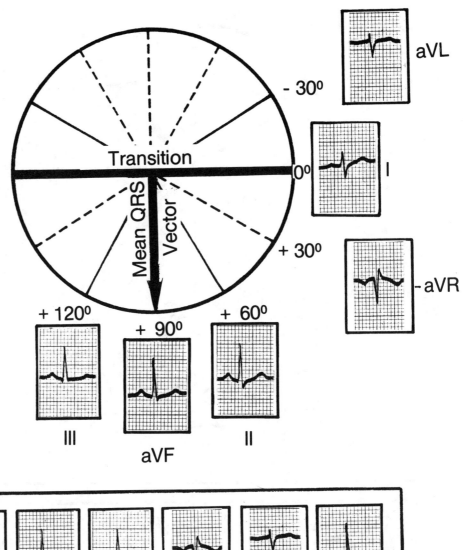

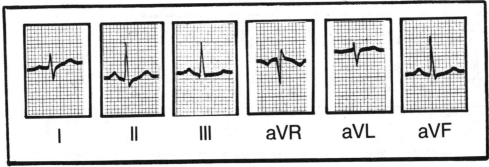

FIGURE 1-35.

The transition is at 0° (lead I). Lead aVL is negative; leads − aVR, II, aVF, and III are positive. The mean QRS vector is, therefore, perpendicular to lead I at 90° (lead aVF).

B. Normal Mean QRS Vector, Left Axis Deviation (LAD), Right Axis Deviation (RAD)

In the normal adult (Figure 1-36), the mean QRS vector is usually between 0° and 90°. That is, the mean QRS vector is normally between leads I and aVF. There is a shaded area between −30 and 0° and between +90 and +105°. Many cardiologists feel that a mean QRS vector falling within these shaded areas is still within the limits of normal. Beyond −30° is *abnormal left axis deviation (LAD)* and beyond +105° is *abnormal right axis deviation (RAD)*. Study Figure 1-36 well and then review Figures 1-24 to 1-35, and determine which mean QRS vectors are normal and which are abnormal. As you can see by Figure 1-36 there is a wide range of normality. As a general rule the mean QRS vector is more rightward in early life and more leftward with increasing age. Some of the pathologic entities responsible for abnormal mean QRS vectors will be discussed later on.

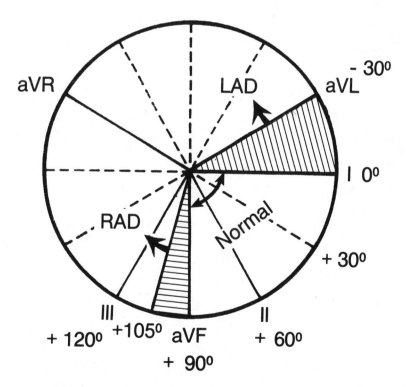

FIGURE 1-36. *Normal and abnormal ranges for the mean QRS vector: LAD, Left axis deviation; RAD, right axis deviation.*

Normal	*0 to +90°*
LAD	*0 to −90°*
Abnormal LAD	*−30 to −90°*
RAD	*+90 to 180°*
Abnormal RAD	*+105 to 180°*
Extreme RAD	*−90 to 180°*

> After you have reviewed the material you have just studied, stop the tape and answer the review questions on the next page.

Review Questions

DIRECTIONS. Provide the information requested in each of the following.

1. What is meant by abnormal left axis deviation (LAD) of the mean QRS vector?

2. What is meant by abnormal right axis deviation (RAD) of the mean QRS vector?

DIRECTIONS. Based on the normal and abnormal ranges for the mean QRS vector studied in Figure 1-36, determine whether the mean QRS vectors in Figures 1-24 through 1-35 are normal (N) or abnormal (A), and circle the appropriate letter.

N A 3. Figure 1-24

N A 4. Figure 1-25

N A 5. Figure 1-26

N A 6. Figure 1-27

N A 7. Figure 1-28

N A 8. Figure 1-29

N A 9. Figure 1-30

N A 10. Figure 1-31

N A 11. Figure 1-32

N A 12. Figure 1-33

N A 13. Figure 1-34

N A 14. Figure 1-35

> After answering the above questions, restart the tape and check your responses with the analyses given on the tape. The answers are also found on page 120.

> The "rule of thumb" for the *normal* mean QRS vector in the frontal plane is presented in Table 1-2, page 97. To quickly determine the quadrant in which the mean QRS vector is located, using leads I and aVF, refer to pages 123-126.

C. Determination of Mean T Vector in the Frontal Plane

The mean T vector is determined in the same manner as the mean QRS vector. In Figure 1-37 the T waves are positive in leads aVL, I, − aVR, II, transitional in aVF, and negative in III. The transition for the T wave is along lead aVF. The mean T vector is perpendicular to the transition on the positive side, at 0° (large arrow).

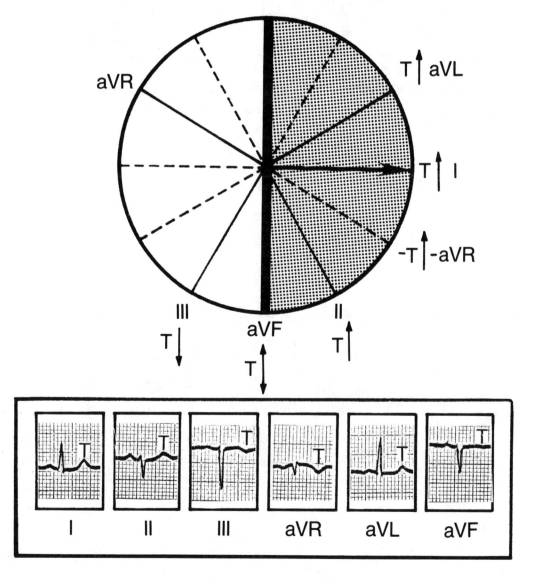

FIGURE 1-37.   Mean T vector at 0°.

> After you have reviewed the material you have just studied, stop the tape and answer the review questions on the following pages.

Review Questions

DIRECTIONS. In the electrocardiograms below, determine the mean T vector. The mean T vector, in the frontal plane, is determined in the same manner as the mean QRS vector.

1.

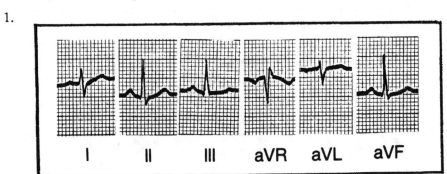

FIGURE 1-38.

Mean T vector:

2.

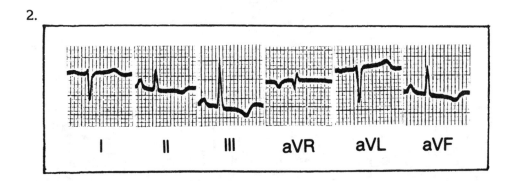

FIGURE 1-39.

Mean T vector:

3.

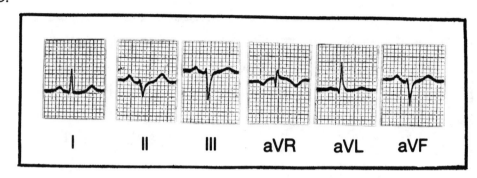

FIGURE 1-40.

Mean T vector:

4.

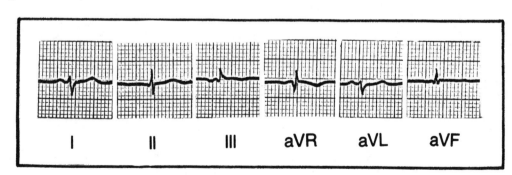

FIGURE 1-41.

Mean T vector:

5.

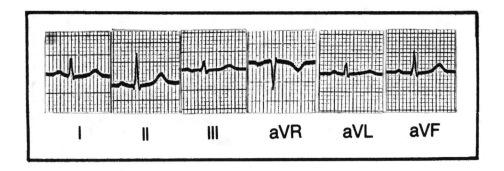

FIGURE 1-42.

Mean T vector:

> After determining the mean T vector in Figures 1-38 through 1-42, restart the tape and listen to the solutions. The analyses are presented in this guide on the following pages. The answers may also be found on page 120.

Solutions to Review Questions
(Figures 1-38 to 1-42)

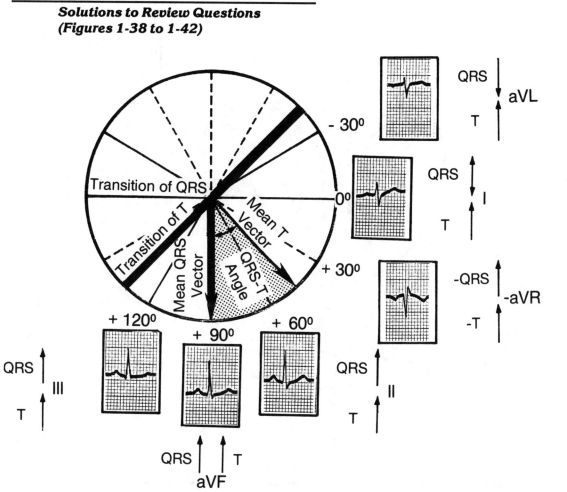

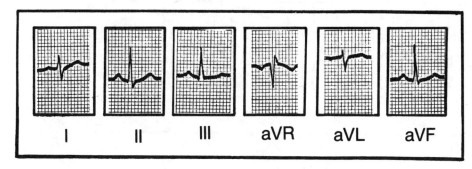

FIGURE 1-38.

All the T waves are positive; remember to invert lead aVR. The transition, therefore, bypasses all the leads, and the mean T vector falls between +30 and +60°. Note the angle of 45° between the mean QRS vector and mean T vector. The QRS-T angle is usually 45° or less in the normal and rarely exceeds 60°.

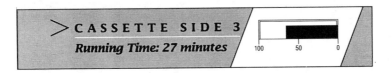

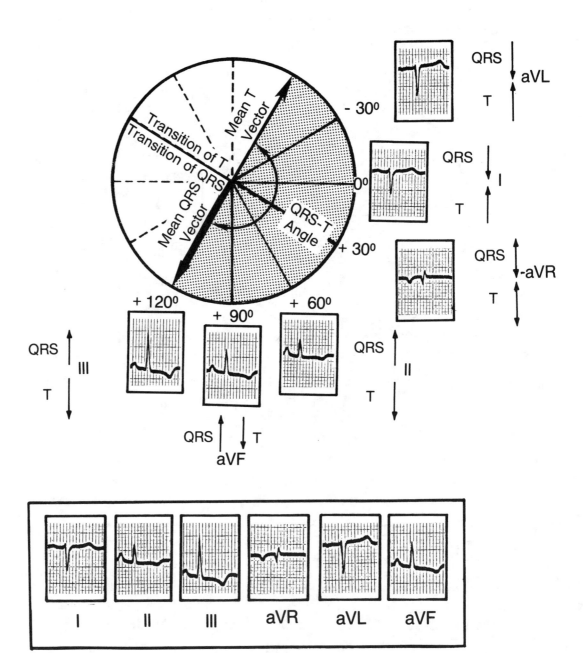

FIGURE 1-39.

The transitional zone for both the QRS and T wave is at lead aVR. In all other leads the QRS deflections are opposite the T deflections, an orientation resulting in a very wide QRS-T angle (180°).

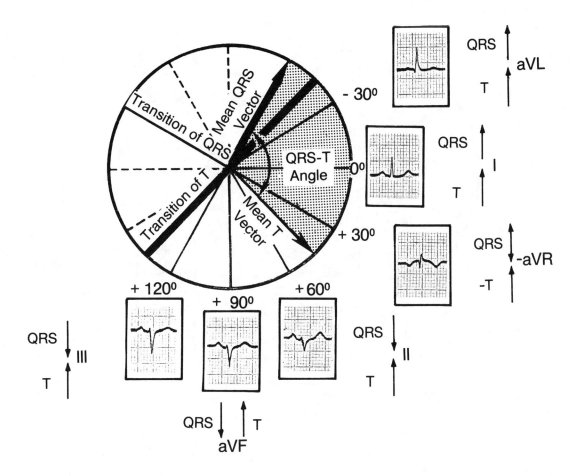

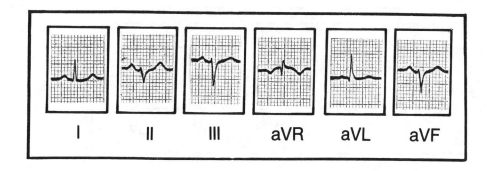

FIGURE 1-40.

Once again we find that all the T waves are positive, with the mean T vector at 45°. Owing to the marked left axis deviation (LAD) of the QRS (−60°), a wide angle is noted between the mean QRS vector and the mean T vector (105°).

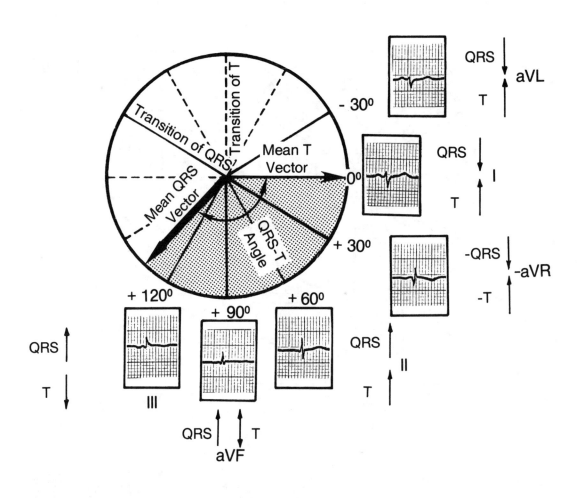

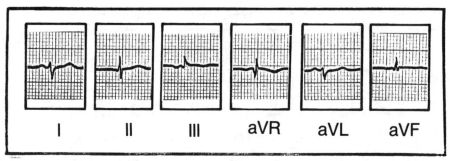

FIGURE 1-41.

The T waves in leads aVL, I, − aVR, and II are positive. The T wave is transitional in lead aVF and negative in lead III. With the transition at aVF, the mean T vector is at 0°. Note the abnormally wide QRS-T angle.

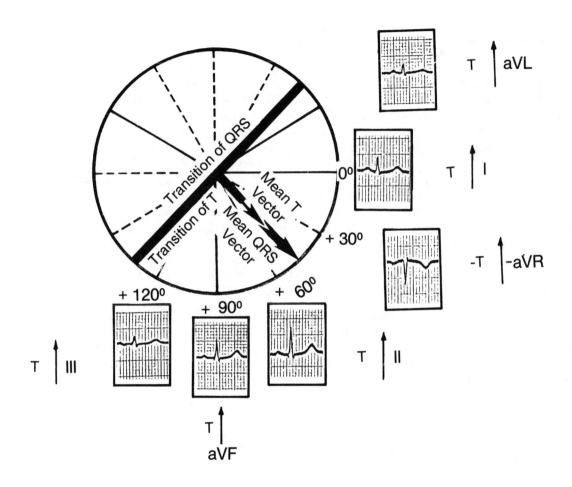

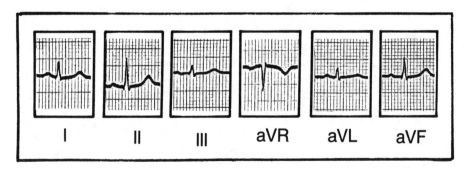

FIGURE 1-42.

All the QRS complexes are positive, as are all the T waves. The mean QRS vector and mean T vector are superimposed, thereby forming a very narrow, if any, angle between them.

> At this point stop the tape and read the next page.

D. The QRS-T Angle

The angle formed between the mean QRS vector and the mean T vector is a sensitive method for relating the forces of ventricular depolarization with the forces of ventricular repolarization. In the normal adult the QRS-T angle is rarely wider than 60° and is often less than 45°. This most important relationship is illustrated in Figures 1-38 to 1-42. Study these electrocardiograms. In each, the mean QRS and mean T vectors have already been determined. In Figure 1-38 the mean QRS vector is at 90° and the mean T vector is at 45°. The QRS-T angle is, therefore, normal at 45°. In Figure 1-39 the mean QRS vector at 120° and the mean T vector at − 60° produce a very wide QRS-T angle, 180°. In Figure 1-40 the mean QRS vector is at − 60° and the mean T vector os at approximately 45°. The QRS-T angle is therefore abnormally wide. In Figure 1-41 the QRS-T angle is abnormally wide with a mean QRS vector beyond 120° and a mean T vector at 0°. In Figure 1-42 all the QRS complexes and T waves are in the same direction, producing a normal, very narrow (if any) QRS-T angle. The "rule of thumb" for the *normal* QRS-T angle in the frontal plane is presented in Table 1-2, page 97.

Not only the width of the QRS-T angle but also the orientation of the mean T vector in relation to the mean QRS vector are important. If the mean QRS vector is horizontal, the mean T vector is to the right of the mean QRS vector. If the mean QRS vector is vertical, the mean T vector is to the left of the mean QRS vector. If this relationship does not hold, the QRS-T angle may be abnormal, although its width be within 60°.

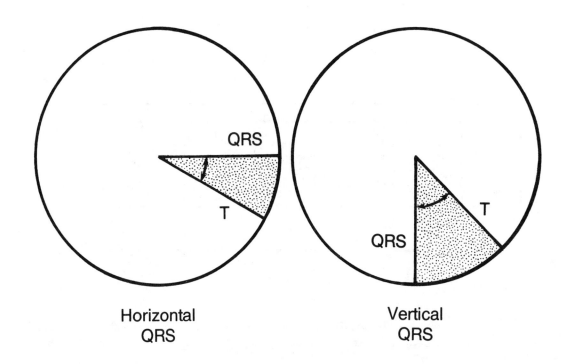

Horizontal
QRS

Vertical
QRS

> Return to Figures 1-38 through 1-42 and determine the QRS-T angle. Then restart the tape and check your analyses with those given as you follow in the guide.

E. The Mean P Vector in the Frontal Plane

To find the mean P vector, use the same approach as for the mean QRS and T vectors. The transitional zone is first calculated, then the mean P vector. In Figure 1-43 note that the P waves are upright (positive) in leads I, II, and III. The transition, therefore, bypasses these three leads; the mean P vector is perpendicular to the transition and is found along the axis of lead II at 60°. The range for the mean P vector is usually rather narrow in the normal electrocardiogram. The outer limits of normal are between 0 and +90°, usually between +15 and +75°, indicated by the arrows outside the circle in Figure 1-43.

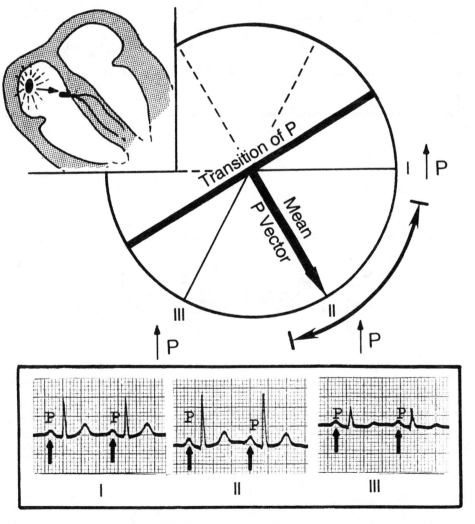

FIGURE 1-43.   The mean P vector at 60°.

> After you have reviewed the material you have just studied, stop the tape and answer the review questions on the next page.

Review Questions

DIRECTIONS. Calculate the mean P vector, and determine the normality or abnormality of the electrocardiograms below.

1.

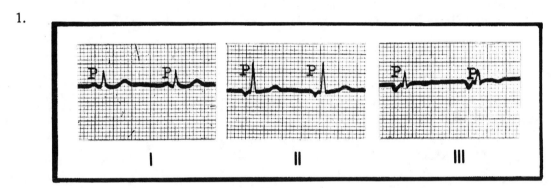

FIGURE 1-44.

Mean P vector:

2.

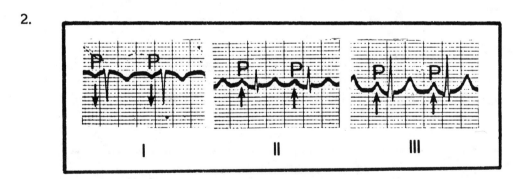

FIGURE 1-45.

Mean P vector:

> After determining the mean P vector in Figures 1-44 and 1-45, restart the tape and check your responses with the analyses given on the tape as you follow in the guide. The answers may also be found on page 121.

Solutions to Review Questions
(Figures 1-44 and 1-45)

Because of the narrow range of normality, pay very close attention to the positivity and negativity of the P waves. A P wave which is negative in lead II, but positive in lead I, is a leftward P (Figure 1-44), and one which is negative in lead I is a rightward P (Figure 1-45).

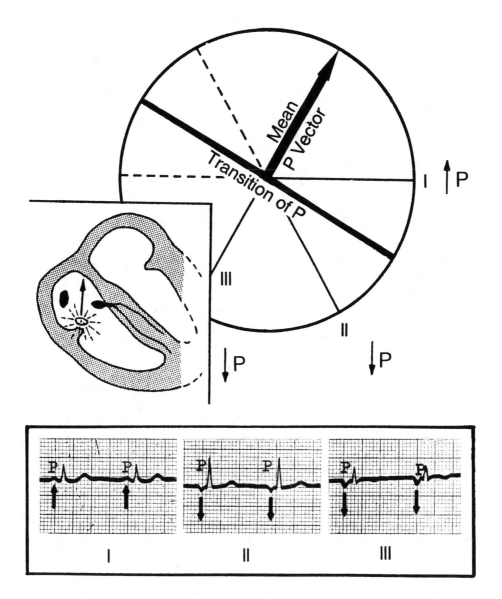

FIGURE 1-44.

The P wave is positive in lead I but negative in leads II and III. The transition is, therefore, between leads I and II, resulting in an abnormal left axis deviation of the mean P vector. The origin of the impulse is not from the S-A node but from some other focus; it is from an ectopic focus, representing an abnormal sequence of atrial depolarization.

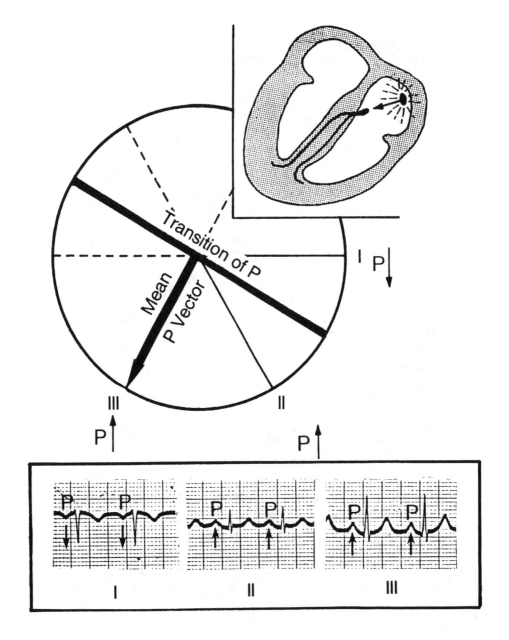

FIGURE 1-45.

The P wave is negative in lead I but positive in leads II and III. The transition is, therefore, between leads I and II; the mean P vector is deviated abnormally to the right. This electro-cardiogram is from a patient with known dextrocardia. This is an exception to the general rule, for the origin of the impulse may be in the S-A node. It is only that the heart is not in the usual location. (The heart is on the right side rather than the left.)

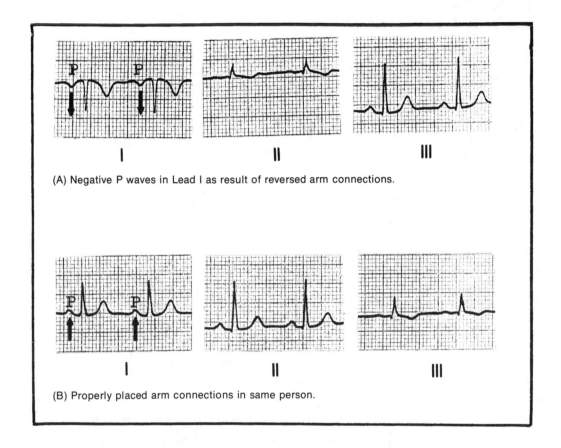

(A) Negative P waves in Lead I as result of reversed arm connections.

(B) Properly placed arm connections in same person.

FIGURE 1-46.

Another cause of a negative P wave in lead I is the misplacement of the electrodes (right arm electrode on the left arm and left arm electrode on the right arm). In fact, this misplacement is the most common cause of a negative P wave in lead I; this is a favorite examination question. Dextrocardia is far rarer as a cause of the negative P wave in lead I. Note that in this electrocardiogram (Figure 1-46A), as well as in the previous one (Figure 1-45), both the P wave and the QRS complex in lead I are predominantly negative. Always recheck the arm connections when encountering this situation. Figure 1-46B shows properly placed connections on the same person.

DETERMINATION OF THE HEART RATE FROM THE ELECTROCARDIOGRAM

Figure 1-47 illustrates the time and amplitude markings on electrocardiographic paper. The large and small boxes are used to determine the height and duration of all the inscriptions on the electrocardiogram. Each small box is 0.04 sec. in duration and 1 mm. in height. Each large box is 0.2 sec. in duration and 5 mm. in height. The usual standardization on the electrocardiogram of 1 millivolt (mv.) results in a deflection of 2 large boxes (10 mm.). This standardization is used on all electrocardiograms in this course, allowing comparison of electrocardiograms whether enlarged or reduced in size.

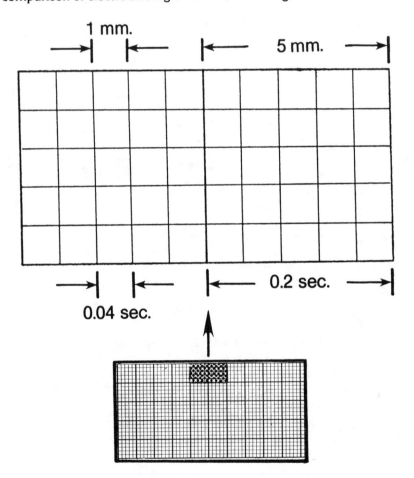

Small Box = 1 mm. = 0.04 sec.
Large Box = 5 mm. = 0.2 sec.

FIGURE 1-47.   Time and amplitude markings on electrocardiographic paper.

> The electrocardiographic standardization is illustrated on page 127.

The usual electrocardiographic speed is 25 mm. per second (5 large boxes per second). At this speed, when the rate is 300 per minute, the interval is 1 large box (0.2 sec.) between 2 complexes. When the heart rate is 150 per minute, the interval is 2 large boxes (0.4 sec.) between 2 complexes. Figure 1-48 illustrates this relationship and 3 heart rate determinations are presented.

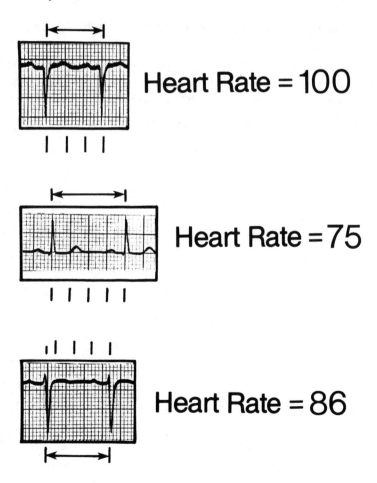

FIGURE 1-48.   Determination of heart rate from the electrocardiogram.

> Another method for the electrocardiographic determination of heart rate is illustrated on page 128.

NORMAL SINUS
RHYTHM

In order to describe the rhythm of the heart as normal sinus rhythm (the impulse originating in the sinoatrial node), which is the normal rhythm of the heart, the following conditions must be met:

1. Normal Mean P Vector (to the left and inferior-upright P waves in leads I and aVF or I and II.

2. Each P wave must be followed by a QRS complex and each QRS complex must be preceded by a P wave.

3. The normal P-R interval (from the beginning of the P wave to the beginning of the QRS complex) is rarely greater than 0.2 sec. (one large box) in duration. The normal range is 0.12 to 0.2 sec. and is constant from beat to beat.

4. The rate is constant between 60 and 100 beats per minute.

> Normal sinus rhythm may be illustrated using a ladder diagram as shown on page 129.

> After you have reviewed the material you have just studied, stop the tape and answer the review questions on the following pages.

CUMULATIVE REVIEW

DIRECTIONS. Provide the information requested.

1. Define sinus rhythm.

DIRECTIONS. The next series of electrocardiograms (Figures 1-49 to 1-53) contains at least one abnormality or technical error, which can easily be spotted by applying the information acquired so far. Analyze each electrocardiogram using the following steps:

1. Leads I + III = lead II.
    Leads aVR + aVL + aVF = 0.

2. Calculate the mean P vector.

3. Calculate the mean QRS vector.

4. Calculate the mean T vector and determine the QRS-T angle.

2.

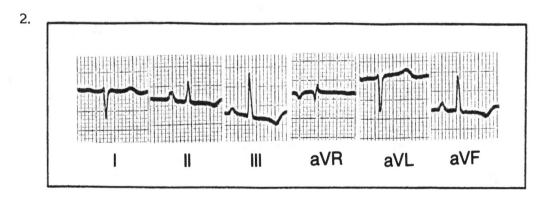

FIGURE 1-49.

Analysis:

3.

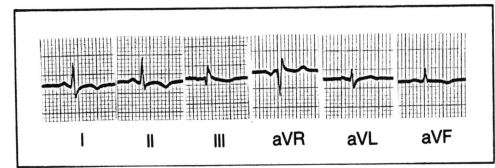

FIGURE 1-50.

Analysis:

4.

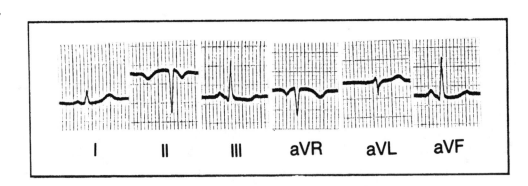

FIGURE 1-51.

Analysis:

5.

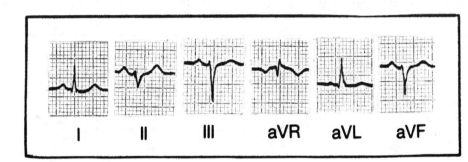

FIGURE 1-52.

Analysis:

6.

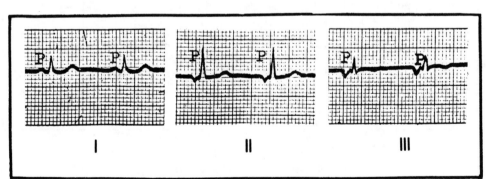

FIGURE 1-53.

Analysis:

> After answering these questions, restart the tape and check your responses with the analyses given on the tape as you follow in the guide. The answers will also be found on page 121.

Solutions to Review Questions
(Figures 1-49 to 1-53)

The abnormality or technical error is described in the legend to each electrocardiogram.

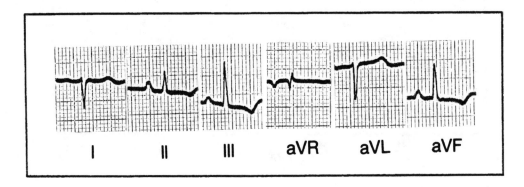

FIGURE 1-49.   Abnormal right axis deviation (RAD) and abnormally wide QRS-T angle.

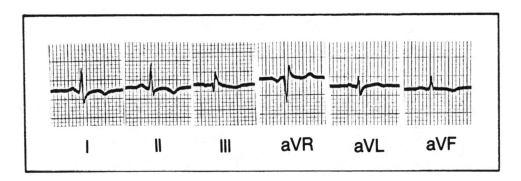

FIGURE 1-50.   Abnormally wide QRS-T angle.

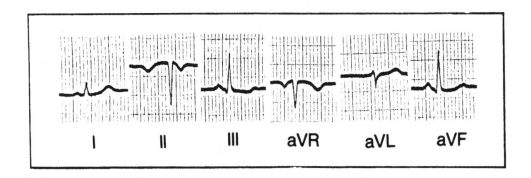

FIGURE 1-51.   Lead II has been mounted upside down. Even if you did not recognize this on sight, you would soon see that leads I + III do not add up to lead II.

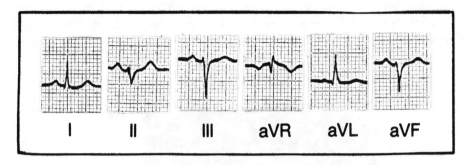

FIGURE 1-52.   Abnormal left axis deviation (LAD) and abnormally wide QRS-T angle.

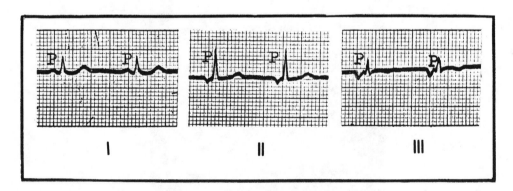

FIGURE 1-53.   The mean P vector is abnormal. The site of origin of the impulse is not in the S-A node; this is an ectopic atrial pacemaker.

THE HORIZONTAL
PLANE VECTOR

The six electrocardiographic leads studied heretofore—I, II, III, aVR, aVL, and aVF—are leads in the *frontal* plane. The boundaries of the frontal plane are superior, inferior, right, and left (Figure 1-54).

Superior

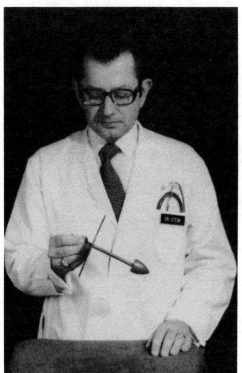

Right

Left

Inferior

FIGURE 1-54.   Boundaries of the frontal plane.

When the mean QRS, T, and P vectors were indicated by an arrow, only two dimensions in space could be described. This is seen in Figure 1-55.

A. The arrow points to the left and inferior.
B. The arrow points to the left and superior.
C. The arrow points to the right and inferior.
D. The arrow points to the right and superior.

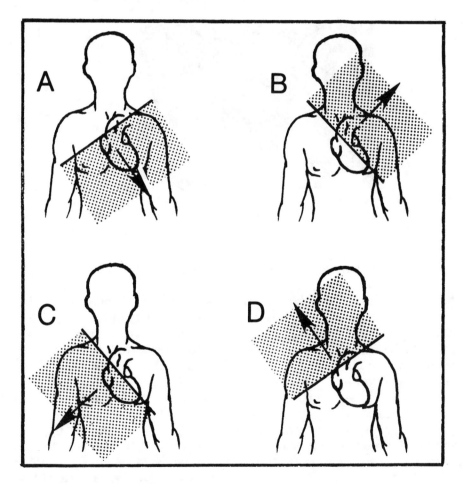

FIGURE 1-55.   *Describe each arrow in two dimensions.*

In order to provide the third dimension in space to describe the cardiac vectors, the *horizontal* plane must be added. The boundaries of the horizontal plane are anterior, posterior, right, and left (Figure 1-56).

FIGURE 1-56.   Boundaries of the horizontal plane.

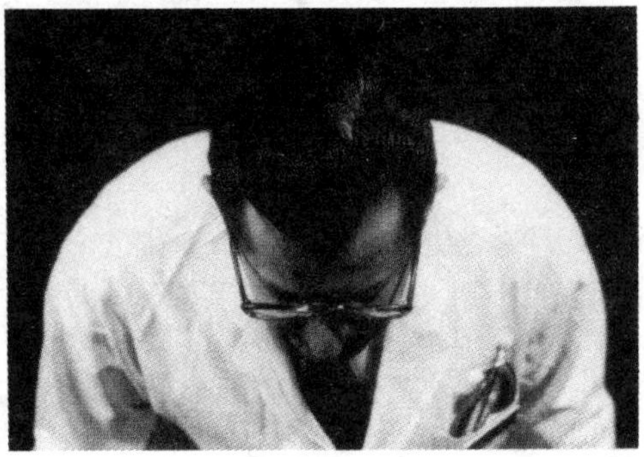

Einthoven had no difficulty with the frontal plane. There was very little difference in the deflection recorded whether the electrode was placed on the finger, wrist, or elbow, or on the toe, ankle, or knee of the arm or leg. The frontal plane has convenient projections from the body in the form of arms and legs. It was found that as long as the electrode is at least 15 cm. distant from the heart, moving the electrode still further away records little change on the electrocardiogram. As the electrode is brought very close to the heart—for example, to 3 cm.—a small change in position will result in major changes in the deflections recorded on the electrocardiogram. In the frontal plane, the extremities permit the placement of the electrodes at least 15 cm. from the heart. However, there are no anterior-posterior projections from the chest and from the back to take us 15 cm. from the heart in the horizontal plane. Any position on the chest for recording the horizontal vector is within this critical distance. Einthoven, therefore, in the early days of electrocardiography, abandoned attempts to measure this anterior-posterior vector. It was years later, after many trials, that the chest, or precordial, leads were established and placed in the positions shown in Figure 1-57A as V_1 to V_6. Still later, measurements of the cardiac vectors in the horizontal plane were shown to be possible.

Although the six precordial leads do not lie in the same horizontal plane (Figure 1-57A), an approximation of the horizontal projection of a QRS loop is illustrated in Figure 1-57B. With the addition of the horizontal plane (precordial leads), you will soon be ready to determine the mean spatial vectors in three dimensions.

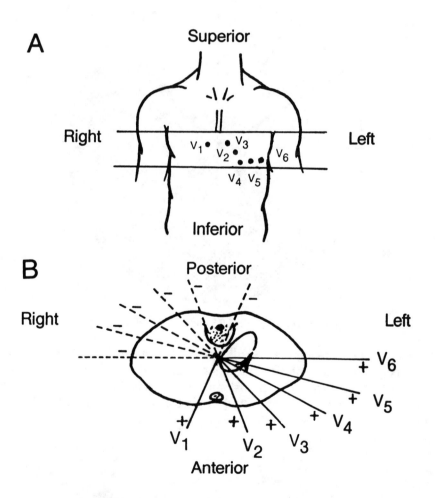

FIGURE 1-57.   A, Positions of the precordial electrodes. Electrode positions are as follows:

V_1 Fourth intercostal space to the right of the sternum
V_2 Fourth intercostal space to the left of the sternum
V_3 Midway between V_2 and V_4
V_4 Fifth intercostal space—midclavicular line
V_5 Anterior axillary line—horizontal level of V_4
V_6 Midaxillary line—horizontal level of V_4
B, QRS loop in the horizontal plane.

While studying the QRS complex in the frontal plane, we were accustomed to drawing a line representing the transitional zone, and another line with an arrow perpendicular to it representing the mean QRS vector. We were working with lines since we were limited to only two possible dimensions. An example of this is seen in Figure 1-58. The two-dimensional description of this arrow representing the mean QRS vector is left and inferior.

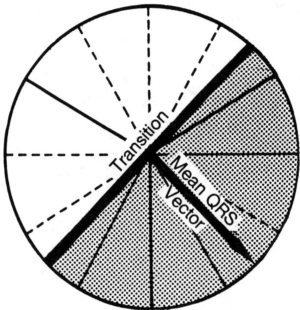

FIGURE 1-58.   Mean QRS Vector—left and inferior.

We had not really been looking at a transitional *line,* but at a *disk* dividing the body into positive and negative areas. The circumference of this disk viewed on end appeared to be a line (Figure 1-59A). In a three-dimensional view, as seen in Figure 1-59B, the disk and arrow are tilted slightly posteriorly to show that we are not actually looking at a line, but at a disk.

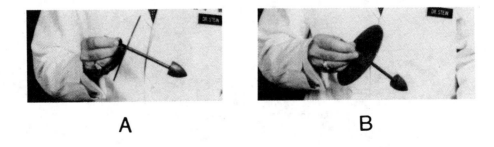

A   B

FIGURE 1-59.   A, In two dimensions, the disk is seen as a line with an arrow. B, In three dimensions, the full disk is seen with the posterior tilt of the arrow.

The vector model, seen in Figure 1-60, may be used to visualize better the cardiac vector in three dimensions. The lines in Figure 1-60A representing the *frontal* plane, are leads I, II, and III. The precordial leads in Figure 1-60B representing the *horizontal* plane are leads V_1 to V_6. The zero on the frontal plane and the zero on the horizontal plane line up, and they line up with the center point of the disk. *We can rotate the disk only through this zero point,* which limits the motion of the disk. We cannot move this disk up and down as we do with a piston. Although inaccuracies are present, since the body is neither a cylinder nor a circle, this method facilitates the understanding of the general vectorial concept in three dimensions.

Other possible sources of error should be noted. For example, the precordial leads (Figure 1-57A) are arbitrarily placed in certain fixed positions on the chest, without regard to the "lie" of the heart. Also, there are wide variations in sizes and shapes of chests among patients.

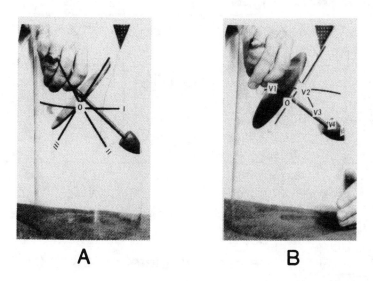

FIGURE 1-60. Vector model, with frontal (A) and horizontal (B) leads.

DETERMINATION OF MEAN SPATIAL QRS VECTOR IN THREE DIMENSIONS

Determine the mean QRS vector in the frontal plane using leads I, II, III, aVR, aVL, and aVF. After plotting the transitional zone and mean QRS vector, check your work with Figure 1-62. The horizontal plane will then be analyzed. Figures 1-62 to 1-65 all relate to Figure 1-61.

On inspection of the electrocardiogram, we see that all six leads are positive, remembering to invert lead aVR. The transitional zone bypasses all of the leads and the mean QRS vector falls between leads II and aVR, to the *left* and *inferior* in the frontal plane.

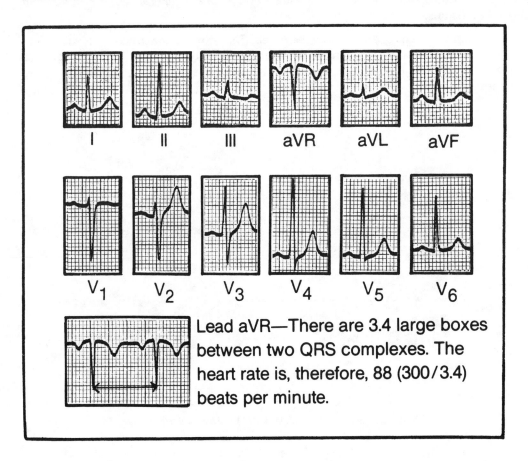

Lead aVR—There are 3.4 large boxes between two QRS complexes. The heart rate is, therefore, 88 (300/3.4) beats per minute.

FIGURE 1-61.   *Refer to Figures 1-62 and 1-65 to help visualize the mean QRS vector in three dimensions.*

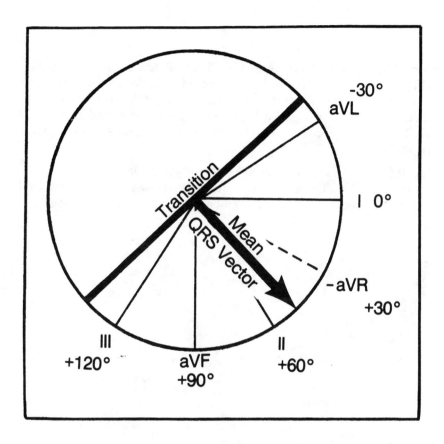

FIGURE 1-62.   Mean QRS vector in frontal plane, to left and inferior.

The disk and arrow (Figure 1-63), held to the left and inferior, do not actually appear as a disk and arrow, but rather as a line and an arrow. The area facing the arrow is positive and the area away from the arrow, on the other side of the transition, is negative.

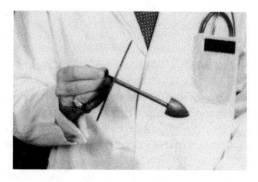

FIGURE 1-63.   Disk and arrow indicating the mean QRS vector to the left and inferior in the frontal plane.

Using our vector model in Figure 1-64A we see leads I, II, and III, and the vector is to the *left* and *inferior*. In Figure 1-64B, on the other side of the model, we have a representation of the horizontal plane. *If there were no anterior-posterior rotation,* if the vector were simply to the *left and inferior*, V_1 would be *negative*. (V_1 is the only precordial lead on the negative side of the disk. The arrow side of the disk is the positive side.) Leads V_2, V_3, V_4, V_5, and V_6 would all be positive.

To review for emphasis (Figure 1-64A), if the vector were only to the left and inferior, V_1 (Figure 1-64B) would be negative since it faces away from the arrow side of the disk. On the other hand, leads V_2 to V_6 would all be positive since they all face the arrow side of the disk.

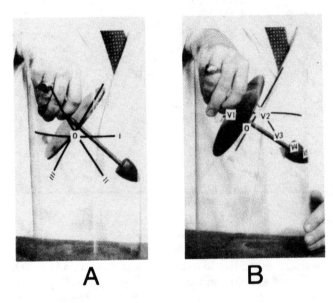

A   B

FIGURE 1-64.   *Vector model, with frontal (A) and horizontal (B) leads.*

Is this the case in Figure 1-61? No. On looking at Figure 1-61, notice that *not only* V_1 but *also* V_2 is negative. Leads V_3, V_4, V_5, and V_6 are *positive*. The transition in the horizontal plane is between V_2 and V_3. How do we make our model reflect the electrocardiographic inscription? Note again that the fixed point on this model is the 0, which is aligned with the center of the disk. The disk and arrow cannot be moved up or down but must be rotated anteriorly or posteriorly. We must tilt the disk so that the arrow faces *posteriorly* (Figure 1-65). In this position both leads V_1 and V_2 face the negative side of the disk, away from the arrow. Leads V_3, V_4, V_5, and V_6 are positive.

The mean QRS vector, as seen from Figure 1-61, described in three dimensions, is to the *left, inferior, and posterior.* This describes the mean spatial QRS vector of the normal adult (Figure 1-65).

To summarize, whether the mean QRS vector is *left and inferior, left and superior, right and inferior, or right and superior* is determined from the frontal plane leads, I, II, III, aVR, aVL, and aVF. Whether the mean QRS vector is *anterior* or *posterior* must be determined from the *horizontal plane leads:* V_1 to V_6.

The vector approach, despite the inaccuracies pointed out earlier, affords us a unifying concept in our understanding of the electrocardiogram. By visualizing the distribution of electrical potential in a three-dimensional way, a single picture, as seen in Figure 1-65, actually indicates what we may find on the twelve-lead electrocardiogram.

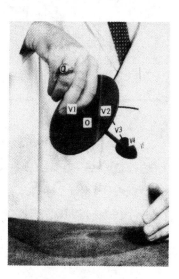

FIGURE 1-65.   The mean QRS
vector, in three dimensions, is to the
left, inferior, and posterior.

> Older terms, less commonly used today, described the electrical position of the heart. These included the terms horizontal, vertical, semihorizontal, semivertical, and intermediate. It is much more common to state that the mean electrical axes are 0°, 45° or 90° than to refer to those hearts as horizontal, intermediate or vertical, respectively. Please refer to pages 130 and 131 for the illustration of the terms clockwise and counterclockwise rotation.

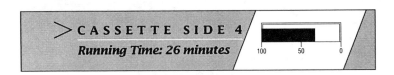

Analyze Figure 1-66 following the steps used in Figure 1-61. After you have determined the mean QRS vector in three dimensions, check your work with Figures 1-67 and 1-68.

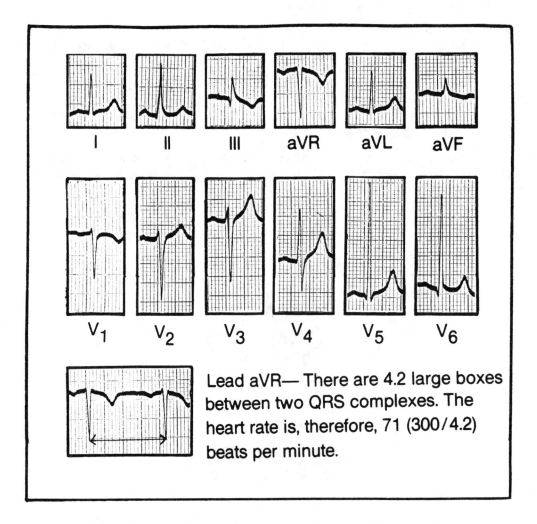

Lead aVR— There are 4.2 large boxes between two QRS complexes. The heart rate is, therefore, 71 (300/4.2) beats per minute.

FIGURE 1-66. Refer to Figures 1-67 and 1-68 for visualization of the mean QRS vector in three dimensions.

Analyzing the electrocardiogram (Figure 1-66), we see that once again all six leads are positive, remembering to invert lead aVR. The transitional zone bypasses all of the leads, the mean QRS vector falls between leads II and −aVR. This is diagrammed in Figure 1-67, as you have seen many, many times before. The mean QRS vector, in the frontal plane, is to the left and inferior.

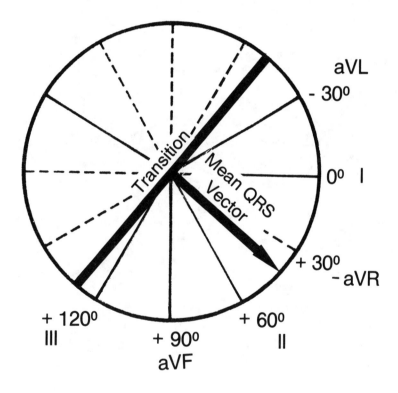

FIGURE 1-67.   Mean QRS vector in frontal plane, to left and inferior.

With the mean QRS vector to the left and inferior in the frontal plane (Figure 1-68A), we now turn out attention to the precordial leads for its orientation in the horizontal plane (Figure 1-68B). Leads V_1, V_2, and V_3 are negative, and V_4, V_5, and V_6 are positive. The transition in the precordial leads falls between V_3 and V_4. We must, therefore, rotate our disk so that the arrow faces more and more posteriorly. Here, too, the mean QRS vector is to the left, inferior, and posterior; it is more posterior, however, than in Figure 1-61.

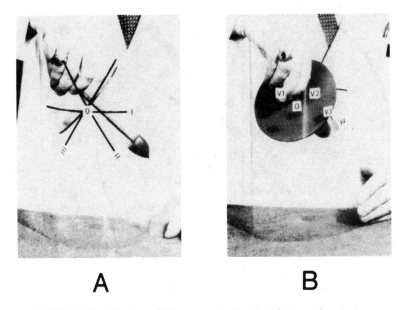

A   **B**

FIGURE 1-68.   The mean QRS vector is to the left, inferior, and posterior.

In Figure 1-69 the transition is at lead I and the mean QRS vector is at 90°. The mean QRS vector in this frontal plane is neither to the left nor to the right. The arrow is pointing directly inferiorly (Figure 1-70). This frontal plane mean QRS vector is also illustrated on our vector model in Figure 1-71.

If the mean QRS vector were directly inferior—neither anterior nor posterior (Figure 1-72A), leads V_1 and V_2 would both be negative and leads V_3 to V_6 would all be positive. The electrocardiogram (Figure 1-69), however, shows the transition to be between V_3 and V_4. In order to make V_3 negative on the vector model we must tilt the arrow posteriorly. The mean QRS vector is, therefore, inferior and posterior (Figure 1-72B).

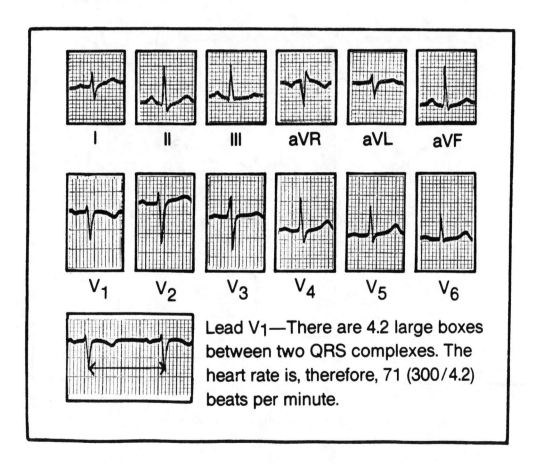

FIGURE 1-69.   *Refer to Figures 1-70 to 1-72 to help you describe the mean spatial QRS vector.*

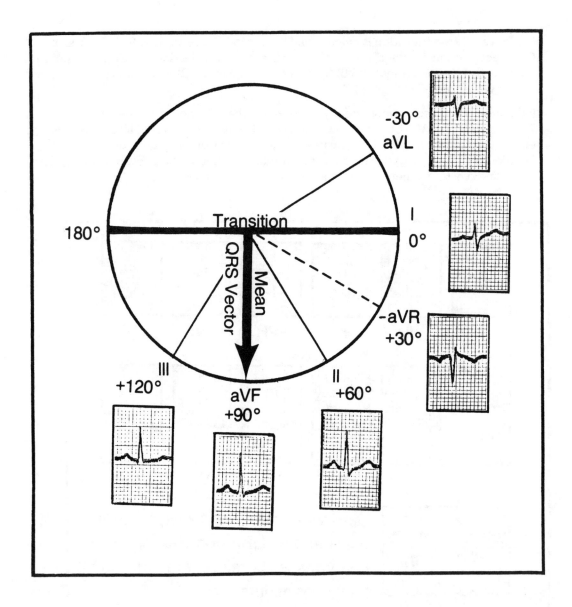

FIGURE 1-70.   Mean QRS vector inferior, at 90°, in the frontal plane.

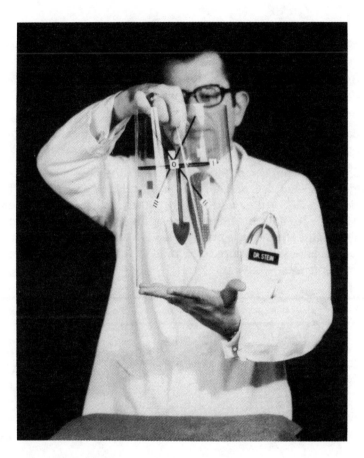

FIGURE 1-71. *Mean QRS vector inferior, at 90°, in the frontal plane.*

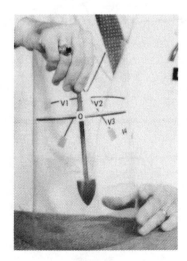

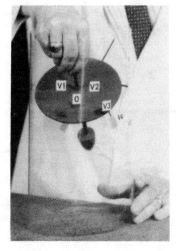

A   B

FIGURE 1-72. *Vector model for illustration of the mean QRS vector.*

Figure 1-73 is from a patient with chronic lung disease and cor pulmonale with enlargement of the right atrium and right ventricle. These entities will be studied in Chapter 2. For the present, evaluate the mean QRS vector as in previous examples.

In the frontal plane, the transition is at lead aVL, with the positive area in the upper part of the circle (Figure 1-74). The mean QRS vector is to the *right* and *superior.*

The mean QRS vector, on our vector model (Figure 1-75A), is again seen to be to the right and superior, with leads I, II, and III all negative, all facing away from the arrow side of the disk. If the mean QRS vector were merely to the right and superior, lead V_1 would be positive and leads V_2 to V_6 would fall on the negative side of the disk. Figure 1-73, however, reveals that the transition is between leads V_2 and V_3. We must tilt the disk so that the arrow points anteriorly (Figure 1-75C) and the mean spatial QRS vector is to the *right, superior,* and *anterior.*

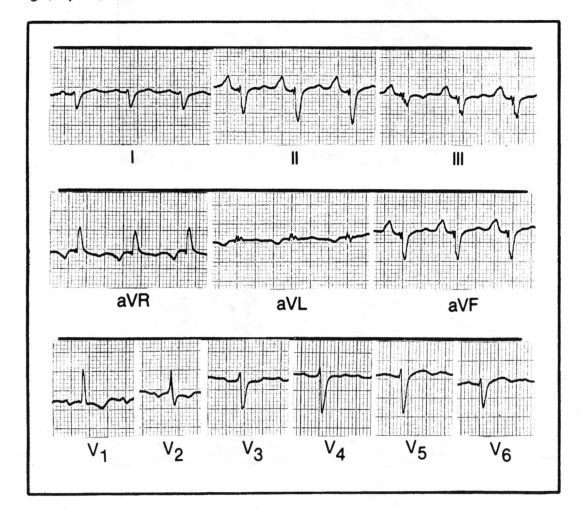

FIGURE 1-73. Calculate the mean spatial QRS vector. Refer to Figures 1-74 and 1-75.

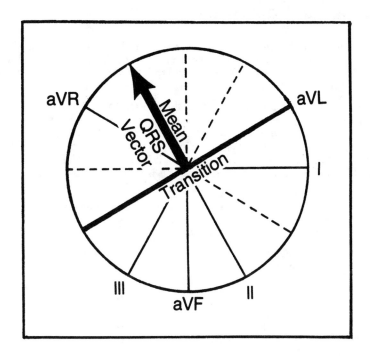

FIGURE 1-74.   *The mean QRS vector in the frontal plane is to the right and superior.*

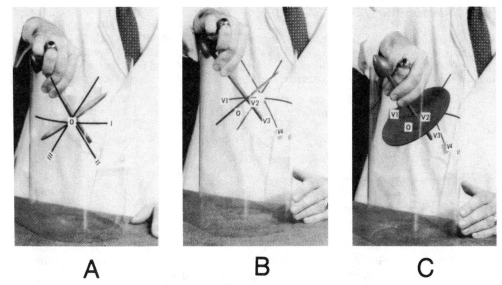

FIGURE 1-75.   *Vector model for illustration of mean spatial QRS vector.*

Mean T Vector in the Horizontal Plane, The S-T Segment, and the Q-T Interval

Using the steps outlined for the mean QRS vector, the mean T vector may be studied in the horizontal plane. This is important for the determination of the horizontal QRS-T angle, which rarely exceeds 60° in the normal adult. The "rules of thumb" for the *normal* mean QRS vector and normal QRS-T angle in the horizontal plane are presented in Table 1-2, page 97.

The S-T segment, representing the early phase of the ventricular repolarization process, is very important in clinical medicine and will be discussed again in later chapters. The S-T segment is usually isoelectric—neither elevated nor depressed (the same as the baseline for the electrocardiogram). An S-T segment which is not isoelectric, however, does not automatically indicate abnormality. When a mean S-T vector is measurable, it is usually parallel to the mean T vector (the S-T segment follows the T wave in direction). This is commonly seen in the presence of large T waves and will be covered in a later chapter.

Another measurement of importance is the *Q-T interval* (review Figure 1-22), from the beginning of the QRS complex to the end of the T wave. This interval is related to the heart rate. The mean Q-T intervals for various heart rates are as follows:

Heart Rate (beats per minute)	*Q-T Interval* (sec.)
40	0.46
60	0.39
80	0.35
100	0.31
120	0.29
140	0.26
160	0.25

In summary, we have discussed the development of the Einthoven triangle, the triaxial system, and the hexaxial system including leads I, II, III, aVR, aVL, and aVF. These six frontal plane leads were assigned degrees around the circle from lead aVL at −30° to III at +120°. The summations, leads I + III = II and aVR + aVL + aVF = 0, were studied, as were depolarization, repolarization, and the conduction system of the heart, and electrocardiographic waves, intervals, and segments. Heart rate and sinus rhythm were discussed. The six horizontal plane leads, V₁ to V₆ were studied. The spatial vector concept was emphasized in the study of the QRS, T, and P, as well as the special relationship between the QRS and T, known as the QRS-T angle. The Q-T interval was found to be related to heart rate. Items such as size of QRS complexes and P waves, although important, have not been discussed, since they will be studied in future chapters.

Based on information in this chapter, electrocardiograms will be analyzed as to: rhythm, rate, P-R interval, mean QRS vector, QRS interval, mean T vector, QRS-T angle, S-T segment, and Q-T interval.

REVIEW AND ANALYSIS OF ELECTROCARDIOGRAMS: "RULES OF THUMB"

Following is Table 1-2 which will serve as a general review of this chapter and as a key for the stepwise analysis of electrocardiograms. "Rules of thumb" are also included.

**TABLE 1-2.   Review and Stepwise Analysis
of Electrocardiograms Including "Rules of Thumb"**
(Based on information in Chapter 1)

The aim of all the many hours of study has been to emphasize a few, but very basic, concepts to facilitate an understanding of the electrocardiogram. You should, at this point, review all of the material; an additional hour now will same many in the future. Much of what has been covered may be summarized in a few simple steps. Several "rules of thumb" are also included here. As with any summary in which vast amounts of material are condensed into basic rules, you may find some exceptions, but, in general, they work quite well. Any electrocardiograms not strictly fitting the criteria summarized below should be analyzed more carefully; the electrocardiogram may still be within the outer limits of normal.

1. **Leads I + III = Lead II**
    Leads aVR + aVL + aVF = 0
    These are electrical truths and hold for all inscriptions on the electrocardiogram. If these do not add up, recheck the electrocardiogram—for example, for mismounting. Remember it is the *area* which adds up; the height and depth of the complexes may be used as good approximations.

2. **Calculate the mean P vector** to see if it falls within the narrow limits of normal. In order to describe the rhythm of the heart as *sinus rhythm* (the impulse originating in the sinoatrial node), which is the normal rhythm of the heart, the following conditions must be met.
    a.   The mean P vector must be normal.
    b.   Each P wave must be followed by a QRS complex and each QRS complex must be preceded by a P wave.
    c.   The P-R interval (from the beginning of the P wave to the beginning of the QRS complex) is rarely greater than 0.20 sec. (one large box) in duration in the normal adult. The normal range is 0.12 to 0.20 sec., and constant from beat to beat.
    d.   The rate is constant, between 60 and 100 beats per minute. In a regular rhythm divide the number of large boxes (0.20 sec.) between two complexes into 300 to determine the rate per minute.
    "Rule of thumb" for normal P vector: The normal P waves must be positive (upright) in leads I and aVF. Leads I and II may be used, as an approximation, if aVF is not given.

3. **Calculate the mean QRS vector.** The QRS complex should be 0.10 sec. (2½ small boxes), or less, in duration.
    "Rule of thumb" for normal mean QRS vector in the frontal plane: The QRS deflections must be *positive* in leads I and aVF. Leads I and II may be used, as an approximation, if aVF is not given. *"Rule of thumb" for normal mean QRS vector in the horizontal plane:* When the mean QRS vector is normal (leftward and inferior in orientation), leads V_1, V_2 and often V_3 are predominantly negative and leads V_4, V_5, and V_6 are predominantly positive leads.

4. **Calculate the mean T vector and determine the QRS-T angle.**
    "Rule of thumb" for normal QRS-T angle in the frontal plane: The T waves should follow the QRS complexes, in direction, in leads I and aVF. For example, when the QRS is positive in lead I, the T wave should also be positive. When the QRS is negative, the T wave should also be negative. Leads I and II may be used if aVF is not given. This is, at best, an approximation. The actual calculation is always better than the "rule of thumb."
    "Rule of thumb" for normal QRS-T angle in the horizontal plane: The T waves should follow the QRS complexes, in direction, from leads V_3 to V_6 or at least from V_4 to V_6.

    In most normal persons the QRS complexes are predominantly positive from leads V_3 or V_4 to V_6. The T waves are predominantly positive from V_2 or V_3 to V_6. A variant of this, in the normal, will be seen later in the course.

5. **Evaluation of the S-T segment.**
    The S-T segment in the normal adult is usually isoelectric (same as baseline for the electrocardiogram), neither elevated nor depressed. An S-T segment which is not isoelectric, however, does not automatically indicate abnormality. When a mean S-T vector is measurable it is usually parallel to the mean T vector (the S-T segment follows the T wave in direction). This is commonly seen in the presence of large T waves and will be studied in a later chapter.

6. **Q-T interval.**

Heart Rate (beats per minute)	Q-T Interval (sec.)	Heart Rate (beats per minute)	Q-T Interval (sec.)
40	0.46	120	0.29
60	0.39	140	0.26
80	0.35	160	0.25
100	0.31		

Note: "Rules of thumb" are given as an aid; they must never be a substitute for a thorough knowledge of the subject.

TABLE 1-2 (cont'd)

After gaining experience analyzing the normal electrocardiograms in this chapter, following the six steps previously outlined, you will be able to shorten the written analysis by mentally checking the electrical truths and combining the determination of the QRS-T angle and evaluation of the S-T segment under one heading, using the following form.

1. **Rhythm and Rate**
   P-R Interval
   P Wave Abnormalities
   Abnormalities of Rhythm
2. **QRS Complex**
   Duration
   Mean QRS Vector, Mean Electrical Axis or "Axis"
   Abnormalities
3. **S-T Segment and T Wave (Ventricular Repolarization)**
   QRS-T Angle
   Abnormalities
4. **Q-T Interval**

Impression and Comment

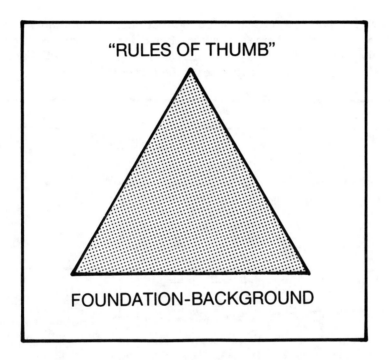

FIGURE 1-76.   Whenever "rules of thumb" are given caution must be exercised. "Rules of thumb" must never be used without falling back upon the foundation of knowledge. They are merely the tip of the iceberg, and exceptions will be found. Always be ready to analyze completely any electrocardiogram for which questions arise. Keep reviewing the basis for the "rules."

> After you have reviewed Chapter 1, stop the tape and begin the post-test on the following page.

P O S T · T E S T

DIRECTIONS. This post-test consists of four normal electrocardiograms. Following the outline in Table 1-2, analyze them as to: summation of leads, mean P vector, rhythm, rate, P-R interval, mean QRS vector, QRS interval, mean T vector, QRS-T angle, S-T segment, and Q-T interval. Write your analyses in the spaces indicated.

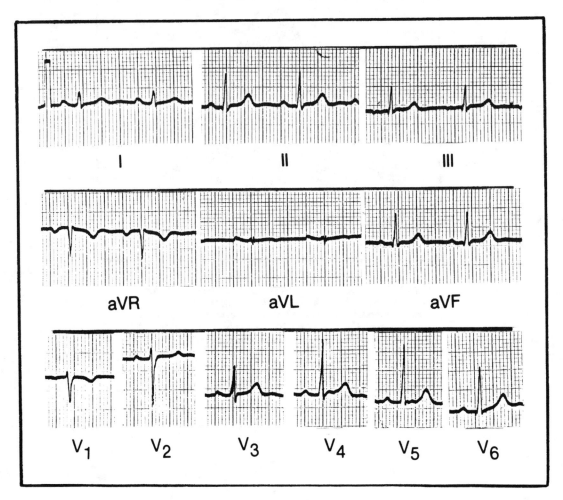

FIGURE 1-77. Normal.

1. Analysis:

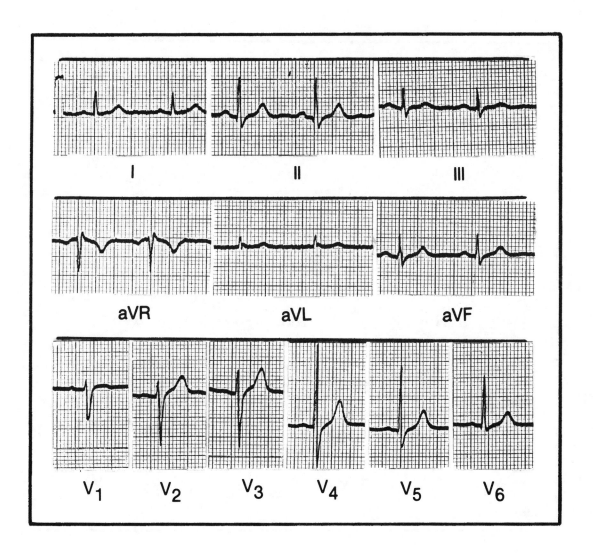

FIGURE 1-78. Normal.

2. Analysis:

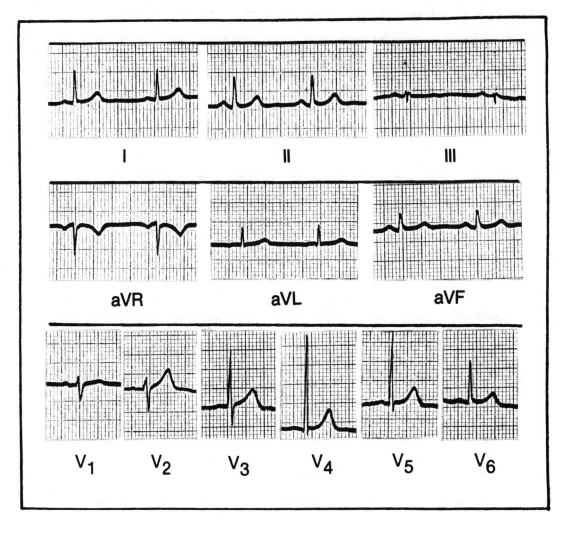

FIGURE 1-79. Normal.

3. Analysis:

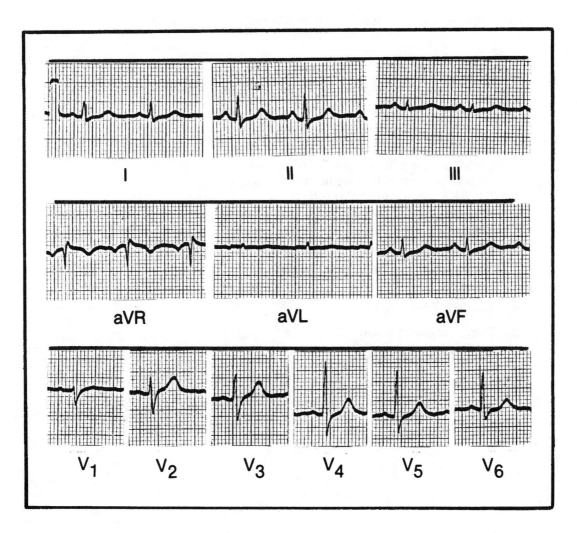

FIGURE 1-80. Normal.

4. Analysis:

> After completing your analyses, restart the tape for the solutions, which are also found on the next four pages.

ANSWERS TO
POST-TEST

The analyses are based on the steps outlined in Table 1-2.

Figure 1-77: Analysis 1

1. Leads I + III = lead II
   Leads aVR + aVL + aVF = 0

2. The mean P vector is normal at 30°.
   Each P wave is followed by a QRS complex.
   Each QRS complex is preceded by a P wave.
   The P-R interval is normal at 0.16 sec.
   The heart rate is 75 beats/min.
   The rhythm is normal sinus rhythm.

3. The QRS complex is normal in duration.
   The mean QRS vector is normal at 60°.
   The mean QRS vector is to the left, inferior, and posterior, which is normal.

4. The QRS-T angle is normal.

5. The S-T segment is normal.

6. The Q-T interval is normal.

Impression: The electrocardiogram is normal.

Figure 1-78: Analysis 2

1. Leads I + III = lead II
   Leads aVR + aVL + aVF = 0

2. The mean P vector is normal at 60°.
   Each P wave is followed by a QRS complex.
   Each QRS complex is preceded by a P wave.
   The P-R interval is normal at 0.16 sec.
   The heart rate is 70 beats/min.
   The rhythm is normal sinus rhythm.

3. The QRS complex is normal in duration.
   The mean QRS vector is normal at approximately 45°.
   The mean QRS vector is to the left, inferior, and posterior, which is normal.

4. The QRS-T angle is normal.

5. The S-T segment is normal.

6. The Q-T interval is normal.

Impression: The electrocardiogram is normal.

> This electrocardiogram was also number 10 on the pretest. Compare your analyses on the pretest and post-test.

Figure 1-79: Analysis 3

1. Leads I + III = lead II
   Leads aVR + aVL + aVF = 0

2. The mean P vector is normal at approximately 60°.
   Each P wave is followed by a QRS complex.
   Each QRS complex is preceded by a P wave.
   The P-R interval is normal at 0.16 sec.
   The heart rate is approximately 65 beats/min.
   The rhythm is normal sinus rhythm.

3. The QRS complex is normal in duration.
   The mean QRS vector is normal at approximately 20°.
   The mean QRS vector is to the left, inferior, and posterior, which is normal.

4. The QRS-T angle is normal.

5. The S-T segment is normal.

6. The Q-T interval is normal.

Impression: The electrocardiogram is normal.

Figure 1-80: Analysis 4

1. Leads I + III = lead II
   Leads aVR + aVL + aVF = 0

2. The mean P vector is normal at approximately 60°.
   Each P wave is followed by a QRS complex.
   Each QRS complex is preceded by a P wave.
   The P-R interval is normal at 0.16 sec.
   The heart rate is approximately 85 beats/min.
   The rhythm is normal sinus rhythm.

3. The QRS complex is normal in duration.
   The mean QRS vector is normal at approximately 50°.
   The mean QRS vector is to the left, inferior, and posterior, which is normal.

4. The QRS-T angle is normal.

5. The S-T segment is normal.

6. The Q-T interval is normal.

Impression: The electrocardiogram is normal.

> On the following pages are additional normal electrocardiograms for review and practice.

REVIEW
ELECTROCARDIOGRAMS

The remaining normal electrocardiograms (Figures 1-81 through 1-86) are presented for your continued practice in the complete analysis of the normal electrocardiogram using the steps outlined in Table 1-2.

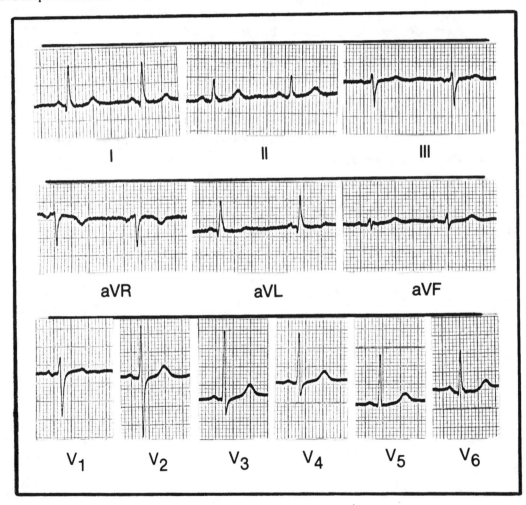

FIGURE 1-81. Normal.

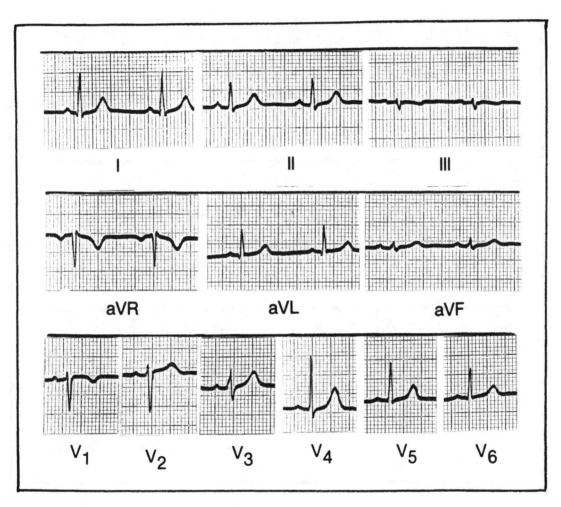

FIGURE 1-82. Normal.

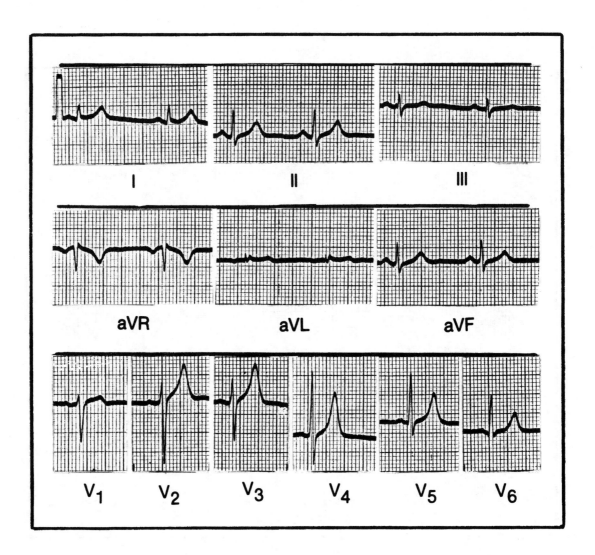

FIGURE 1-83.   Normal.

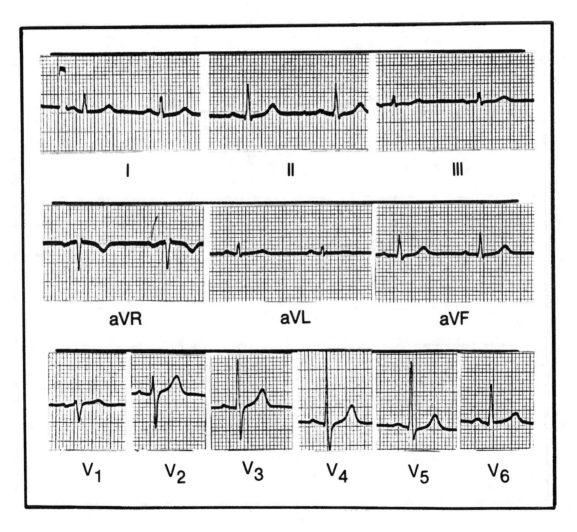

FIGURE 1-84. Normal.

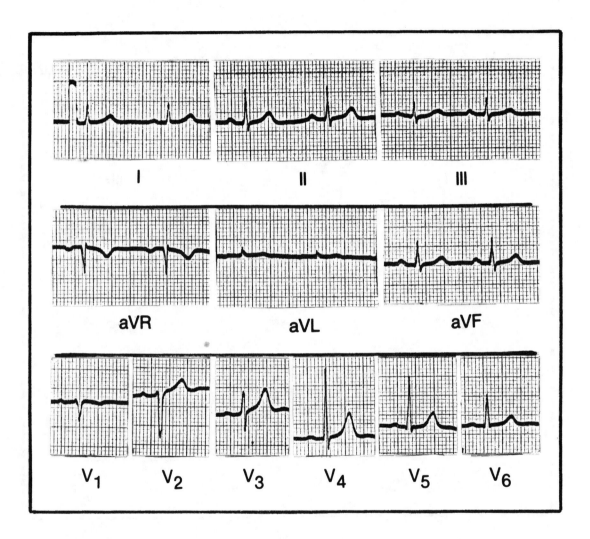

FIGURE 1-85.   Normal.

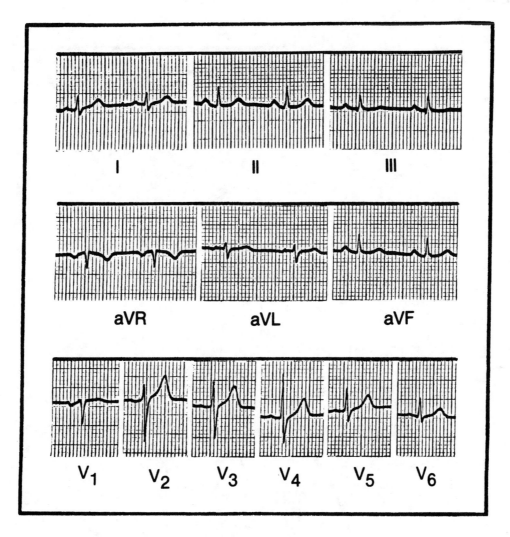

FIGURE 1-86.   Normal.

> On the following pages are the solutions to the pretest as well as to the review
> questions.

ANSWERS TO PRETEST

1.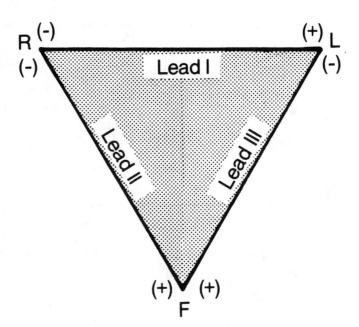

2. Lead I + lead III = lead II
3. Leads aVR + aVL + aVF = 0
4.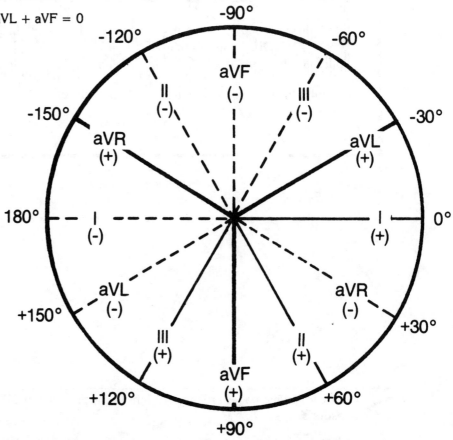

5.

6. A mean QRS vector beyond −30° indicates abnormal left axis deviation (LAD).

7. A mean QRS vector beyond +105° indicates abnormal right axis deviation (RAD).

8. The P wave is positive in lead I but negative in leads II and III. The transition is therefore between leads I and II and the mean P vector is deviated abnormally to the left at approximately $-60°$.

9. QRS-T angle is 180°.

10. Analysis (following stepwise outline of Table 1-2, p. 97).

Figure 1-78

1. Leads I + III = lead II
   Leads aVR + aVL + aVF = 0

2. The mean P vector is normal at 60°.
   Each P wave is followed by a QRS complex.
   Each QRS complex is preceded by a P wave.
   The P-R interval is normal at 0.16 sec.
   The heart rate is 70 beats/min.
   The rhythm is normal sinus rhythm.

3. The QRS complex is normal in duration.
   The mean QRS vector is normal at approximately 45°.
   The mean QRS vector is to the left, inferior, and posterior, which is normal.

4. The QRS-T angle is normal.

5. The S-T segment is normal.

6. The Q-T interval is normal.

Impression: The electrocardiogram is normal.

ANSWERS TO
REVIEW QUESTIONS

From Page 18

1. Lead I
   a. extremity: left arm (+)
   b. extremity: right arm (−)

2. Lead II
   a. extremity: left leg (+)
   b. extremity: right arm (−)

3. Lead III
   a. extremity: left leg (+)
   b. extremity: left arm (−)

4.

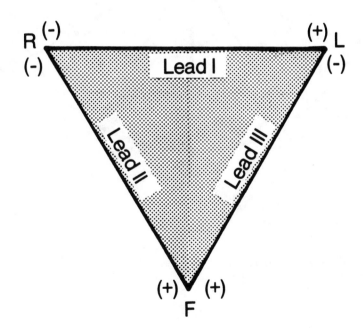

From Page 29

1.

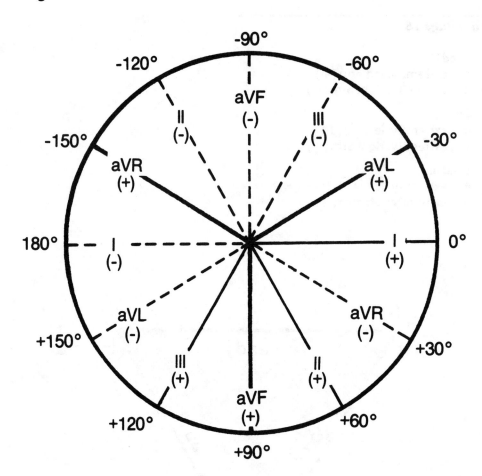

2. Lead I + lead III = lead II
3. Leads aVR + aVL + aVF = 0

From Page 33

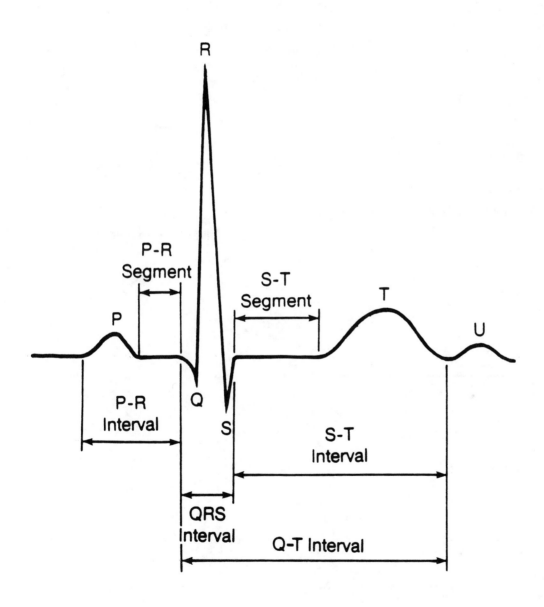

From Pages 40-43

1. 0°
2. 60°
3. beyond 120°
4. beyond −30°
5. approximately 110°

6. −60°
7. approximately 45°
8. approximately 45°
9. 90°

From Page 54

1. QRS vector which is beyond −30°
2. QRS vector which is beyond 105°
3. N
4. A
5. N
6. N
7. N

8. A
9. A
10. A (slightly beyond +105°)
11. A
12. N
13. N
14. N

From Pages 56-58

1. approximately 45°
2. −60°
3. approximately 45°

4. 0°
5. approximately 45°

From Page 66

1. −60° (abnormal)

2. 120°. A mean P vector of 120° is abnormal; however, the electrocardiogram is from a patient with dextrocardia (heart on *right* rather than left side). The origin of the impulse is in the S-A node. For *this patient* it is a normal mean P vector.

From Pages 73-75

1. Sinus rhythm is the normal rhythm of the heart, originating in the S-A node. The criteria are as follows: (a) the mean P vector is normal; (b) each P wave is followed by a QRS complex and each QRS complex is preceded by a P wave; (c) the P-R interval is between 0.12 and 0.2 sec. and constant from beat to beat; and (d) the heart rate is constant at 60 to 100 beats/min.

2. Abnormal RAD, abnormally wide QRS-T angle.

3. Abnormally wide QRS-T angle.

4. Lead I + lead III ≠ lead II (lead II is mounted upside down).

5. Abnormal LAD, abnormally wide QRS-T angle.

6. Abnormal mean P vector (ectopic atrial pacemaker).

NOTES AND REFERENCES

From Page 32:
Types of QRS Complexes

Although not all of the ventricular complexes contain Q, R, and S waves, they are commonly called QRS complexes. The ventricular complexes may also be described using large and small letters indicating the large or small sizes of the waves. For example, the complex in No. 1 may be described as QRS or qRs since the q and s waves are small relative to the R wave. Similarly, No. 2 may be described as RS or Rs, etc. The use of large and small letters is especially helpful in a written description when not accompanied by the actual electrocardiogram.

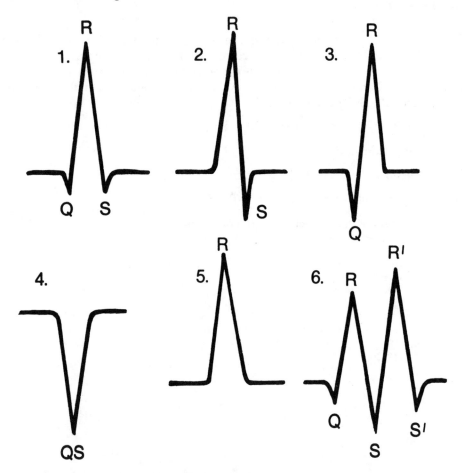

1. QRS; Q wave—negative deflection before the R wave
   R wave—positive deflection
   S wave—negative deflection after the R wave.
2. RS; no Q wave present.
3. QR; no S wave present.
4. QS; totally negative complex, no R wave present.
5. R; no Q or S waves present.
6. QRSR′S′, a second positive deflection after an S wave in an R′ (R prime), which, in turn, may be followed by a second negative deflection, an S′ (S prime).

From Page 54:   Mean QRS Vector—
Normal and Abnormal

A method for rapid determination of the quadrant in which the mean QRS vector is located, using leads I and aVF, is illustrated below.

In the normal adult the mean QRS vector is usually between 0 and 90°, that is, the mean QRS vector is normally between leads I and aVF (shaded area). From 0 to − 90° is *left axis deviation (LAD)* and from 90 to 180° is *right axis deviation (RAD)*. The area from − 90 to 180° has usually been described as *extreme right axis deviation*. As noted on page 53, *abnormal* LAD is beyond − 30° and *abnormal* RAD is beyond +105°.

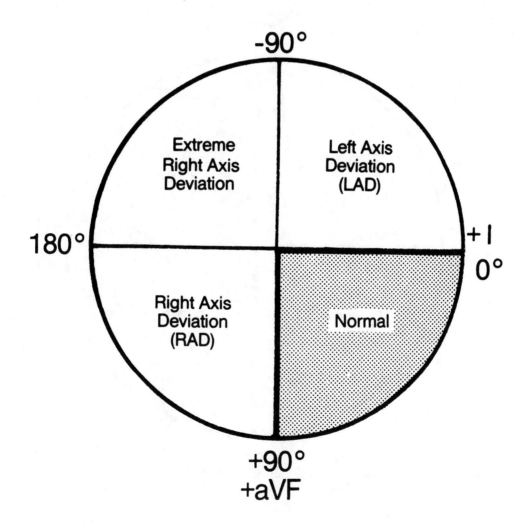

Since leads I and aVF are at right angles to each other, the quadrant in which a mean QRS vector is located may be easily found by using these two leads. The entire left (shaded) half of the circle is *positive* for lead I. Therefore, if the QRS complex is *positive* in lead I, the mean QRS vector is either normal or deviated to the left. If the QRS complex is *negative* in lead I, we have right axis or extreme right axis deviation.

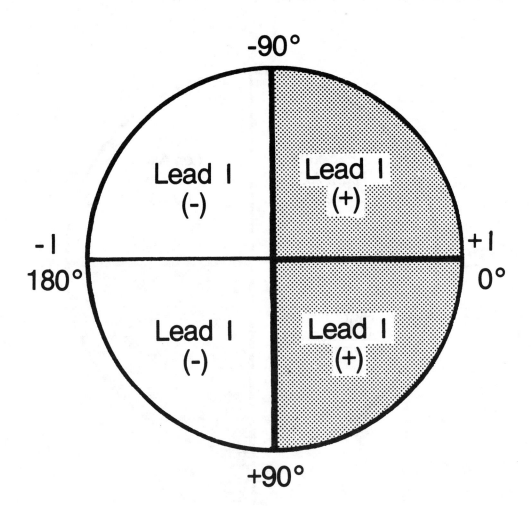

The entire lower half (shaded) of the circle is *positive* for lead aVF and the upper half is *negative* for lead aVF. Therefore, if the QRS complex is *positive* in lead aVF, the mean QRS vector is either normal or deviated to the right. If the QRS complex is *negative,* we have left axis deviation or extreme right axis deviation.

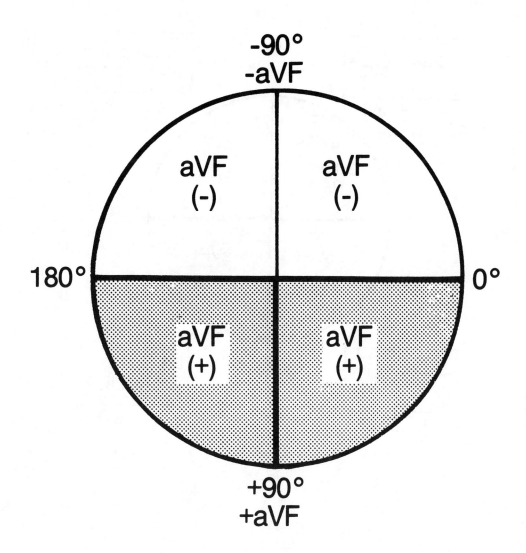

By utilizing both leads I and aVF, we can localize the quadrant containing the mean QRS vector. If both leads I and aVF are *positive,* the mean QRS vector is normal (shaded area). Describe leads I and aVF in left axis deviation, right axis deviation, and extreme right axis deviation.

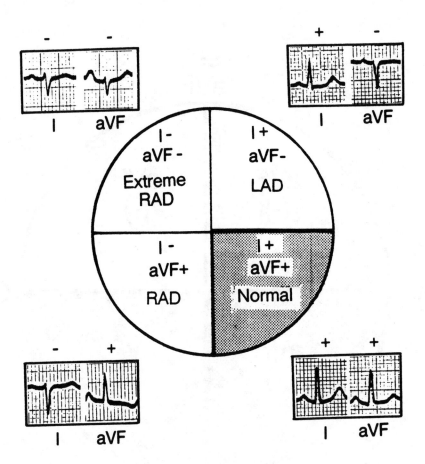

From Page 70:
Electrocardiographic Standardization

The usual standardization on the electrocardiogram of 1 mv. results in a deflection of 2 large boxes (10 mm.). This standardization is essential in order to properly evaluate the size of the deflections and has been used on the electrocardiograms in this course.

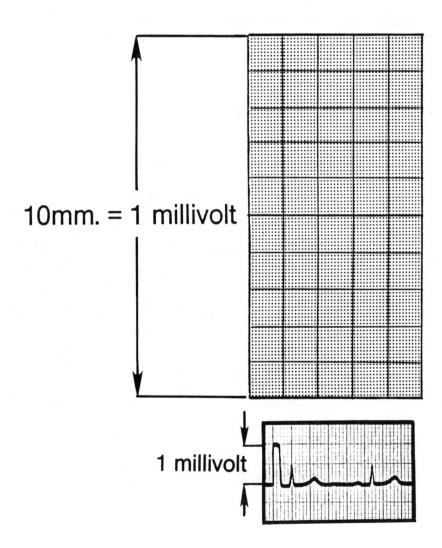

10mm. = 1 millivolt

1 millivolt

From Page 71:   Heart Rate
Determination—Another Method

Another method of determining heart rate is to utilize the 3-sec. markers (15 large boxes = 3 sec.) at the upper border of the electrocardiographic paper. Count the number of QRS complexes in a 6-sec. period and multiply by 10 for the rate per minute. Within the 6-sec. period above there are 6 QRS complexes. Therefore, the heart rate is 6 × 10 = 60 beats per minute. This method is especially useful when the rhythm is not regular.

Very often the electrocardiographic paper has been cut down so that the marks are not evident. In that case, count 30 large boxes and the number of QRS complexes within the 30 boxes and multiply by 10.

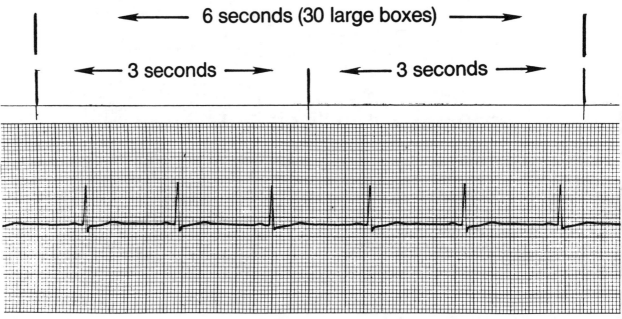

No. ECG 100

QRS Complexes in 6 sec. x 10 = Heart Rate

From Page 72:   Ladder Diagrams (Laddergrams)

The ladder diagram or laddergram is a useful aid in the study of normal and abnormal rhythms of the heart. It is a method of visually displaying the timing of events. The ladder consists of at least three tiers. A represents atrial depolarization, the P wave. V represents ventricular depolarization, the QRS complex. A-V represents the atrioventricular conduction across the atrioventricular junction. The sinoatrial node is at the top of the A tier. A laddergram of normal sinus rhythm is illustrated below.

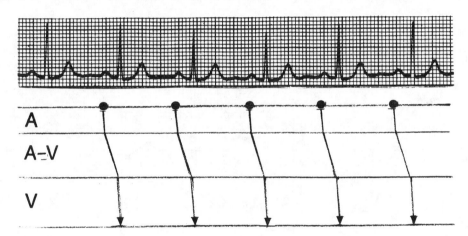

The dot (●) representing the site of impulse formation and the arrow (↓) showing the direction of the impulse have been added for graphic completeness, but are not critical since the slope of the lines provides this information. Note the slowing of the impulse at the A-V level.

From Page 87:   Clockwise and Counterclockwise Rotation

It had been thought that the electrocardiographic manifestations described below were the result of anatomic rotation; actually, very little rotation occurs. The terms *clockwise and counterclockwise rotation* are still in use, but should be used in an electrical sense only.[1-1]

Normal. The transition from predominantly S waves to predominantly R waves occurs in lead V_3 or V_4 or between them.[1-2] In this electrocardiogram the transition occurs between leads V_3 and V_4.

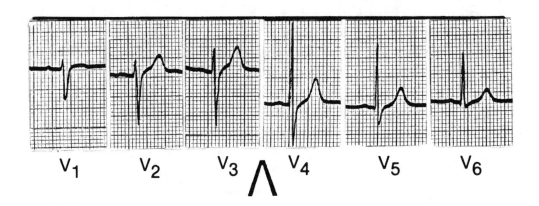

Clockwise rotation. The transition occurs beyond lead V_4. In this electrocardiogram the transition occurs between leads V_4 and V_5. Schamroth refers to clockwise rotation when rS or RS patterns are present in all or most of the precordial leads.[1-1]

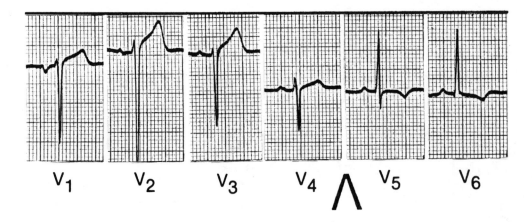

Counterclockwise rotation. The transition occurs before lead V_3. In this electrocardiogram the transition occurs between leads V_1 and V_2.

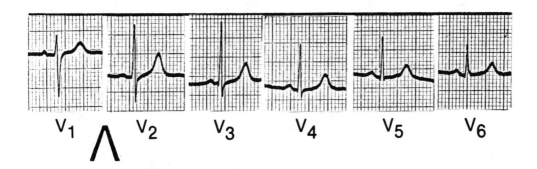

Other terms, less commonly used today, described the electrical position of the heart. These include the terms horizontal, vertical, semihorizontal, semivertical, and intermediate. It is much more common to state that the mean electrical axes are 0°, 45°, or 90° than to refer to those hearts as horizontal, intermediate, or vertical, respectively.

References

1-1. Schamroth, L.: The 12 Lead Electrocardiogram. Oxford, Blackwell Scientific Publications, 1989, pp. 11-12.

1-2. Marriott, H.J.L.: Practical Electrocardiography, 8th Ed. Baltimore, Williams & Wilkins, 1988, pp. 44-46.

2

RIGHT VENTRICULAR HYPERTROPHY (INCLUDING RIGHT AND LEFT ATRIAL ENLARGEMENT)

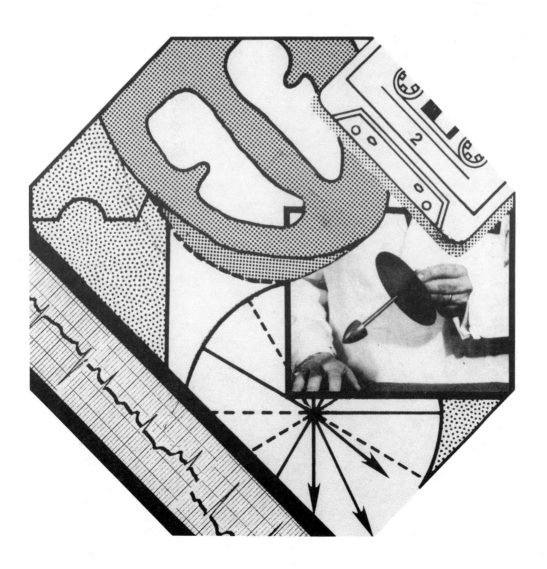

CHAPTER 2:
CONTENTS

INTRODUCTION

The diagnosis of right ventricular hypertrophy is frequently difficult to make electrocardiographically in the adult. The left ventricle if dominant, and even a very hypertrophied right ventricle may be overshadowed by a normal left ventricle. A normal electrocardiogram does not therefore rule out right ventricular hypertrophy. There are, however, certain findings on the electrocardiogram which help us make the diagnosis.

The presumptive, or indirect evidence, of right ventricular hypertrophy has often helped in the absence of direct electrocardiographic evidence. In addition to right atrial enlargement, left atrial enlargement will be studied since it may accompany right ventricular hypertrophy, for example, in the presence of mitral stenosis. The word "hypertrophy" is commonly used. Admittedly, hypertrophy is not the only cause of an enlarged right ventricle, and differentiation is often difficult on the electrocardiogram. "Enlargement" is a more inclusive term. Both terms are used in this study.

In clinical practice some causes of right ventricular hypertrophy (congenital and acquired) encountered include pulmonic stenosis, atrial septal defect, transposition of the great vessels, tetralogy of Fallot, chronic obstructive pulmonary disease, primary pulmonary hypertension, mitral stenosis, and tricuspid insufficiency.

O B J E C T I V E S

Upon completion of this chapter, you should be able to:

1. Recognize the electrocardiographic manifestations of right ventricular hypertrophy with respect to the following factors:

   (a) right axis deviation; (b) increase in the magnitude of the mean QRS vector; (c) repolarization abnormalities (abnormalities of the S-T segments and T waves); and (d) presumptive evidence of right ventricular hypertrophy.

2. State the major electrocardiographic criterion for the diagnosis of right ventricular hypertrophy, and list three additional criteria.

3. State the characteristics of the ischemia pattern on the electrocardiogram.

4. State the definition of strain pattern on the electrocardiogram.

5. Recognize the validity of the terms ischemia pattern and strain pattern.

6. State three factors demonstrating the importance of age (children versus adults) in the criteria for the electrocardiographic diagnosis of right ventricular hypertrophy.

7. Explain why right and left atrial enlargement is studied together with right ventricular hypertrophy.

8. Recognize the principal electrocardiographic characteristics of a mean spatial QRS vector which is to the right, inferior, and anterior.

9. Recognize the importance of the relationship between right axis deviation and right ventricular hypertrophy.

10. List the criteria for the electrocardiographic diagnosis of right and left atrial enlargement.

11. State the significance of an R wave which is the main ventricular deflection in lead V_1.

12. State what is meant by right axis deviation of the mean QRS vector.

13. List the magnitude criteria for the electrocardiographic diagnosis of right ventricular hypertrophy in children.

P R E T E S T

DIRECTIONS: This pretest consists of four electrocardiograms. Write a brief analysis of each in the space provided.

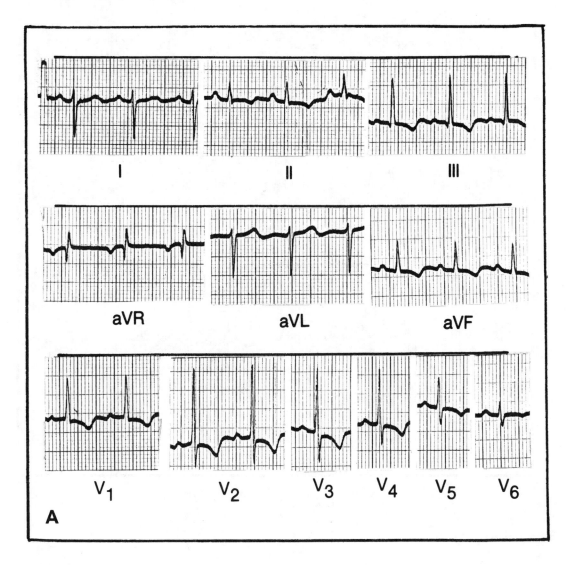

FIGURE 2-3A.

1. Analysis:

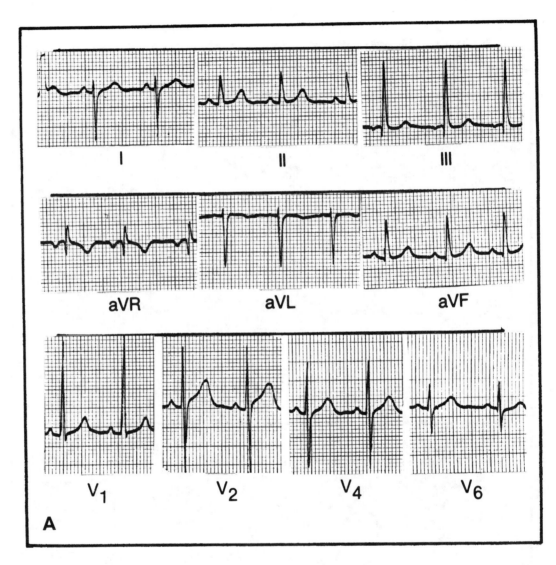

FIGURE 2-7A.

2. Analysis:

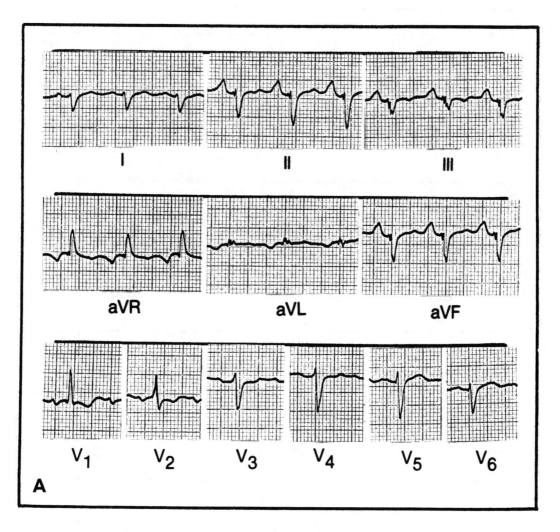

FIGURE 2-9A.

3. Analysis:

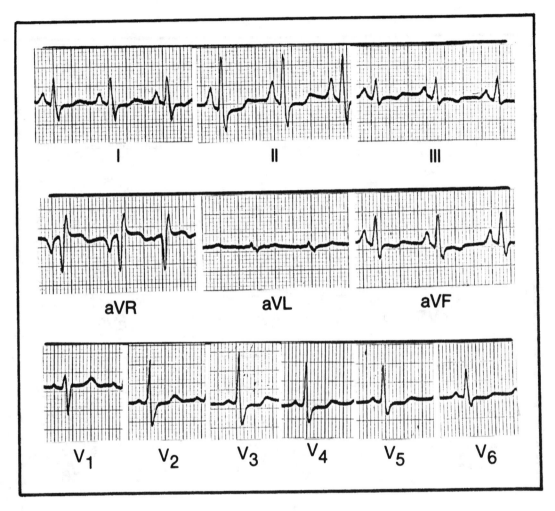

FIGURE 2-16.

4. Analysis:

> Solutions to the pretest will be indicated later in this chapter.

> When you have finished your analyses, start Cassette Side 5 and continue on the next page.

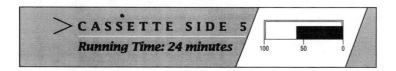

CASSETTE SIDE 5
Running Time: 24 minutes

100   50   0

DIAGNOSTIC CRITERIA OF RIGHT VENTRICULAR HYPERTROPHY

Electrocardiographic diagnosis of right ventricular hypertrophy is made on the basis of (A) right axis deviation of the mean QRS vector; (B) magnitude of the mean QRS vector; (C) repolarization abnormalities, that is, abnormalities of the S-T segments and T waves; and (D) presumptive evidence in the form of right atrial enlargement and left atrial enlargement in the presence of mitral stenosis.

A. *Right Axis Deviation (RAD)*

In the normal adult, as already learned, the left ventricle is dominant (Figure 2-1A), and the mean spatial QRS vector is usually oriented to the *left, inferiorly,* and *posteriorly.* In the newborn (Figure 2-1B), the right ventricle, located anteriorly and to the right of the left ventricle, is dominant and the mean QRS vector, reflecting this dominance, is usually to the *right, inferior,* and *anterior.*

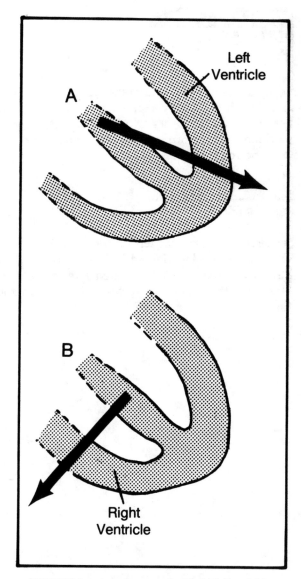

FIGURE 2-1.   A, In the normal adult the left ventricle is dominant, and the mean QRS vector is usually to the left, inferior, and posterior. B, In early life the right ventricle is dominant and the mean QRS vector is usually to the right, inferior, and anterior.

Abnormal right axis deviation (RAD) of the mean QRS vector refers to a vector beyond + 105°. This is illustrated in Figure 1-36.

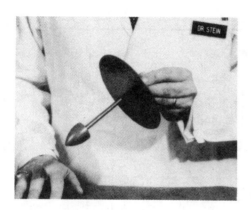

A. Infancy

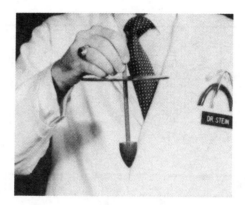

B. Youth

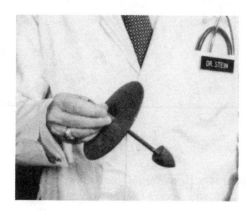

C. Adulthood

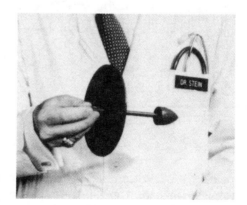

D. Old Age

FIGURE 2-2.   *Changes in the mean QRS vector from birth to old age.*

The mean QRS vector, which in infancy is to the *right, inferior,* and *anterior,* becomes ever more *leftward* and ever more *posterior* throughout life. The left ventricle early becomes, and remains throughout life, the dominant ventricle. Therefore, progression to, or persistence of, the pattern seen in infancy should cause you to immediately stop and evaluate the patient for right ventricular hypertrophy. The importance of serial electrocardiograms must be emphasized, for you may see subtle changes providing the clue to progressive hypertrophy of the right ventricle.

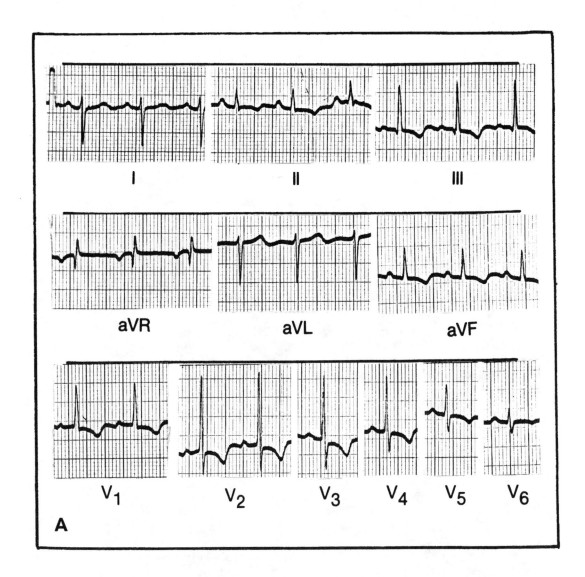

FIGURE 2-3A.   Right ventricular hypertrophy.

In Figure 2-3A, the QRS complexes in lead I are almost entirely negative, with positive QRS complexes in leads II and III. The transitional zone falls along the axis of lead aVR, with the mean QRS vector at $+120°$, clearly in the area of right axis deviation. This is diagrammed in Figure 2-4. Leads V_1 to V_5 are predominantly positive with the transition at V_6. Therefore, the three-dimensional mean QRS vector, in addition to being to the *right* and *inferior,* is also *anterior* (Figure 2-5). From a vectorial point of view, these findings, which are characteristic of the hypertrophied right ventricle, are in such contrast to the normal findings (compare and contrast this electrocardiogram with the normal in Figure 2-3B) that they stand out sharply upon inspection of the electrocardiogram.

The two electrocardiographic characteristics of a mean spatial QRS vector oriented to the *right* and *anteriorly* are:

1. QRS deflections in lead V_1 are *negative.*
2. QRS deflections in leads V_1 and V_2 are *positive.*

> The analysis of Figure 2-3A both in the text and on the tape is the solution to item 1 on the pretest.

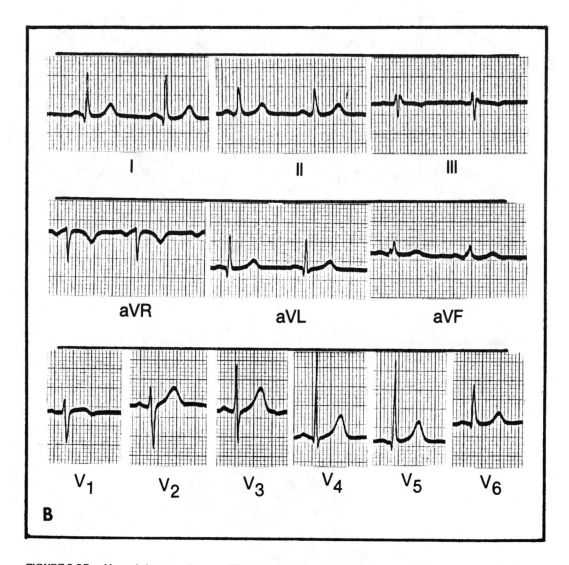

FIGURE 2-3B.   Normal electrocardiogram. When studying the abnormal always go back, compare, and contrast with the normal.

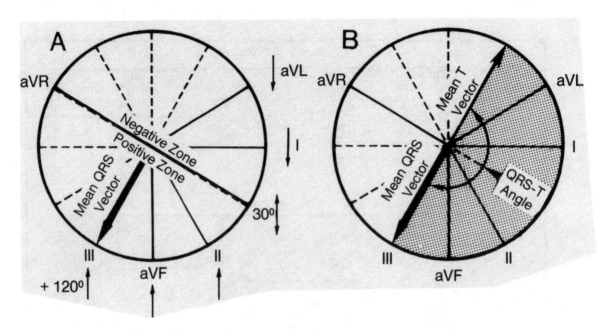

FIGURE 2-4.   A, The mean QRS vector in Figure 2-3A is to the right and inferior at + 120°, in the frontal plane. B, In Figure 2-3A, in addition to the abnormally oriented QRS vector, the QRS-T angle is also abnormal.

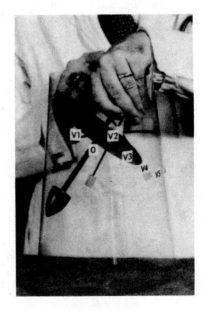

FIGURE 2-5.

The addition of the precordial leads permits us to see that the mean QRS vector, in addition to being to the *right* and *inferior,* is also *anterior.* In the face of frank right axis deviation, lead V_1 may be positive without anterior or posterior rotation of the mean QRS vector; however, if V_2 is also positive the mean QRS vector is rotated anteriorly.

B. Magnitude of the Mean Spatial QRS Vector

In the adult with right ventricular hypertrophy, the magnitude of the QRS deflections frequently is not increased. In fact, in emphysematous patients, with marked right ventricular hypertrophy, the QRS deflections may actually be small.

Although this course deals principally with adult electocardiography, examples of congenital heart disease in children are included. The question often arises as to the diagnosis of right ventricular hypertrophy in young children who *normally* have right ventricular preponderance. Table 2-1 gives one set of suggested criteria. It is in circumstances such as these that the criteria in this table may be helpful. In addition, Figure 2-17, from Nadas and Fyler, gives the R-S ratio in lead V_1 from birth to 13 years. For instance, if at birth the algebraic sum of the R and S waves in lead V_1 is 25 mm., which is well outside the normal range, right ventricular hypertrophy may be strongly suspected.

In the adult when the R wave is the *main ventricular deflection* in lead V_1, regardless of size, right ventricular hypertrophy enters into the differential diagnosis. Other causes of an R wave (or R'), as the main ventricular deflection in lead V_1, include true posterior myocardial infarction, right bundle branch block (RSR'), and the Wolff-Parkinson-White syndrome, type A. These will be studied later in the course.

C. Ventricular Repolarization (S-T Segment and T Wave) Abnormalities

Figure 2-3A not only illustrates a mean QRS vector which is abnormally oriented to the right, inferiorly, and anteriorly, but the QRS-T angle is also abnormal. This is diagrammed in Figure 2-4B. Note also the depression of the S-T segments, especially in leads V_2 to V_4. The wide QRS-T angle has often been referred to as an "ischemia" pattern, and S-T segment abnormalities together with a wide QRS-T angle, in the hypertrophied ventricle, as a "strain" pattern. These are not proper terms since these repolarization abnormalities are *secondary* (explained in Chapter 4) and not *primary* abnormalities. These repolarization abnormalities are expected with hypertrophy. The term *ischemia* in this course will refer only to *primary* repolarization abnormalities. The term "ventricular repolarization abnormalities," covering both the wide QRS-T angle and the abnormal S-T segment, is a better term. This will be repeated and reemphasized in the study of left ventricular hypertrophy in Chapter 3.

In order to be able to recognize right ventricular hypertrophy electrocardiographically, we will examine a number of electrocardiograms. In each figure, part A represents the hypertrophied right ventricle, and part B is the normal for comparison.

In Figure 2-6A the QRS complex is predominantly negative in lead I and positive in leads II and III. The mean QRS vector is to the *right* and *inferior* in the frontal plane. In leads V_1 and V_2 the QRS deflections are positive. The mean QRS vector is therefore not only to the right and inferior, but also *anterior*. Note the repolarization abnormalities; the QRS-T angle is wide, with S-T segment abnormalities.

None of the deflections is unusually large, but three important findings of right ventricular hypertrophy are present.
1. Right axis deviation (mean QRS vector oriented to the right).
2. The R wave is the main ventricular deflection in lead V_1. See criteria for the adult in Table 2-1.
3. Repolarization abnormalities (wide QRS-T angle and S-T segment abnormalities).

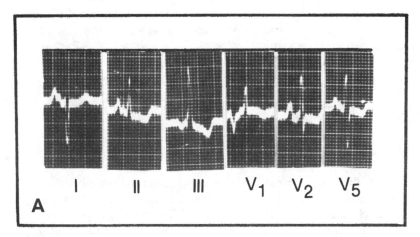

FIGURE 2-6A.   Right ventricular hypertrophy in a patient with mitral stenosis. (Electrocardiogram reduced in size.)

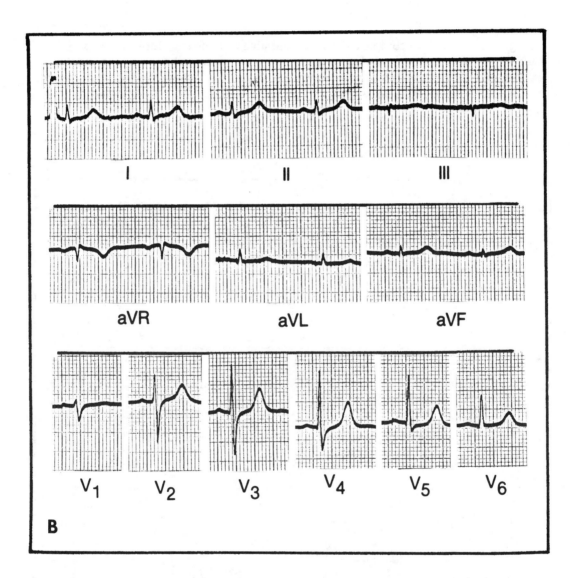

FIGURE 2-6B.   Normal electrocardiogram. How do the findings here differ from those in the electrocardiogram in Figure 2-6A?

In Figure 2-7A the QRS complex in lead I is negative with the transition at lead aVR. The QRS in lead V_1 is positive and of great magnitude. The mean QRS vector is to the *right, inferior,* and *anterior,* in contrast to the normal (Figure 2-7B), where the mean QRS vector is to the *left, inferior,* and *posterior.*

This patient, who had congenital heart disease, has an R wave magnitude greater than 25 mm. in lead V_1, which would permit an electrocardiographic diagnosis of right ventricular hypertrophy even at birth (see Figure 2-17).

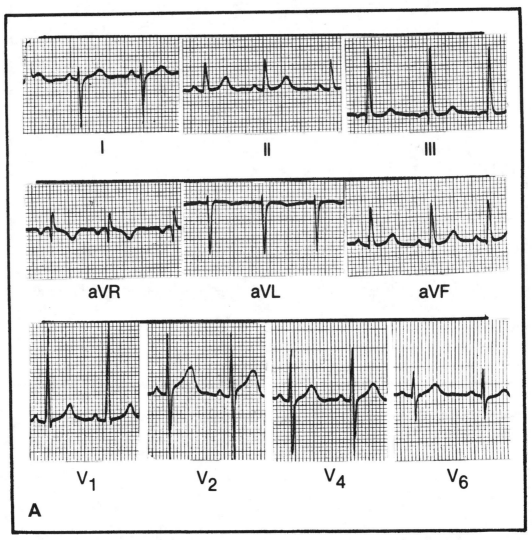

FIGURE 2-7A. *Right ventricular hypertrophy in a patient with congenital heart disease.*

> The analysis of the Figure 2-7A both in the text and on the tape is the solution to item 2 on the pretest.

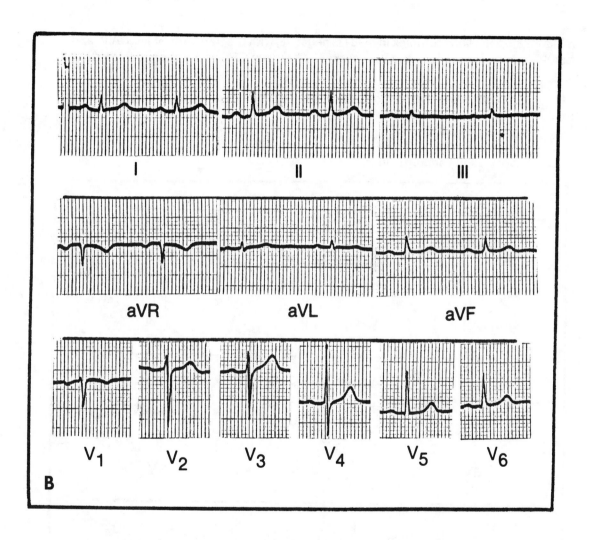

FIGURE 2-7B.   Normal electrocardiogram. Compare with the electrocardiogram in Figure 2-7A.

In Figure 2-8A the QRS complex in lead I is negative, with the transition at lead aVR, and the QRS complex in leads V_1 and V_2 is positive. The mean QRS vector therefore is to the *right, inferior,* and *anterior.*

Although the complexes are not large, the important findings of right ventricular hypertrophy in the adult are once again seen:

1. Right axis deviation.
2. The R wave in lead V_1 is the main ventricular deflection.
3. Repolarization abnormalities.

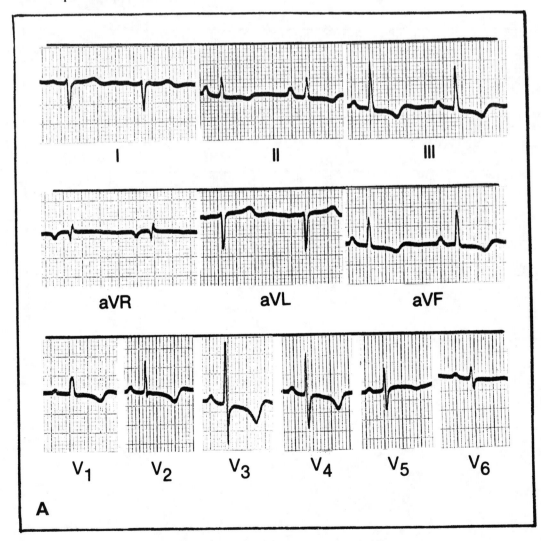

FIGURE 2-8A. Right ventricular hypertrophy in an adult.

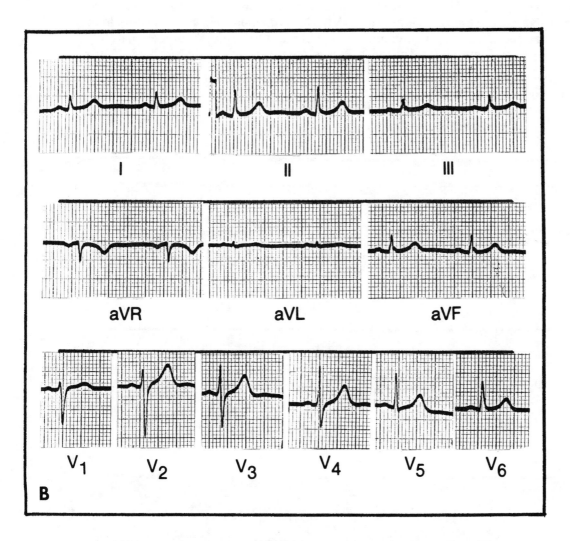

FIGURE 2-8B.   Normal electrocardiogram. Compare with electrocardiogram in Figure 2-8A.

Figure 2-9A, from a patient with advanced chronic obstructive lung disease with cor pulmonale, was studied earlier (see Figure 1-73); this electrocardiogram emphasizes the importance of understanding the vectorial forces. In the previous electrocardiograms representing right ventricular hypertrophy in this chapter, lead I was negative while leads II and III were positive. Here we have an electrocardiogram in which leads I, II, and III are all negative and the transition is near lead aVL. This is diagrammed in Figure 2-10. In the precordial leads, V_1 and V_2 are predominantly positive and the rest are predominantly negative (review Figure 1-75). The mean QRS vector is to the *right, superior,* and *anterior.*

Again the criteria, so far learned, for right ventricular hypertrophy are met:
1.   Right axis deviation.
2.   The R wave in lead V_1 is the main ventricular deflection.
3.   Repolarization abnormalities.

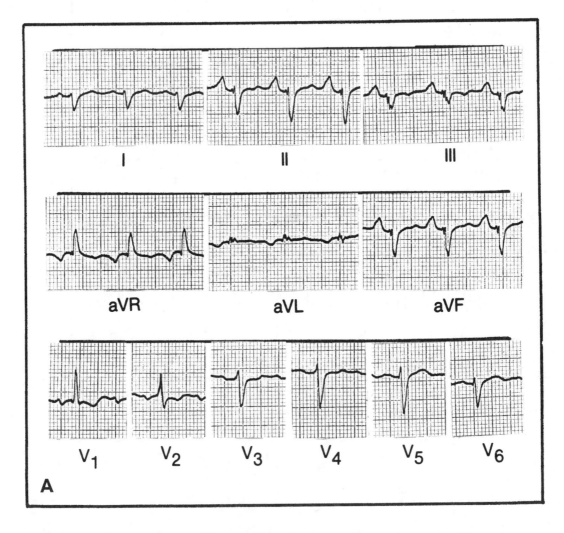

FIGURE 2-9A.   *How does the mean QRS vector differ in this electrocardiogram, representing right ventricular hypertrophy, from the mean QRS vectors seen in the previous electrocardiograms representing right ventricular hypertrophy in this chapter? This is diagrammed in Figure 2-10.*

> The analysis of Figure 2-9A both in the text and on the tape is the solution to item 3 on the pretest.

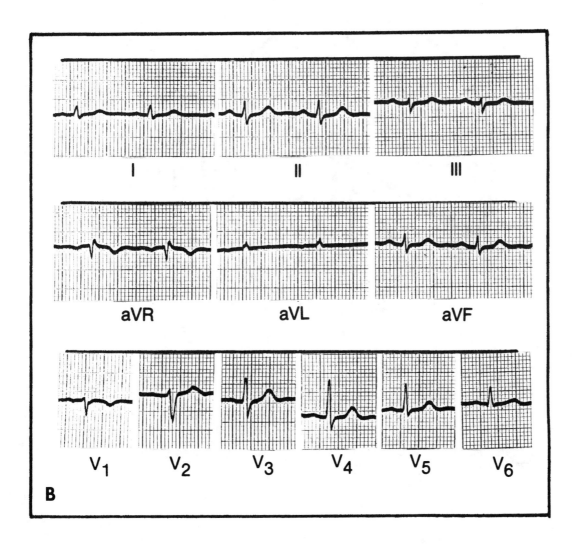

FIGURE 2-9B.   Normal electrocardiogram. Compare with electrocardiogram in Figure 2-9A.

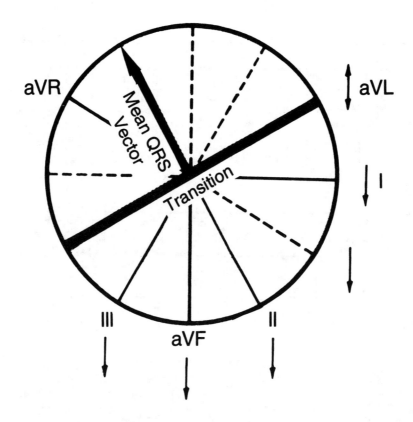

FIGURE 2-10.   The mean QRS vector in Figure 2-9A is to the right and superior in the frontal plane.

The hypertrophied right ventricle does not occur in a vacuum. It is often accompanied by the enlargement of the right atrium and, at times, by enlargement of the left atrium, as seen in mitral stenosis.

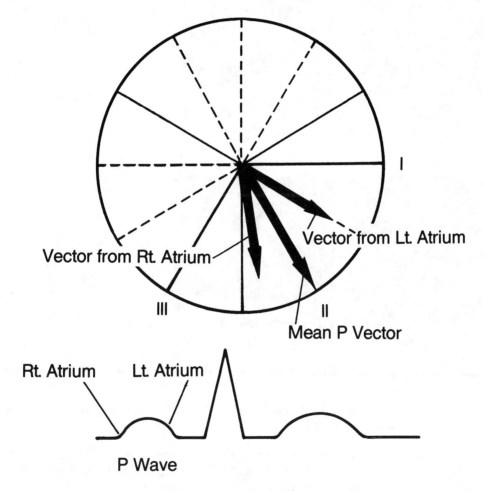

FIGURE 2-11.

The mean P vector, representing both atria, is usually in the area of lead II, with the P waves positive in leads I and aVF and often in lead III as well (see Figure 1-43). Figure 2-11 illustrates, in addition to the mean P vector, the right and left atrial vectors. The earlier right atrial vector is more rightward and anteriorly oriented compared with the left atrial vector, which is more leftward and posteriorly oriented.

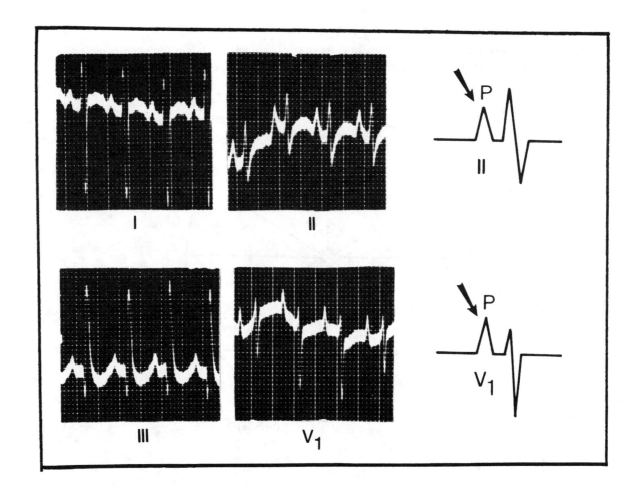

FIGURE 2-12.   *Electrocardiographic manifestations of right atrial enlargement in a young patient with congenital heart disease. (Electrocardiogram enlarged.)*

The right atrial vector is earlier, more rightward, and anterior compared to the left atrial vector. The right atrial vector faces leads II and III. Enlargement of the right atrium therefore results in the following electrocardiographic manifestations:

1. Tall, peaked P waves in leads II and III or even in leads I, II, and III.

2. Since the right atrial vector is also anterior, the early part of the P wave, or even the entire P wave, may be positive and of great magnitude in lead V_1 or leads V_1 and V_2.

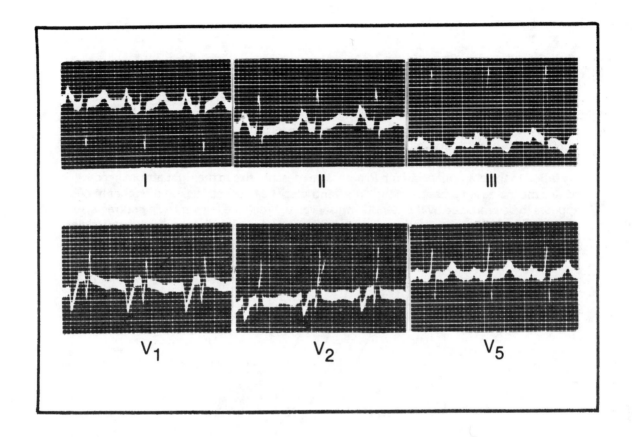

FIGURE 2-13.   Electrocardiographic manifestations of left atrial enlargement. (Electrocardiogram enlarged.)

Left atrial depolarization starts later than right atrial depolarization. The left atrial vector is more leftward and posterior compared with the right atrial vector and faces leads I and II. *Enlargement of the left atrium* therefore results in the following electrocardiographic manifestations:

1. Broad, notched, and sometimes tall P waves in leads I and II or even in leads I, II, III. The notching is due to the fact that the right atrial inscription is seen first, in the early part of the P wave, which is followed by the delayed depolarization of the enlarged left atrium.

2. The vector is posteriorly oriented, so that the latter part, sometimes the entire P wave, may be negative and of great magnitude in lead V_1.

Rarely, if ever, is the P wave deflection in the normal electrocardiogram greater than 3 mm. in any lead. If a P wave of this magnitude is found, atrial enlargement must be considered.

Biatrial enlargement, together with right ventricular enlargement, is not uncommon (mitral stenosis). Although left atrial enlargement is most prominent in this figure, the enlarged right atrium is represented by the early peaking of the P waves, especially in leads I and II. The initial Q wave, seen here in leads V_1 and V_2, together with the other findings, provides additional evidence of right ventricular hypertrophy.

Figure 2-14 is a representation of the enlargement of both atria and the right ventricle which may be found in patients with mitral valve stenosis. We will start at the left atrium. Between the left atrium and the left ventricle is the mitral valve. If the mitral orifice is significantly narrowed (stenotic), the left atrium enlarges, since it cannot supply blood properly to the left ventricle. As the pressure in the left atrium rises, it is reflected backwards into the pulmonary veins. This increased pressure in the pulmonary circuit is, in turn, reflected backwards into the right ventricle, whose pressure must increase to supply blood to the pulmonary circuit. Progressive pressure rise in the right atrium accompanies the increased pressure in the right ventricle. The left ventricle, on the other hand, appears to be protected by the stenotic mitral valve. When the left ventricle contracts, blood enters the aorta, and if there is no significant aortic valve disease, the left ventricle may remain relatively normal in size or even smaller than normal.

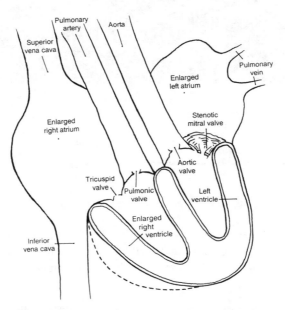

FIGURE 2-14. *The hypertrophied right ventricle is not infrequently accompanied by an enlarged right atrium and an enlarged left atrium (as seen in mitral stenosis).*

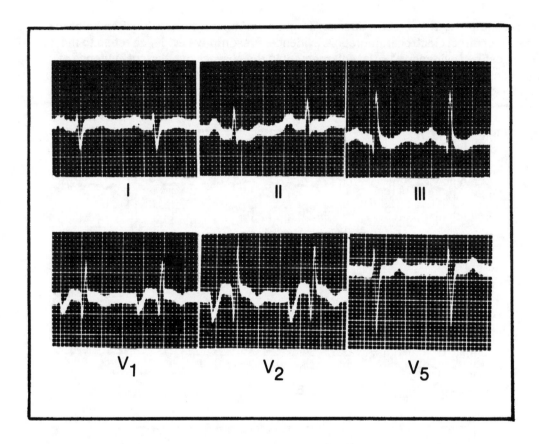

FIGURE 2-15. Adult with mitral stenosis. List all the criteria for (1) right ventricular and (2) left atrial enlargement. (Electrocardiogram enlarged.)

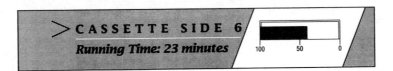

D. "Presumptive" Evidence of Right Ventricular Hypertrophy

The presumptive, or indirect, evidence of right ventricular hypertrophy often helps in the absence of direct electrocardiographic evidence. Presumptive evidence refers to the clearly defined evidence of atrial enlargement in the *absence* of clear-cut evidence of right ventricular enlargement. The assumption is that atrial enlargement, right or left, is not an isolated finding.

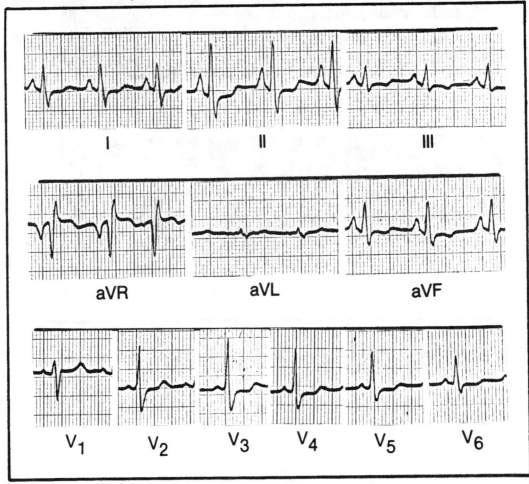

FIGURE 2-16.   *Elderly patient with chronic obstructive lung disease and cor pulmonale. What is the "presumptive" evidence which makes you suspicious of right ventricular hypertrophy? Note the tall, peaked P waves, especially prominent in lead II, representing right atrial enlargement, and good "presumptive" evidence of right ventricular enlargement. In the absence of tricuspid stenosis, which is rare as a single lesion, enlargement of the right atrium signifies enlargement of the right ventricle.*

> The analysis of Figure 2-16 in the legend and the text and on the tape is the solution to item 4 on the pretest.

TABLE 2-1.   Right Ventricular Hypertrophy

Once the basic concepts of the vectorial forces of right ventricular and right and left atrial enlargement are understood, the criteria are easily learned. The emphasis in this course has always been on the concept rather than on the "criteria." Do not be a slave to figures; they frequently change in the face of evolving information. The following values are general, especially for infants and children in whom the changes progress rapidly during the first few years.

A. Right Axis Deviation (RAD)
   Evaluate carefully since right axis deviation is normal in the very young.

B. Magnitude of the Mean QRS Vector
   Frontal Plane Leads: I, II, III, aVR, aVL, and aVF.
   Incomplete right bundle branch block (RBBB) pattern. RBBB is discussed and illustrated in Chapter 6.

   $S_I + R_{III}$ and/or $S_{aVL} + R_{aVF} \geq 35$ mm. (principally in children)
   R_{aVR} or $R'_{aVR} = 6$ mm.
   $R_{aVR} > Q_{aVR}$

   The R in lead aVR becomes taller with increased magnitude of the mean QRS vector, especially as the vector becomes more rightward (toward + aVR).

   Horizontal Plane Leads: V_1 to V_6.
   Algebraic sum of R and S waves in lead V_1 more than 15 mm. in height (Figure 2-17). At birth a tall R wave in lead V_1 may still be normal. An R wave in lead V_1 greater than 15 mm., however, may represent an abnormally enlarged right ventricle even in the newborn. In the adult the following criteria may be found.

   $R_{V_1} \geq 7$ mm.
   $S_{V_1} \leq 2$ mm.
   R/S ratio in $V_1 \geq 1$
   qR pattern in V_1

   Increased ventricular activation time with delayed onset of intrinsicoid deflection. (Ventricular activation time and intrinsicoid deflection are illustrated on page 192.)

   R_{V_5} or $R_{V_6} \leq 5$ mm.
   S_{V_5} or $S_{V_6} \geq 7$ mm.
   R/S ratio in V_5 or $V_6 \leq 1$

C. Repolarization Abnormalities
   (Wide QRS-T Angle and S-T Segment Abnormalities)
   The terms "ischemia" and "strain" are commonly used to describe repolarization abnormalities of hypertrophy; what is meant is that there is a wide QRS-T angle (ischemia) plus S-T segment abnormalities yielding a "strain" pattern. These are not proper terms since these repolarization abnormalities are *secondary* (explained in

> Ventricular activation time (V.A.T.) and the intrinsicoid deflection are explained and illustrated on page 192.

TABLE 2-1 (cont'd)

Chapter 4) and not *primary* abnormalities. These repolarization abnormalities are expected with hypertrophy. "Ischemia" is a term more appropriately used with *primary* repolarization abnormalities. The term "ventricular repolarization abnormalities," covering both the wide QRS-T angle and the abnormal S-T segment, is a better term.

Note: In an adult, if the R wave is the main ventricular deflection in lead V₁, regardless of size, the possibility of right ventricular enlargement must be considered. This finding alone does not always point to the enlarged right ventricle. In your differential diagnosis should be:

a.   True posterior wall myocardial infarction.
b.   Right bundle branch block (RSR').
c.   The Wolff-Parkinson-White syndrome, type A.

These will be studied later.

D. Presumptive Evidence of Right Ventricular Hypertrophy

Presumptive evidence refers to the clearly defined evidence of atrial enlargement in the *absence* of clear-cut evidence of right ventricular enlargement. Review the criteria for right and left atrial enlargement as explained in Figures 2-12 and 2-13, and remember that a more common cause of left atrial enlargement is left ventricular enlargement. In the adult the normal right ventricular wall is only one third as thick as the left ventricular wall. Even a 100% increase in the thickness of the right ventricle will not cause it to be as thick as the predominant left ventricle. As a result, even marked hypertrophy of the right ventricle may not be manifest on the clinical electrocardiogram. On the other hand, clear evidence of right atrial enlargement, in the absence of tricuspid valve stenosis, is good presumptive evidence of right ventricular enlargement.

Right Atrial Enlargement

See Figure 2-12 for explanation and illustration of tall, peaked P waves in leads II, III, and V₁.

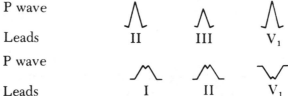

Left Atrial Enlargement

See Figure 2-13 for explanation and illustrations of broad, notched P waves in leads I, II, and V₁.

⟩ Additional criteria will be found on pages 193 and 194.

TABLE 2-1(cont'd)

Right Ventricular Hypertrophy
Principal Criteria—Review

In right ventricular hypertrophy the mean QRS vector shifts *rightward* and *anteriorly,* inscribing both the *negative* QRS complex in lead I and the *positive* QRS complex in lead V_1. Ventricular repolarization (ST-T) abnormalities commonly accompany right ventricular hypertrophy. Another criterion is *presemptive evidence* of right ventricular hypertrophy. This refers to evidence of right atrial enlargement in the *absence* of electrocardiographic evidence of right ventricular hypertrophy. Right atrial enlargement rarely occurs alone.

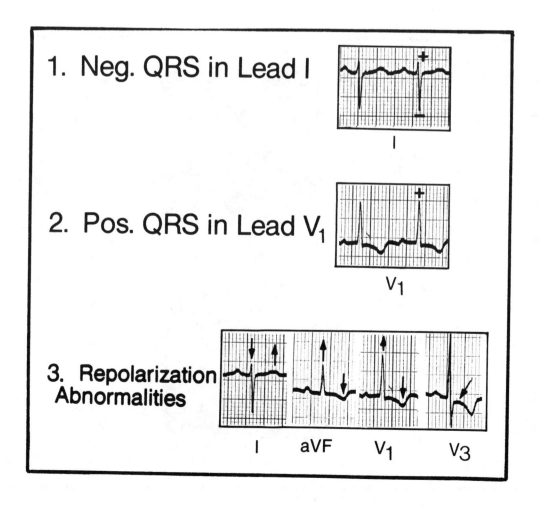

TABLE 2-1 (cont'd)

Right Atrial Hypertrophy
Principal Criteria—Review

In right atrial enlargement we see tall, early peaked P waves in

Lead II, often also in leads III and aVF

Lead V_1 or leads V_1 and V_2

Note: When evidence of right atrial enlargement is found in the electrocardiogram, it is good *presumptive evidence* of right *ventricular* hypertrophy, since right atrial enlargement rarely occurs alone.

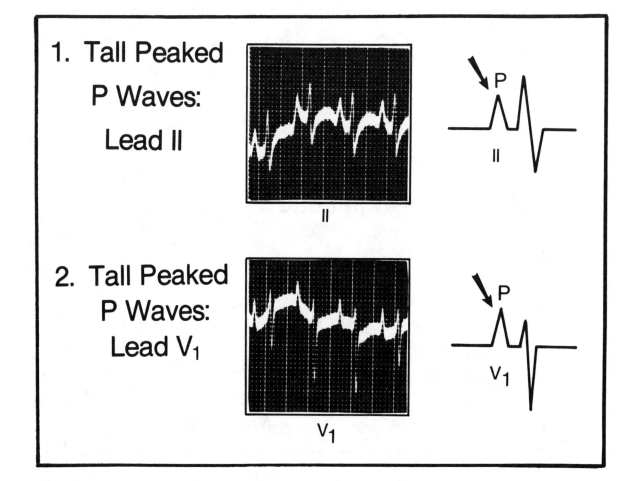

1. Tall Peaked P Waves: Lead II

2. Tall Peaked P Waves: Lead V_1

TABLE 2-1 (cont'd)

Left Atrial Enlargement
Principal Criteria—Review

In left atrial enlargement the following types of P waves may be seen:
Lead I—Broad, notched P waves
Lead V_1—Negative P waves of increased magnitude:

A. Broad and notched.
B. Entirely negative.
C. Second part of diphasic P wave, markedly negative.

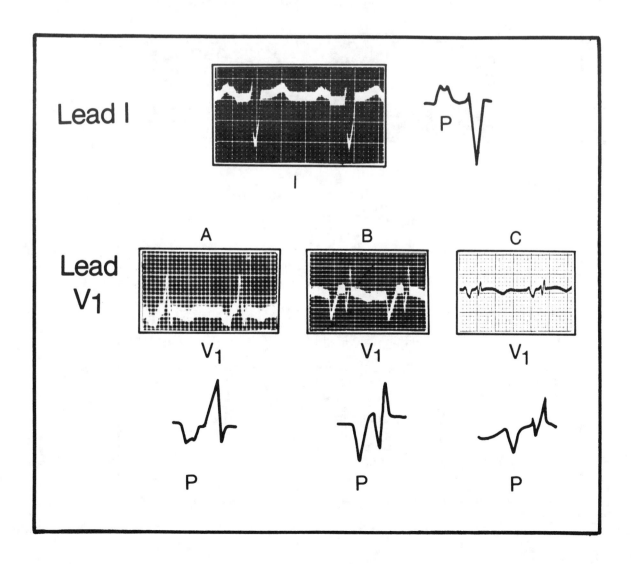

TABLE 2-1 (cont'd)

Biatrial Enlargement

Biatrial enlargement has features of both right and left atrial enlargement. In leads I and II we have the early peaking of the P wave of right atrial enlargement and the notching of left atrial enlargement. In lead V_1 we see the prominent first half of the diphasic P wave of right atrial enlargement and the significantly negative second half, representing left atrial enlargement.

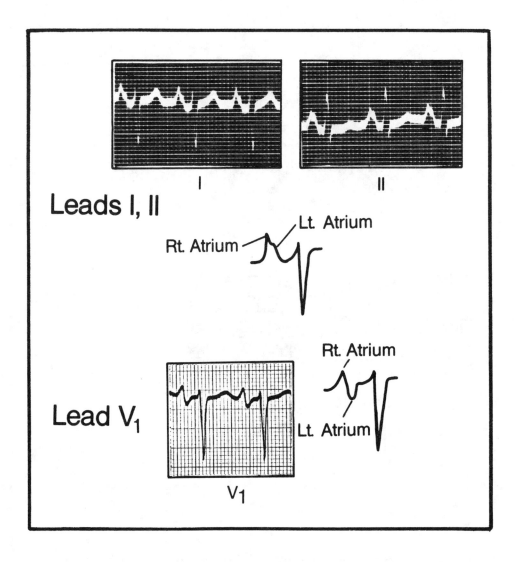

Figure 2-17, from Nadas and Fyler, gives the algebraic sum of the R and S waves in lead V_1 from birth to 13 years. For example, as noted earlier in this chapter, if at birth the algebraic sum of the R and S waves is 25 mm., which is well outside the normal range, right ventricular hypertrophy is strongly suggested.

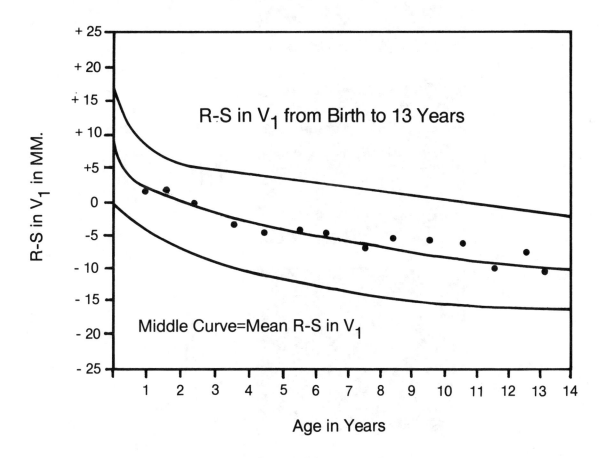

FIGURE 2-17.   The algebraic sum of R and S waves in lead V_1 from birth to 13 years. The progression of the mean QRS vector in the horizontal plane, from anterior to posterior, is reflected in the R-S sum in lead V_1. (From Nadas, A.S., and Fyler, D.C.: Pediatric Cardiology, 3rd Ed. Philadelphia, W.B. Saunders, 1972.)

REVIEW
ELECTROCARDIOGRAMS

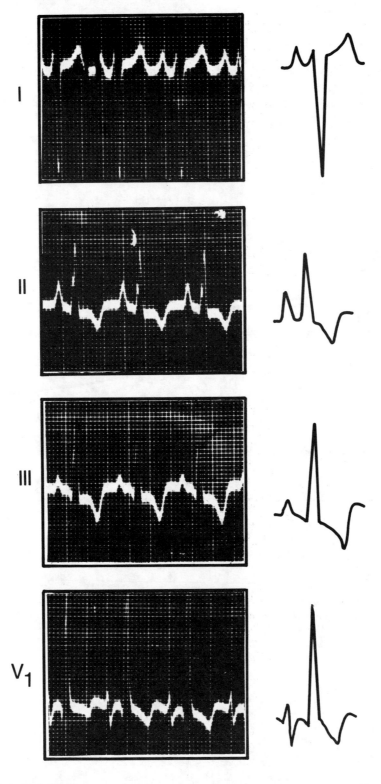

I

II

III

V₁

FIGURE 2-18.   Right ventricular hypertrophy in a young patient with congenital heart disease. (Electrocardiogram enlarged.)

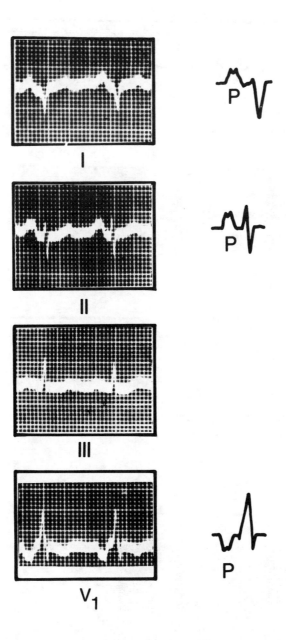

I

II

III

V₁

FIGURE 2-19.   Adult with mitral stenosis. Describe the characteristics of right ventricular and left atrial enlargement. (Electrocardiogram enlarged.)

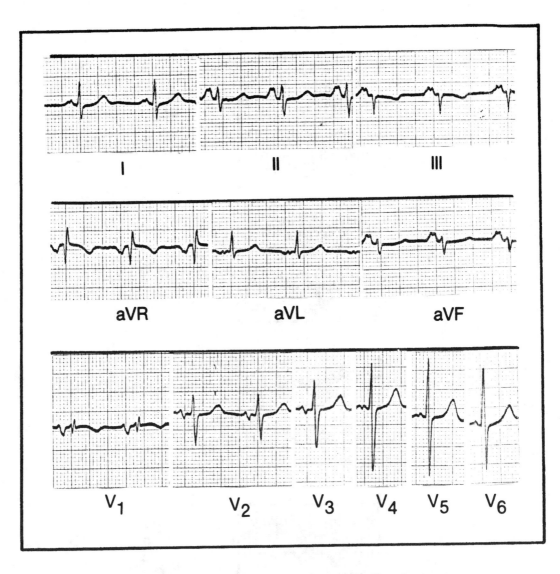

FIGURE 2-20.   Review all the electrocardiographic evidence of chamber enlargement.

> After you have analyzed Figure 2-20 refer to page 194 for definition of systolic and diastolic overload of the right ventricle.

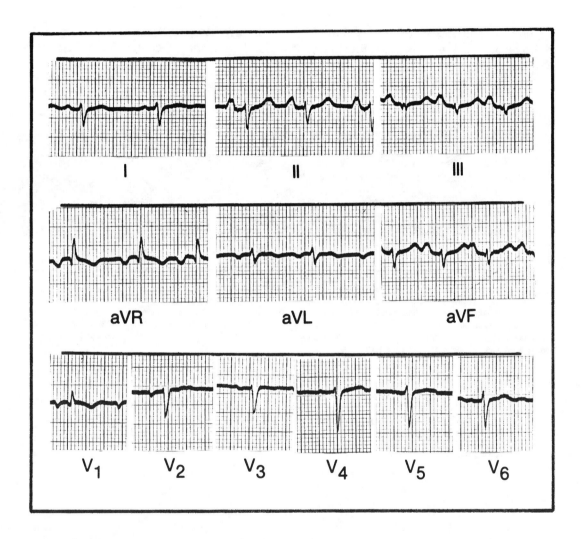

FIGURE 2-21.   *Right ventricular hypertrophy, in a patient with chronic lung disease and cor pulmonale. Note that, although it is small, the R wave is the main ventricular deflection in lead V₁. What is the orientation of the mean QRS vector?*

Figures 2-22 to 2-35 are examples of right ventricular hypertrophy. Practice analyzing them by detailing all the criteria for right ventricular hypertrophy, including: (a) right axis deviation; (b) increase in the magnitude of the mean QRS vector; (c) repolarization abnormalities; and (d) "presumptive" evidence.

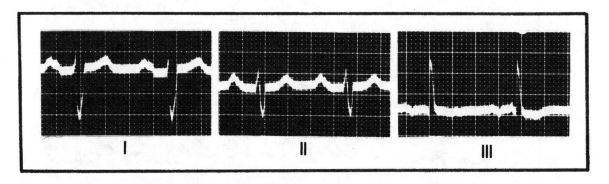

FIGURE 2-22.   Right ventricular hypertrophy. Right axis deviation is a common finding in right ventricular hypertrophy. Also evident is the broad, notched P wave, especially in lead I, and the wide QRS-T angle. The distance from the beginning of the P wave to the beginning of the QRS complex is greater than 0.2 sec. (one large box). This is known as first-degree atrioventricular block and will be observed again later. This patient had mitral stenosis. (Electrocardiogram enlarged.)

Analysis:

    a. right axis deviation:

    b. increase in the magnitude of the mean QRS vector:

    c. repolarization abnormalities:

    d. "presumptive" evidence:

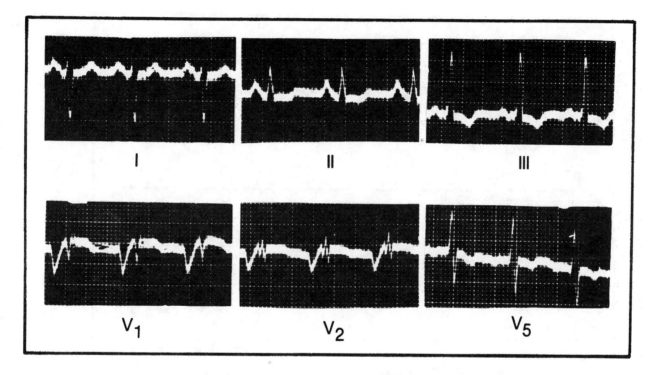

FIGURE 2-23. *Right ventricular hypertrophy. Note right axis deviation, broad and notched P waves, especially in lead I, tall P waves in lead II, deep negative P waves in lead V_1 (the P waves are of greater magnitude than the QRS complexes), and a wide QRS-T angle. Although we have clear evidence of right ventricular enlargement, the QRS vector in the horizontal plane is posterior, as seen from the negative QRS complexes in lead V_1. One does not need all the criteria in each and every case to make the diagnosis. This patient had mitral stenosis with right ventricular and biatrial enlargement. (Electrocardiogram enlarged.)*

Analysis:

    a.   right axis deviation:

    b.   increase in the magnitude of the mean QRS vector:

    c.   repolarization abnormalities:

    d.   "presumptive" evidence:

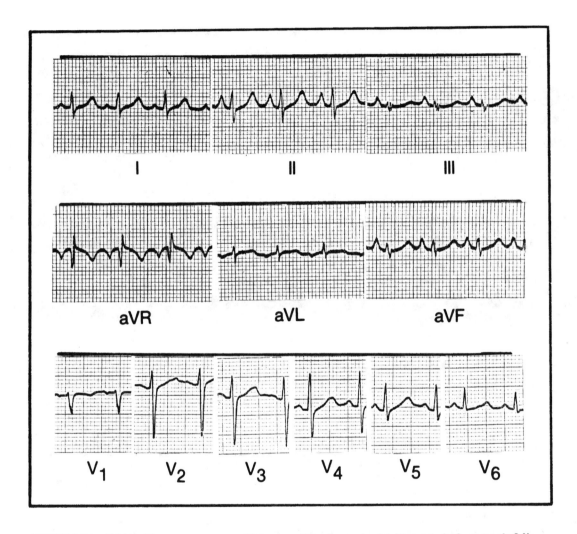

FIGURE 2-24. *What evidence can you assemble to support the diagnosis of right ventricular hypertrophy? Up to this point your diagnosis would be based on "presumptive" evidence. In a later chapter, you will study the "S$_I$ S$_{II}$ S$_{III}$ syndrome," which includes right ventricular hypertrophy in the differential diagnosis.*

Analysis:

    a. right axis deviation:

    b. increase in the magnitude of the mean QRS vector:

    c. repolarization abnormalities:

    d. "presumptive" evidence:

Figure 2-25 emphasizes a concept of great importance, the contribution of serial electro-cardiograms in following a patient. In Figure 2-25A the QRS complex is predominantly positive in leads I, II, and III; the mean QRS vector is within normal limits. The tall peaked P waves in lead II and, to a lesser degree, in leads I and III, represent right atrial enlarge-ment in this elderly patient and constitute good presumptive evidence of right ventricu-lar enlargement.

A year and a half later we no longer had to look for "presumptive" evidence because the QRS deflections in lead I in Figure 2-25B had become predominantly negative; the mean QRS vector had shifted rightward. The importance of serial electrocardiograms must again be emphasized.

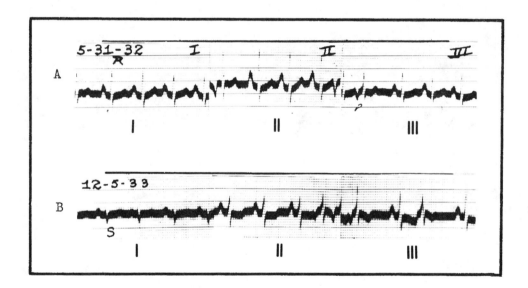

FIGURE 2-25.   Enlargement of the right ventricle (progressive). What changes have occurred in the interim between the two electrocardiograms? Compare and contrast Figure 2-25A with Figure 2-25B. (Electrocardio-gram reduced in size.)

Analysis:

    a.   right axis deviation:

    b.   increase in the magnitude of the mean QRS vector:

    c.   repolarization abnormalities:

    d.   "presumptive" evidence:

In Figure 2-26A the mean QRS vector is within normal limits. Several months later, as seen in Figure 2-26B, the QRS deflections in lead I had become predominantly negative; the mean QRS vector had shifted rightward with the progression of this man's pulmonary disease.

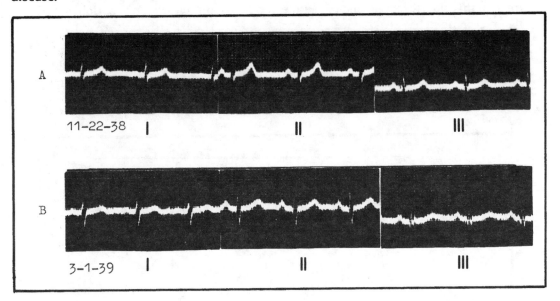

FIGURE 2-26. Axis shift from normal to right with progression of pulmonary disease and cor pulmonale. Compare and contrast Figure 2-26A with Figure 2-26B. (Electrocardiogram reduced in size.)

Analysis:

    a. right axis deviation:
    b. increase in the magnitude of the mean QRS vector:
    c. repolarization abnormalities:
    d. "presumptive" evidence:

In Figure 2-27B not only has the mean QRS vector shifted rightward but the P waves have also become more prominent, especially in lead II, with progression of pulmonary disease and cor pulmonale.

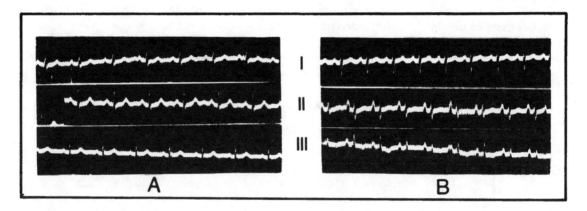

FIGURE 2-27.   Note the rightward shift of the mean QRS vector in B. What P wave changes are noted? This is another example of the importance of serial electrocardiograms in patient follow-up. Compare and contrast Figure 2-27A with Figure 2-27B. (Electrocardiogram reduced in size.)

Analysis:

    a.   right axis deviation:

    b.   increase in the magnitude of the mean QRS vector:

    c.   repolarization abnormalities:

    d.   "presumptive" evidence:

Figure 2-28A represents the "stable" pattern in a patient with long-standing chronic obstructive lung disease. During a clinic visit, this patient stated that he felt well and just wanted renewal of his medication. An astute house officer detected slightly increased shortness of breath and ordered an electrocardiogram as part of the evaluation. Figure 2-28B, showing a rightward shift of the mean QRS vector, was taken at this time. The patient was immediately hospitalized and treated.

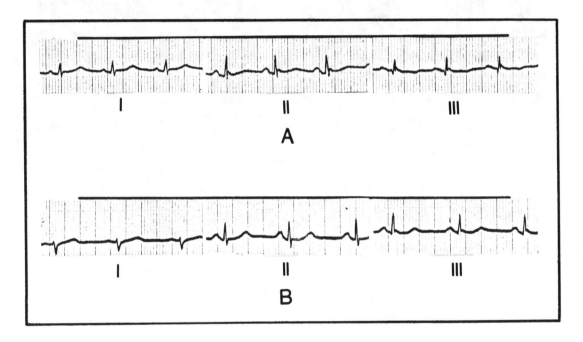

FIGURE 2-28. *A mean QRS vector shift to the right confirmed clinical findings. Compare and contrast Figure 2-28A with Figure 2-28B. (Electrocardiogram reduced in size.)*

Analysis:

    a. right axis deviation:

    b. increase in the magnitude of the mean QRS vector:

    c. repolarization abnormalities:

    d. "presumptive" evidence:

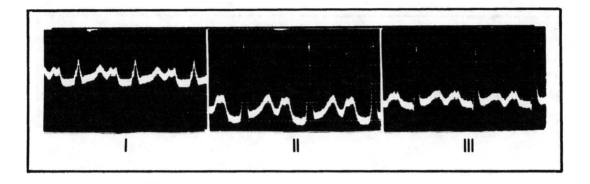

FIGURE 2-29. *This electrocardiogram will be studied again in a later chapter. For the present, analyze the following. (Electrocardiogram enlarged.)*

Analysis:

    a.   size of P waves:

    b.   configuration of P waves:

    c.   duration of P-R interval:

    d.   depression of P-R segment (atrial repolarization): Diagnosis?

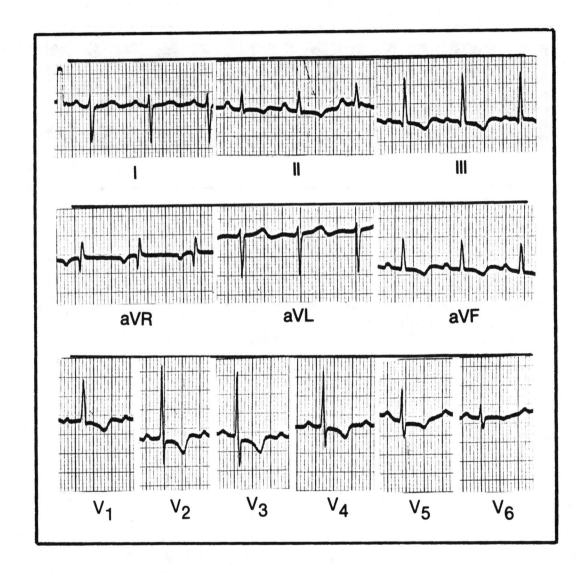

FIGURE 2-30. Right ventricular hypertrophy. Figures 2-30 to 2-35 are labeled "right ventricular hypertrophy." Analyze each using all the criteria learned for right ventricular hypertrophy.

Analysis:

    a. right axis deviation:

    b. increase in the magnitude of the mean QRS vector:

    c. repolarization abnormalities:

    d. "presumptive" evidence:

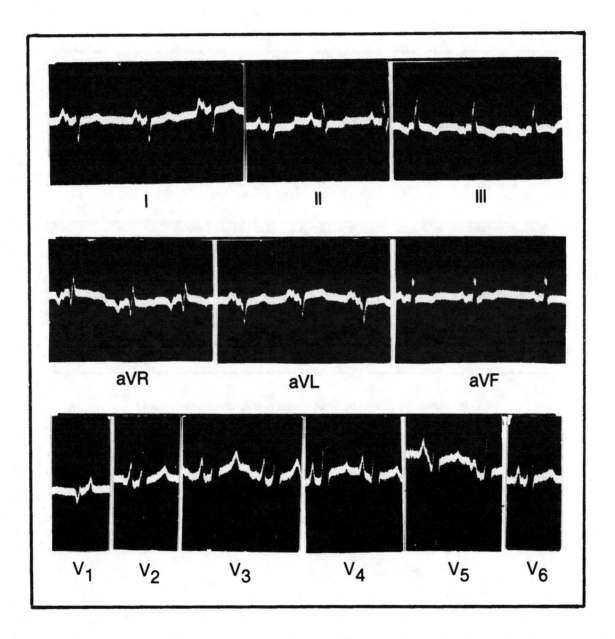

FIGURE 2-31. Right ventricular hypertrophy. (Electrocardiogram reduced in size.)

Analysis:

    a. right axis deviation:

    b. increase in the magnitude of the mean QRS vector:

    c. repolarization abnormalities:

    d. "presumptive" evidence:

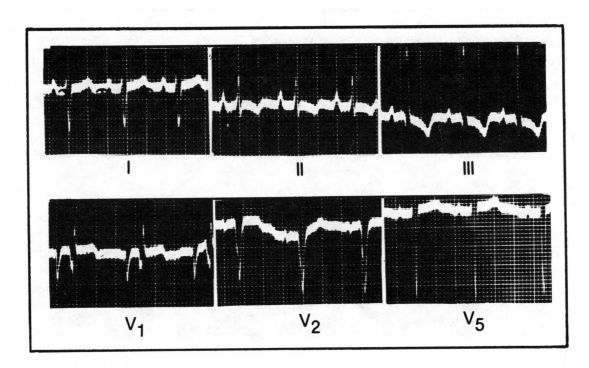

FIGURE 2-32.   Right ventricular hypertrophy. (Electrocardiogram enlarged.)

Analysis:

    a.   right axis deviation:

    b.   increase in the magnitude of the mean QRS vector:

    c.   repolarization abnormalities:

    d.   "presumptive" evidence:

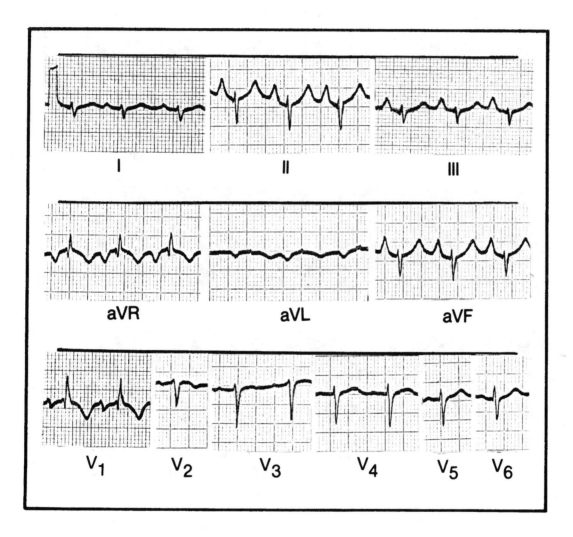

FIGURE 2-33.   *Right ventricular hypertrophy.*

Analysis:

    a. right axis deviation:

    b. increase in the magnitude of the mean QRS vector:

    c. repolarization abnormalities:

    d. "presumptive" evidence:

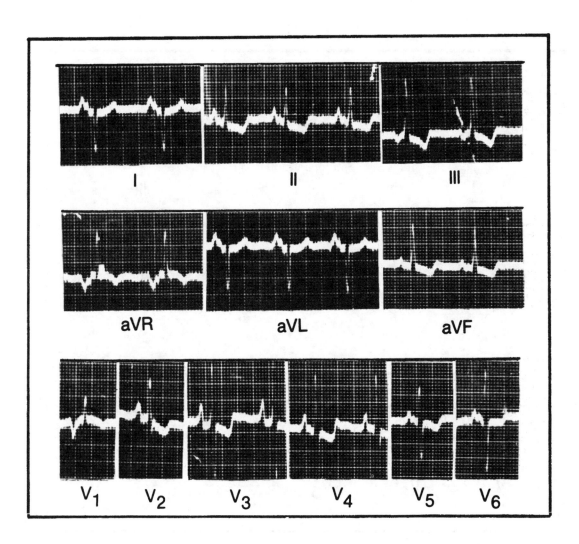

FIGURE 2-34. Right ventricular hypertrophy. (Electrocardiogram reduced in size.)

Analysis:

    a. right axis deviation:

    b. increase in the magnitude of the mean QRS vector:

    c. repolarization abnormalities:

    d. "presumptive" evidence:

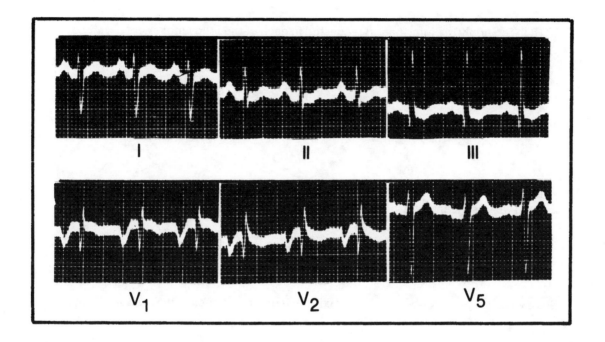

FIGURE 2-35. Right ventricular hypertrophy. (Electrocardiogram enlarged.)

Analysis:

    a.   right axis deviation:

    b.   increase in the magnitude of the mean QRS vector:

    c.   repolarization abnormalities:

    d.   "presumptive" evidence:

> After completing the analyses, proceed to the post-test on the next page.

P O S T · T E S T

DIRECTIONS. Supply the information requested in each of the following:

1. State the major electrocardiographic criterion for the diagnosis of right ventricular hypertrophy, and list three additional criteria.

   a. major criterion:

   b.

   c.

   d.

2. What are the characteristics of an ischemia pattern on the electrocardiogram? Explain what is meant by strain pattern. Should these terms be used?

3. State what is meant by abnormal right axis deviation of the mean QRS vector.

4. List the magnitude criteria for the electrocardiographic diagnosis of right ventricular hypertrophy in the frontal and horizontal plane leads.

5. What is the significance of an R wave in lead V_1 which is the main ventricular deflection in the adult?

6. State two reasons why age is an important factor in the criteria for the electrocardiographic diagnosis of right ventricular hypertrophy.

   a.

   b.

7. Why is right and left atrial enlargement studied together with right ventricular
   hypertrophy?

8. Cite a circumstance in which you see right and left atrial enlargement as well as right
   ventricular hypertrophy.

9. State four possibilities for the differential diagnosis of an R wave which is the main
   ventricular deflection in lead V_1 in an adult.

   a.

   b.

   c.

   d.

> Check your responses on the following pages.

ANSWERS TO
POST-TEST

1. a. major criterion: right axis deviation.
   b. increase in the magnitude of the mean QRS vector.
   c. repolarization abnormalities.
   d. "presumptive" evidence.

2. The wide QRS-T angle has often been referred to as an "ischemia" pattern, and the S-T segment abnormalities together with a wide QRS-T angle, in the hypertrophied ventricle, as a "strain" pattern. These are not proper terms since these repolarization abnormalities are *secondary* abnormalities in hypertrophy (explained in Chapter 4) and not *primary* abnormalities. These repolarization abnormalities are expected with hypertrophy. The term *ischemia* in this course will refer only to *primary* repolarization abnormalities. The term "ventricular repolarization abnormalities," covering both the wide QRS-T angle and the abnormal S-T segment, is a better term.

3. Abnormal right axis deviation is defined as a mean QRS vector which is beyond $+105°$.

4. The magnitude criteria for the electrocardiographic diagnosis of right ventricular hypertrophy are as follows:

   Frontal Plane Leads: I, II, III, aVR, aVL, and aVF.
   Incomplete right bundle branch block (RBBB) pattern. RBBB is discussed and illustrated in Chapter 6.

   $S_I + R_{III}$ and/or $S_{aVL} + R_{aVF} \geq 35$ mm. (principally in children)
   R_{aVR} or $R'_{aVR} = 6$ mm.
   $R_{aVR} > Q_{aVR}$

   The R in lead aVR becomes taller with increased magnitude of the mean QRS vector, especially as the vector becomes more rightward (toward + aVR).

   Horizontal Plane Leads: V_1 to V_6.
   Algebraic sum of R and S waves in lead V_1 more than 15 mm. in height (see Figure 2-17). At birth a tall R wave in lead V_1 may still be normal. An R wave in lead V_1 greater than 15 mm., however, may represent an abnormally enlarged right ventricle even in the newborn. In the adult the following criteria may be found.

   $R_{V_1} \geq 7$ mm.
   $S_{V_1} \leq 2$ mm.
   R/S ratio in $V_1 \geq 1$
   qR pattern in V_1

   Increased ventricular activation time with delayed onset of intrinsicoid deflection. (Ventricular activation time and intrinsicoid deflection are illustrated on page 192.)

   R_{V_5} or $R_{V_6} \leq 5$ mm.
   S_{V_5} or $S_{V_6} \geq 7$ mm.
   R/S ratio in V_5 or $V_6 \leq 1$

5. An R wave in lead V_1 which is the main ventricular deflection in the adult is an important criterion for the diagnosis of right ventricular hypertrophy.

6. a. right axis deviation is *normally* found in the newborn.

   b. an R wave in lead V_1 which is the main ventricular deflection, regardless of its size, is an important criterion in the *adult*.

7. Atrial (both right and left) enlargement is studied together with right ventricular hypertrophy because in various disease states right ventricular hypertrophy is associated with either right atrial or both right and left atrial enlargement.

8. Right and left atrial enlargement as well as right ventricular hypertrophy may be found in mitral valve stenosis.

9. a. right ventricular hypertrophy.
   b. true posterior wall myocardial infarction.
   c. right bundle branch block (RSR′).
   d. the Wolff-Parkinson-White syndrome, type A.

NOTES AND REFERENCES

***From page 163:   Ventricular
Activation Time (V.A.T.) and the
Intrinsicoid Deflection[2-3,2-4]***

Briefly summarized, the ventricular activation time is measured from the onset of the
QRS complex to the peak of the R wave (in seconds). The peak of the R wave is also the
onset of the intrinsicoid deflection. The prolonged ventricular activation time or the
delayed onset of the intrinsicoid deflection has been associated with ventricular hypertrophy or ventricular conduction disburbance. The normal values are:

Lead V_1—up to 0.02 sec.
Lead V_6—up to 0.04 sec.

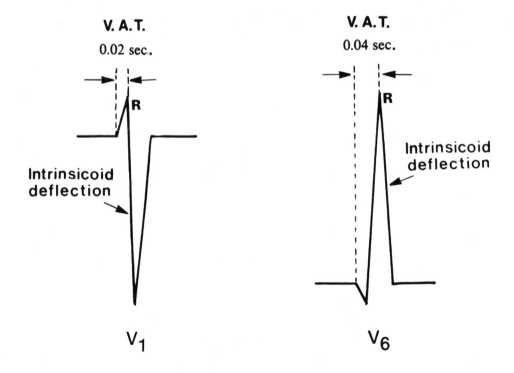

From pages 163-168 (Table 2-1)

As stated in the introduction to Table 2-1, the emphasis in this course is on the concept and not on the "criteria." These criteria attempt to describe the enlarged vector of right ventricular hypertrophy (RVH). The numbers may change in the face of evolving information. The problem with the electrocardiographic recognition of right ventricular hypertrophy is that the left ventricle is dominant in the adult and even a very hypertrophied right ventricle may be overshadowed by the left ventricle. The array of criteria gives evidence that no single criterion or set of criteria have both the *sensitivity* and *specificity* desired in a diagnostic test. Most have much greater specificity than sensitivity.

Sensitivity refers to the ability of a test to yield *positive* findings among those who have the disease. It is a test that is *abnormal* when the patient *has the disease* and may be expressed (as a percentage) as follows:

$$\frac{\text{Persons with RVH and positive on the electrocardiogram}}{\text{Total number tested with RVH}} \times 100$$

Specificity refers to the ability of a test to yield a *negative* finding among those who do not have the disease. It is test that is *normal* when the patient *does not have the disease* and may be expressed (as a percentage) as follows:

$$\frac{\text{Persons without RVH and negative on the electrocardiogram}}{\text{Total number tested without RVH}} \times 100$$

Munuswamy and associates,[2-1] using M-mode echocardiography, studied the sensitivity and specificity of the following six common electrocardiographic criteria for *left atrial enlargement:*

1.   Negative phase of P_{V_1} duration > 0.04 sec.

2.   Notched P wave in any standard lead with interpeak duration > 0.04 sec.

3. P-terminal force in lead V_1 > 0.04 mm./sec. (The P-terminal force in lead V_1 refers to the width (seconds) × depth (mm.) of the terminal part of the P wave.)

4. Depth of negative phase of Pv_1 > 1 mm.

5. Total P wave duration in any standard lead > 0.11 sec.

6. Total P wave duration/P-R interval duration > 1.6

They found that the most *sensitive* criterion was the increased duration of the negative phase of the P wave, > 0.04 sec. in lead V_1 (83%), while the most specific was the notched P wave in any standard lead with an interpeak duration > 0.04 sec. (100%).

Josephson and associates evaluated electrocardiographic criteria for left atrial enlargement with electrophysiologic, echocardiographic, and hemodynamic correlates.[22] They concluded that the electrocardiographic manifestations of left atrial enlargement (a broad notched P wave in lead II and a deep and broad negative P wave in lead V_1) appear to represent an *interatrial conduction defect.* The term *left atrial abnormality* is commonly used.

From Page 172 (Figure 2-20)

So far we have been studying right ventricular hypertrophy due to *systolic overload.* This refers to resistance to right ventricular outflow during systolic contraction as occurs in pulmonary hypertension and pulmonary stenosis.

In diastolic overload the right ventricle is overfilled as occurs in atrial septal defect with a moderate-to-severe left to right shunt. Figure 2-20 is an example of right ventricular hypertrophy with *diastolic overload* characterized by:

1. Incomplete right bundle branch block. There is an RSR′ in lead V_1 and an S wave in lead I with a QRS duration of 0.08 sec. (Right bundle branch block will be studied in Chapter 6).

2. All leads are transitional, including V_6, which, together with the incomplete right bundle branch block, also suggests right ventricular dilatation.

3. Right atrial enlargement is suggested by the tall (3 mm.) initial part of the P waves in lead II.

4. Left atrial enlargement is suggested by the notched, prominent P waves in leads II, III, and aVF and by the biphasic and prominent P waves in leads V_1, V_2, and V_3.

5. Biventricular hypertrophy is also suggested and will be discussed in Chapter 3 (Left Ventricular Hypertrophy), page 247.

References

2-1. Munuswamy, K., et al.: Sensitivity and specificity of commonly used electrocardio-graphic criteria for left atrial enlargement determined by M-mode echocardiogra-phy. Am. J. Cardiol. *53:*829, 1984.

2-2. Josephson, M.E., et al.: Electrocardiographic left atrial enlargement: electrophysio-logic, echocardiographic and hemodynamic correlates. Am. J. Cardiol., *39:*967, 1977.

2-3. Schamroth, L.: The 12 Lead Electrocardiogram. Oxford, Blackwell Scientific Publi-cations, 1989, p. 5.

2-4. Marriott, H.J.L.: Practical Electrocardiography, 8th Ed. Baltimore, Williams & Wilkins, 1988, p. 41.

3

LEFT VENTRICULAR HYPERTROPHY

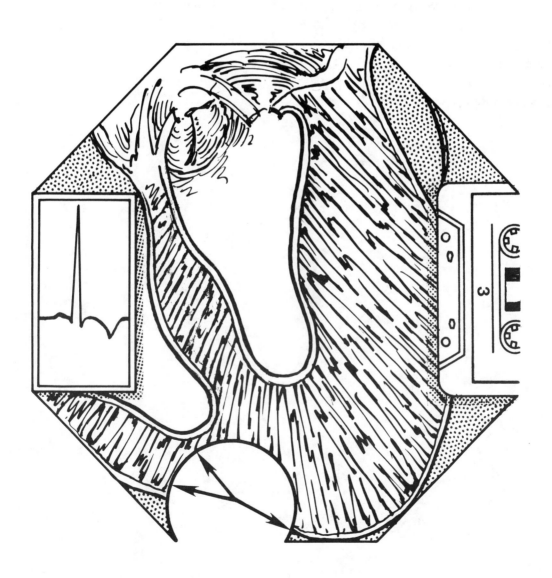

CHAPTER 3:
CONTENTS

INTRODUCTION

In discussing left ventricular hypertrophy we should remember that the *normal left ventricle,* having a wall several times as thick as the normal right ventricle, is the dominant ventricle. Therefore, the normal mean QRS vector, reflecting this dominance, is to the *left, inferior,* and *posterior.* In contrast to right ventricular hypertrophy (see Chapter 2), left ventricular hypertrophy is often accompanied by an *accentuation of the normal vector,* rather than a shift of the vector.

The following factors will be considered in the determination of left ventricular hypertrophy:

a. Increased magnitude of the mean QRS vector.

b. Ventricular repolarization (S-T segment and T wave) abnormalities.

c. Left axis deviation.

In clinical practice some of the causes of left ventricular hypertrophy (congenital and acquired) include systemic hypertension, aortic valve stenosis, hypertrophic cardiomyopathy, aortic regurgitation, mitral regurgitation, coarctation of the aorta, patent ductus arteriosus, and ventricular septal defect.

O B J E C T I V E S

Upon completion of this chapter, you should be able to:

1. Recognize the electrocardiographic manifestations of left ventricular hypertrophy with respect to the following factors: (a) increase in the magnitude of the mean spatial QRS vector; (b) repolarization abnormalities (abnormalities of the S-T segments and T waves); and (c) left axis deviation.

2. State the major electrocardiographic criterion for the diagnosis of left ventricular hypertrophy.

3. Identify the relationship of leftward QRS vectorial shift in left ventricular hypertrophy to rightward shift of the mean QRS vector in right ventricular hypertrophy.

4. Recognize the characteristics of (a) the ischemia pattern and (b) the strain pattern on the electrocardiogram.

5. Identify the reason that repolarization abnormalities *alone* (without magnitude criteria) *should not* be used in the diagnosis of left ventricular hypertrophy.

6. Recognize circumstances in which magnitude criteria may be seen in the horizontal plane and not in the frontal plane in left ventricular hypertrophy.

7. List the magnitude criteria for the electrocardiographic diagnosis of left ventricular hypertrophy in the standard, aV, and chest leads.

8. Recognize the lower limits of the magnitude criteria in the normal electrocardiogram.

9. Recognize the importance of age in the magnitude criteria for the electrocardiographic diagnosis of left ventricular hypertrophy.

P R E T E S T

DIRECTIONS: This pretest consists of four electrocardiograms. Write a brief analysis of each in the space provided.

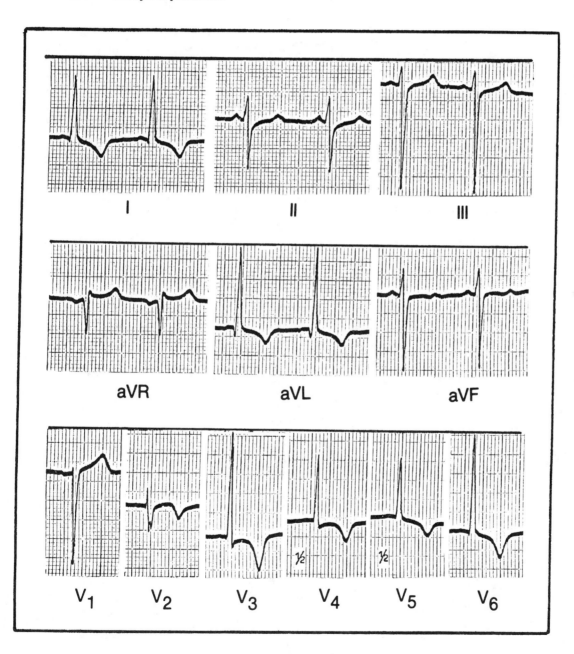

FIGURE 3-4.

1. Analysis:

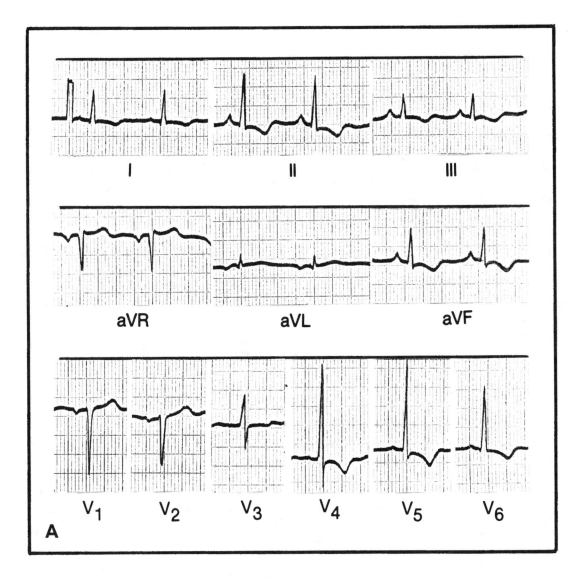

FIGURE 3-5A.

2. Analysis:

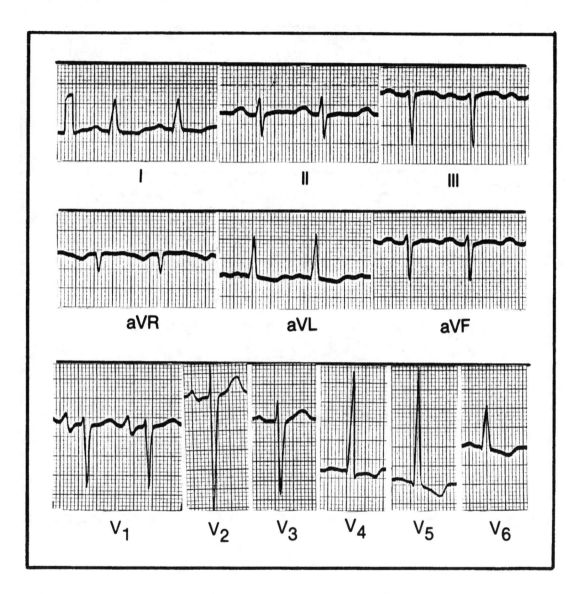

FIGURE 3-6.

3.   Analysis:

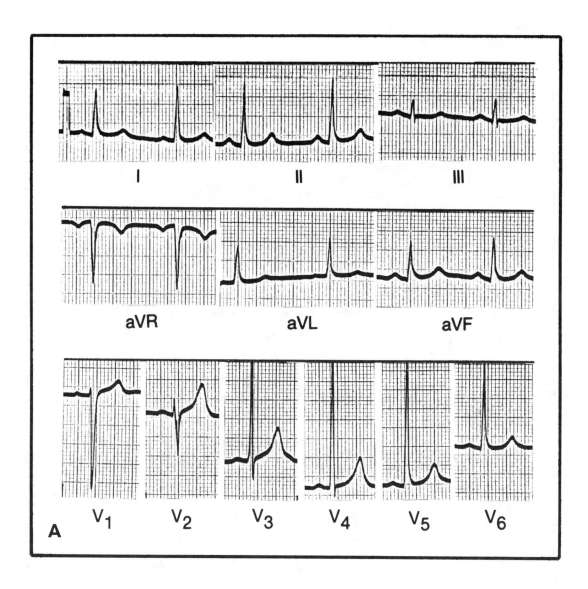

FIGURE 3-9A.

4. Analysis:

> Solutions to the pretest will be indicated later in this chapter.

> When you have completed the pretest start Cassette Side 7 and continue on the next page.

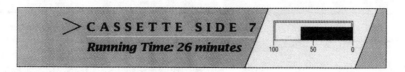

DIAGNOSTIC CRITERIA OF LEFT VENTRICULAR HYPERTROPHY

A. Increased magnitude of the mean QRS vector.

B. Ventricular repolarization (S-T segment and T wave) abnormalities.

C. Left axis deviation.

A. Increased Magnitude of the Mean QRS Vector

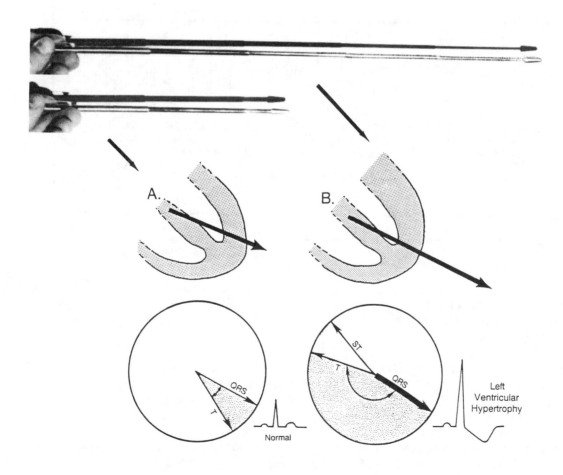

FIGURE 3-1. *Normal left ventricle (A) and hypertrophied left ventricle (B).*

The normally oriented mean QRS vector is increased in magnitude in left ventricular hypertrophy. The pointers, at the top of Figure 3-1, represent the mean QRS vector of left ventricular hypertrophy and the normal mean QRS vector. Accompanying the hypertrophy of the left ventricle are repolarization abnormalities resulting in a wide angle between the mean QRS vector and the mean S-T and T vectors.

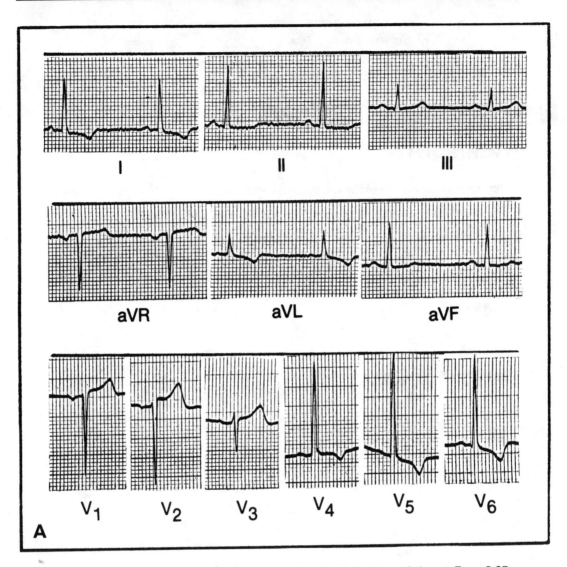

FIGURE 3-2A.   *Left ventricular hypertrophy. Compare the size of the deflections with those in Figure 3-2B, especially in leads V_1, V_2, V_4, V_5, and V_6, and note the increased magnitude of the deflections in Figure 3-2A. The mean QRS vector in each electrocardiogram is to the left, inferior, and posterior.*

B. *Ventricular Repolarization (S-T Segment and T Wave) Abnormalities*

In Figure 3-2A the QRS-T angle is wide, and the S-T segments reveal elevations and depressions. Normally, the S-T segment is isoelectric; it is neither elevated nor depressed (see schematic in Figure 3-1). The wide QRS-T angle is often referred to as an "ischemia" pattern. The wide QRS-T angle plus the abnormal S-T segment (repolarization abnormalities of the ventricle) in the hypertrophied ventricle are often referred to as a "strain" pattern. These are not proper terms since these repolarization abnormalities are *secondary* (explained in Chapter 4) and not *primary* abnormalities. These repolarization abnormalities are expected with hypertrophy. "Ischemia" is a term more appropriately used with *primary* repolarization abnormalities. The term "repolarization abnormalities," covering both the wide QRS-T angle and the abnormal S-T segment, is a better term. The increased magnitude of the mean QRS vector and repolarization abnormalities of the ventricle play an important role in the electrocardiographic diagnosis of left ventricular hypertrophy.

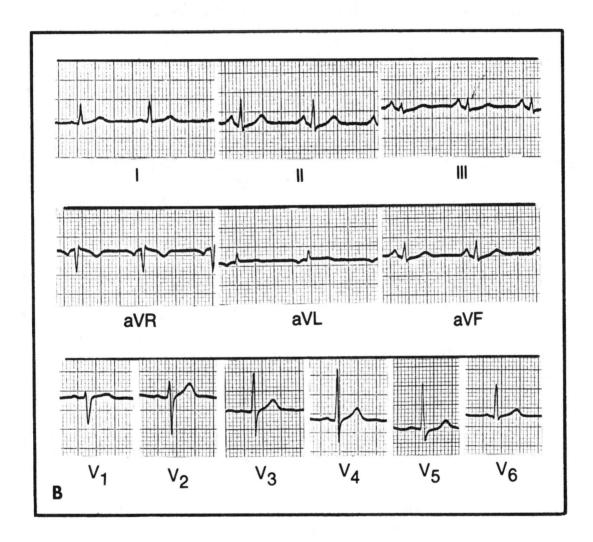

FIGURE 3-2B.   Normal. Compare the QRS deflection size, QRS-T angle, and S-T segments with those in Figure 3-2A.

C. *Left Axis Deviation (LAD)*

Left axis deviation (LAD) refers to a mean QRS vector from 0 to − 90°. *Abnormal* left axis deviation refers to a mean QRS vector from − 30 to − 90° (see Figure 1-36). At one time it was thought strongly suggestive of left ventricular hypertrophy. It is now, however, considered to be a conduction disturbance which may or may not accompany left ventricular hypertrophy. That it may be found alone, without any evidence of left ventricular hypertrophy, is seen in Figure 3-3. Left axis deviation is *not* a major criterion of left ventricular hypertrophy; it is included here because of the frequent association of left axis deviation with left ventricular hypertrophy. This is in contrast to right ventricular hypertrophy, for in right ventricular hypertrophy *right axis deviation* is a major electrocardiographic criterion (see Chapter 2). Some of the causes of left axis deviation will be studied in a later chapter.

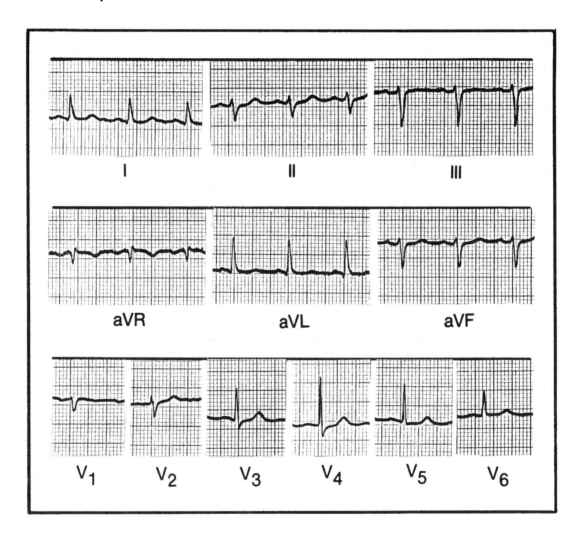

FIGURE 3-3.   Left axis deviation (LAD) in a normal-sized heart.

As in the study of right ventricular hypertrophy, a set of suggested criteria is presented for left ventricular hypertrophy in Table 3-1. Figure 3-4 is then analyzed using these criteria. The expression "suggested criteria" is used since there are numerous sets of criteria in use today. The fact that different sets of criteria are used emphasizes that caution must be exercised and that none contain both the desired sensitivity and specificity. For example, in Table 3-1, a statement is made that the magnitude criteria in the chest leads (leads V_1 to V_6) apply to an adult over the age of 30 years, of normal height and weight. This is important since in the thin and young subjects with normal-sized hearts, magnitude of the QRS complexes may be well within the range for left ventricular hypertrophy. On the other hand, an obese individual with left ventricular hypertrophy may not have QRS complexes greater than normal amplitude. This again emphasizes the importance of knowing your patients. Keep in mind that a normal electrocardiogram does not rule out left ventricular hypertrophy.

The mean QRS vector, increased in magnitude, is the prime electrocardiographic evidence of left ventricular hypertrophy. This is seen best in the precordial leads and will be explained shortly. The diagnosis of left ventricular hypertrophy should not be made in the absence of this increased magnitude.

Although a suggested set of criteria is presented in Table 3-1, the emphasis in this course continues to be on concept. Once the basic concept of the vectorial forces of left ventricular hypertrophy is clear, the specific figures are easily understood. The values given should never be taken as absolute truths; they frequently change in the face of evolving information.

TABLE 3-1.   Left Ventricular Hypertrophy

A. Increased Magnitude of the QRS Vector

Mild QRS complex prolongation may occur with increasing left ventricular hypertrophy, e.g., $0.08 \rightarrow 0.09 \rightarrow 0.10 \rightarrow 0.11$ second.

Frontal Plane Leads: I, II, III, aVR, aVL, and aVF.

$R_I + S_{III}$ and/or $R_{aVL} + S_{aVF} \geq 35$ mm. (in association with left axis deviation)
$R_{aVL} \geq 12$ mm. (especially in presence of a *normally oriented* mean QRS vector)

Horizontal Plane Leads: V_1 to V_6 *(QRS magnitude criteria in an adult over the age of 30 years, of normal height and weight).*

S_{V_1} or $S_{V_2} + R_{V_5}$ or $R_{V_6} \geq 35$ mm.
S_{V_1} or $S_{V_2} \geq 25$ mm.
R_{V_5} or $R_{V_6} \geq 25$ mm. (especially if $R_{V_6} > R_{V_5}$).

B. Repolarization Abnormalities (Wide QRS-T Angle and S-T Segment Abnormalities)

This applies to all leads.

C. Left Axis Deviation (LAD)

This is a conduction disturbance not necessarily associated with the hypertrophied left ventricle. Either may be found independently. It is included here because of the frequent association of LAD with left ventricular hypertrophy.

Once you are thoroughly familiar with these criteria, you will be able to scan electrocardiograms and look for left ventricular hypertrophy in the following order:

a.   Increased magnitude of the mean QRS vector.
b.   Ventricular repolarization abnormalities.
c.   Left axis deviation (LAD).

Note: Clear evidence of *left atrial enlargement* (in absence of mitral stenosis—see Chapter 2) may be the clue that left ventricular hypertrophy is present. Not all of the above criteria are necessary for the electrocardiographic diagnosis of left ventricular hypertrophy. The more the evidence, however, the more secure the diagnosis. The diagnosis should not be made without at least some of the magnitude criteria. Keep in mind that a normal electrocardiogram does not rule out left ventricular hypertrophy.

> Additional criteria will be found on pages 245 to 246.

TABLE 3-1.   (cont'd)

Left Ventricular Hypertrophy
Principal Criteria—Review

In left ventricular hypertrophy the mean QRS vector, which is normally oriented to the left, inferiorly, and posteriorly, is markedly accentuated, inscribing *deep S waves* in the right precordial leads (V_1 and V_2) and *tall R waves* in the left precordial leads (V_5 and V_6). *Increased magnitude of the QRS complex is the major electrocardiographic criterion of left ventricular hypertrophy in the adult.* Because of the posterior orientation of the mean QRS vector in left ventricular hypertrophy, the increased magnitude is seen best in the precordial leads, V_1 to V_6. The diagnosis of left ventricular hypertrophy should not be made without evidence of increased magnitude. *Ventricular repolarization (ST-T) abnormalities* are frequently seen in left ventricular hypertrophy; the *QRS-T angle is wide.* The enlarged left atrium accompanying the hypertrophied left ventricle may be evident on the electrocardiogram; this is seen in lead V_1 below. Left axis deviation may be seen in association with left ventricular hypertrophy, although it is not a major electrocardiographic criterion.

Note: The QRS magnitude criteria apply to *adults* since increased magnitude of the QRS complex without ST-T abnormalities may be seen in a *normal* youth.

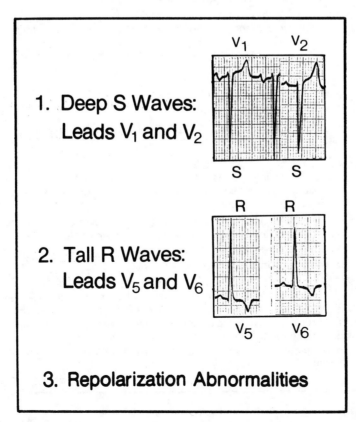

1. Deep S Waves:
   Leads V_1 and V_2

2. Tall R Waves:
   Leads V_5 and V_6

3. Repolarization Abnormalities

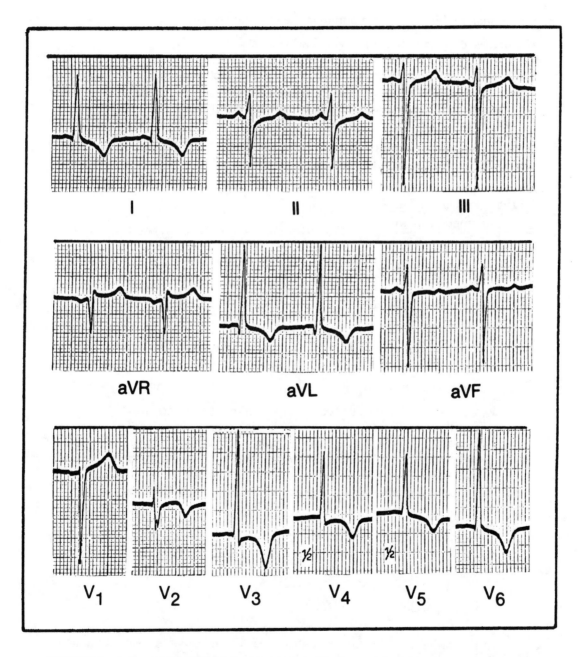

FIGURE 3-4.   Left ventricular hypertrophy. The criteria for the electrocardiographic diagnosis of left ventricular hypertrophy were presented in Table 3-1. The analysis is presented on the following page.

The analysis of Figure 3-4 in the text and on the tape is the solution to item 1 on the pretest.

Let us now analyze this electrocardiogram in the following order:

    a. Increased magnitude of the mean QRS vector.

    b. Ventricular repolarization abnormalities.

    c. Left axis deviation (LAD). As noted, a mean QRS vector beyond $-30°$ is not essential to the diagnosis of left ventricular hypertrophy, although it is frequently associated with it. LAD is generally considered a conduction disturbance and will be studied later.

A. Increased magnitude of the mean QRS vector. Standard leads: I, II, and III. The millimeter measurements are approximate.

R wave in lead I = 17 mm.
S wave in lead III = <u>27 mm.</u>
        summate to 44 mm.

aV leads: aVR, aVL, and aVF

R wave in lead aVL = 22 mm.
S wave in lead aVF = <u>20 mm.</u>
        summate to 42 mm.

Chest leads: V_1 to V_6

S wave in lead V_1 = 24 mm.
R wave in lead V_6 = <u>25 mm.</u>
        summate to 49 mm.

B. The T waves do not follow the QRS complexes in direction. Where the QRS complexes are positive the T waves are generally negative, and vice versa. Therefore, there is a wide QRS-T angle. The S-T segments are not isoelectric and tend to follow the general direction of the T waves, so that we have "repolarization" criteria in addition to "magnitude." Figure 3-1 shows the difference between the normal QRS-T angle and the QRS-T angle and S-T vectors frequently found in the hypertrophied left ventricle.

C. Left axis deviation (LAD) is present (beyond $-30°$).

Note that the precordial V_4 and V_5 are one half standard. Remember therefore to double the size of these leads in making your "magnitude" calculations.

Figure 3-5A, from a patient with known left ventricular hypertrophy, meets the major criteria for left ventricular hypertrophy. Both "magnitude" and "repolarization" criteria are present. A question, however, arises. Since the mean QRS vector is increased in magnitude in the horizontal plane (precordial leads), why do not the frontal plane leads (I, II, III, aVR, aVL, and aVF) show this manifestation of increased vectorial magnitude?

It is possible for a three-dimensional vectorial force of increased magnitude to appear normal in size in one plane (frontal) and large in another plane (horizontal). This is common in left ventricular hypertrophy since the mean QRS vector in the progression of the hypertrophy is often oriented ever more posteriorly. This is explained and illustrated in Figure 3-5B. It is necessary to examine all the leads, in both planes. The "magnitude" criteria do not have to be fulfilled in all the leads, but must be fulfilled in some, to make the electrocardiographic diagnosis of left ventricular hypertrophy. The magnitude criteria are often evident *only* in the precordial leads.

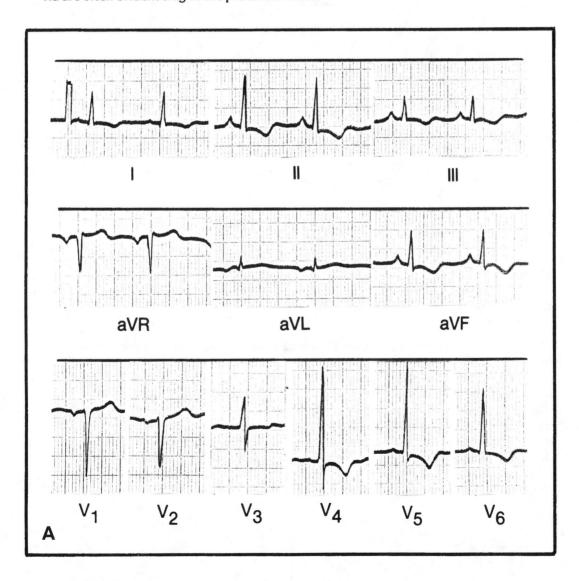

FIGURE 3-5A.   *Enlarged left ventricle. Analyze, following the steps outlined in Figure 3-4 and Table 3-1.*

> The analysis of Figure 3-5A in the text and on the tape is the solution to item 2 on the pretest.

B

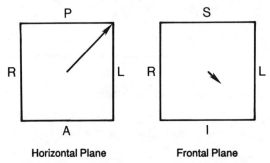

FIGURE 3-5B.   Influence of vectorial position on electrocardiographic deflections.

You will see many electrocardiograms of the enlarged left ventricle (e.g., Figures 3-5A and 3-6) with markedly enlarged QRS deflections in the horizontal plane (leads V_1 to V_6). The frontal plane (leads I, II, III, aVR, aVL, and aVF) QRS deflections, however, are not exceptionally large. How is this possible when all the deflections reflect just one mean QRS vector in space?

The pointers in the upper, middle, and lower panels in Figure 3-5B are the same size. In the upper panel, you see the pointer in its full length—note the size of the shadow. As the pointer is moved posteriorly, or anteriorly, it appears to be shorter (middle panel). In the lower panel, it appears to be still shorter. When you see the pointer on end, it only appears to be short; in reality it may be quite long. So it is with the mean QRS vector. In a markedly posterior (common in the enlarged left ventricle) mean QRS vector, the QRS deflections in the horizontal plane reflect the vector more in its fuller length. The deflections in the frontal plane reflect the vector more on end. The very same, very large mean QRS vectorial force may therefore seem to be large in some leads and small in others. You must look at all the leads and not jump to conclusions from any given lead.

Horizontal Plane   Frontal Plane

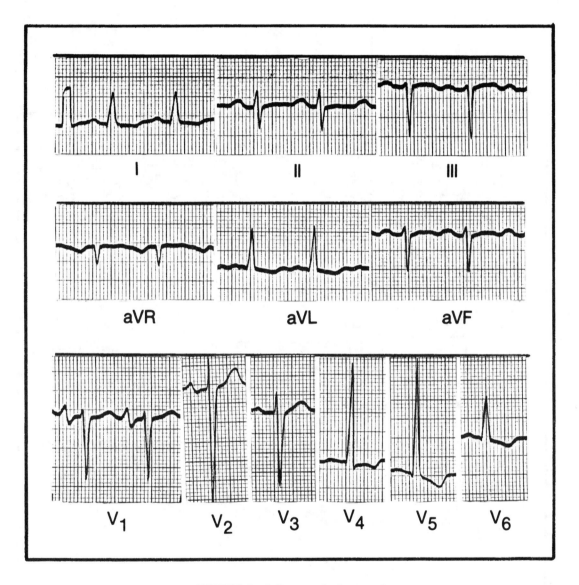

FIGURE 3-6.   Left ventricular hypertrophy.

Review all the criteria stepwise. Why are the voltage criteria so prominent in the chest leads compared with the standard and aVL leads? See explanation in Figure 3-5B. Do the P waves help in elaborating the diagnosis?

All the criteria for left ventricular hypertrophy are met, as follows:

    a.   increased magnitude of the mean QRS vector. This is seen exceptionally well in the precordial leads. Atrial enlargement is also evident from the size and configuration of the P waves in lead V_1.

    b.   repolarization abnormalities. The wide QRS-T angle and S-T segment depression are evident.

    c.   left axis deviation. The mean QRS vector is beyond $-30°$.

The analysis of Figure 3-6 in the text and on the tape is the solution to item 3 on the pretest.

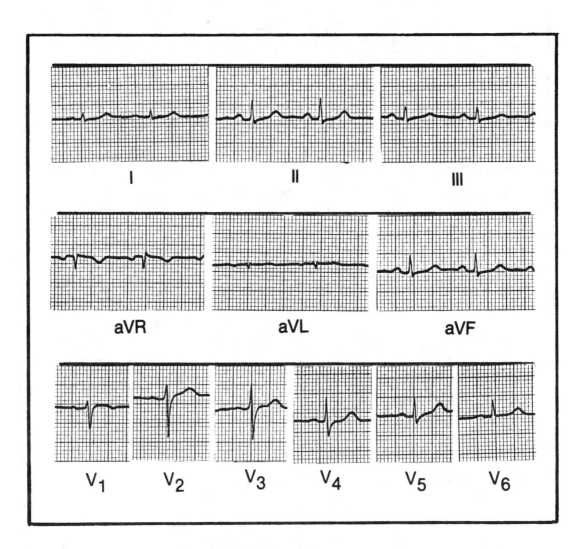

FIGURE 3-7. Normal.

The magnitude criteria for left ventricular and right ventricular hypertrophy have been discussed. Now the question may be asked. What are the lower limits of normal? At what point may the QRS complexes be described as "too small?" These lower limits of normal may be stated as follows:

Frontal plane (leads I, II, III, aVR, aVL, and aVF)
  at least 5 mm. in any lead

Horizontal plane (leads V_1 to V_6)
  at least 10 mm. in any lead

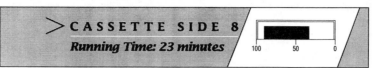

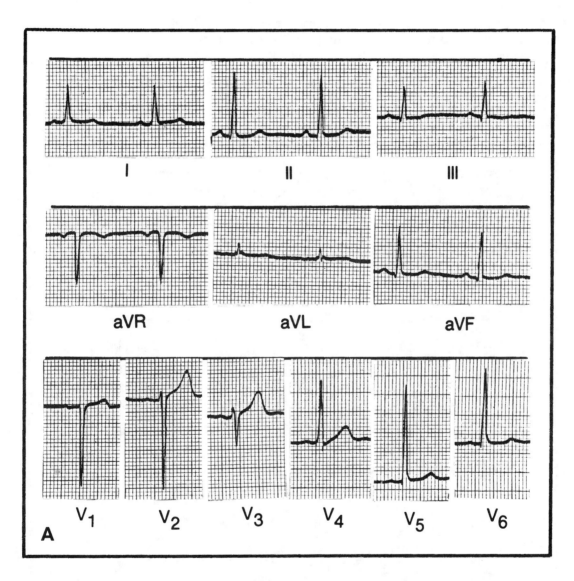

FIGURE 3-8A. Left ventricular hypertrophy.

This electrocardiogram and the next (Figure 3-8B) belong to the same adult patient. Note similarity in QRS deflection amplitude. Have there been any changes in the repolarization phase (S-T segments and T waves)?

In the interim the patient underwent the repair of a defective aortic valve and the insertion of a prosthesis. The patient felt "better" but the electrocardiogram was "worse." Again, emphasis must be placed on

1. sequential study of the electrocardiogram.
2. patient history.

The electrocardiogram must never be dissociated from the patient; it must never be read in a vacuum. You do not tell the patient that he is "worse" because his electrocardiogram is "deteriorating."

It may well be that the repolarization abnormalities in Figure 3-8B reflect a worsened condition of the myocardium following the surgical procedure. The patient may be feeling better because of the positive net effect of heart valve replacement versus continued myocardial deterioration.

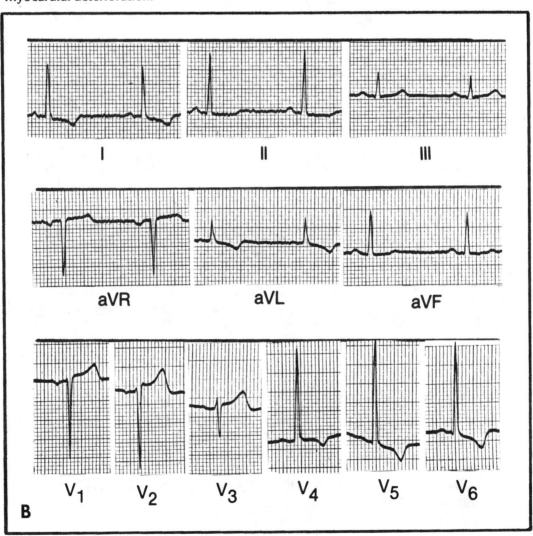

FIGURE 3-8B.   Left ventricular hypertrophy. See discussion of Figure 3-8A.

After you have analyzed Figure 3-8A and B refer to pages 246 and 247 for discussion of systolic and diastolic overload of the left ventricle.

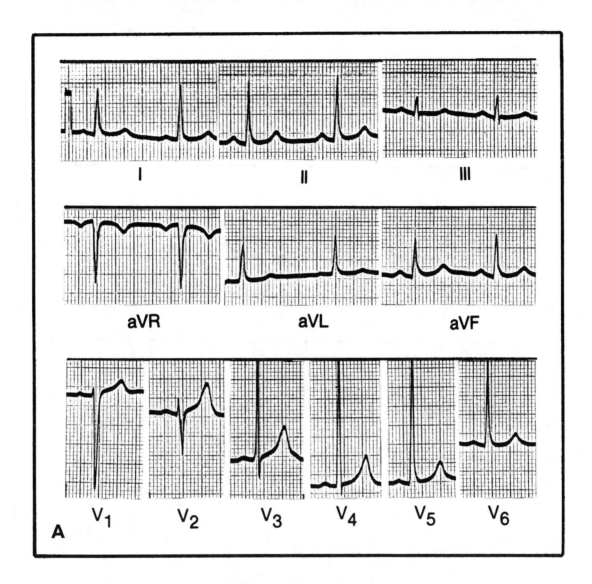

FIGURE 3-9A. *Left ventricular hypertrophy.*

The patient is a young adult with marked hypertension. Do you have the "magnitude" criteria for left ventricular hypertrophy? Do you have the repolarization abnormalities? If the patient were a 16 year old, thin high school student with a small heart on physical examination and on chest X-ray, would you read this electrocardiogram as diagnostic of left ventricular hypertrophy? A mean QRS vector of increased magnitude, in the horizontal plane, without repolarization abnormalities, is not rare among thin and young normal patients. For this reason, when studying the "magnitude" criteria for hypertrophy of the ventricle, it was stated that the patient should be over the age of 30 and of normal height and weight.

On the pretest, since the age and medical history were not given, the diagnosis of left ventricular hypertrophy could not be made with security in the absence of repolarization abnormalities. It could be normal in an adolescent as well as left ventricular hypertrophy with diastolic overload (see Figure 3-8A, page 218, and pages 246 and 247). In the analysis there should be a comment on the magnitude of the QRS complexes in the precordial leads and the need to know the age and medical history.

> The analysis of Figure 3-9A in the text and on the tape is the solution to item 4 on the pretest.

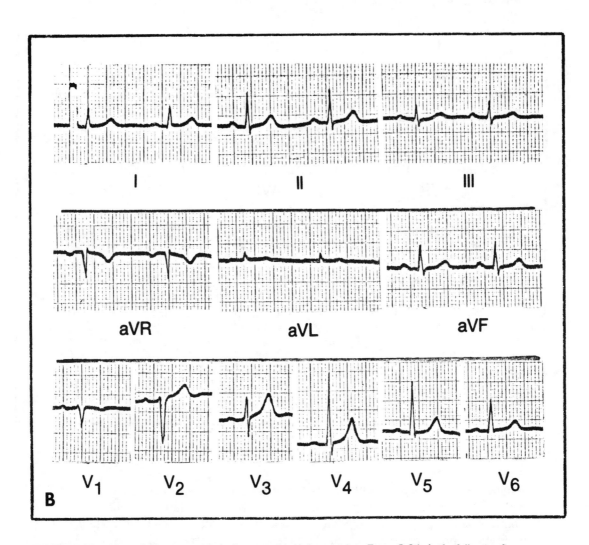

FIGURE 3-9B. Normal. Compare with the hypertrophied left ventricle in Figure 3-9A. In the following figures, part B will be a normal electrocardiogram to help reinforce the criteria of left ventricular hypertrophy.

REVIEW
ELECTROCARDIOGRAMS

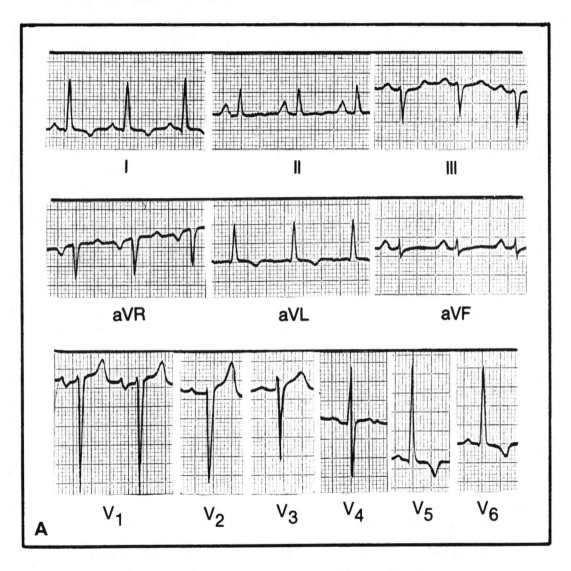

A

FIGURE 3-10A.   *Hypertrophied left ventricle in an elderly patient. Review the criteria and the reasons for the normal-sized QRS complexes in the frontal plane (leads I, II, III, aVR, aVL, and aVF) and large QRS complexes in the horizontal plane (leads V_1 to V_6).*

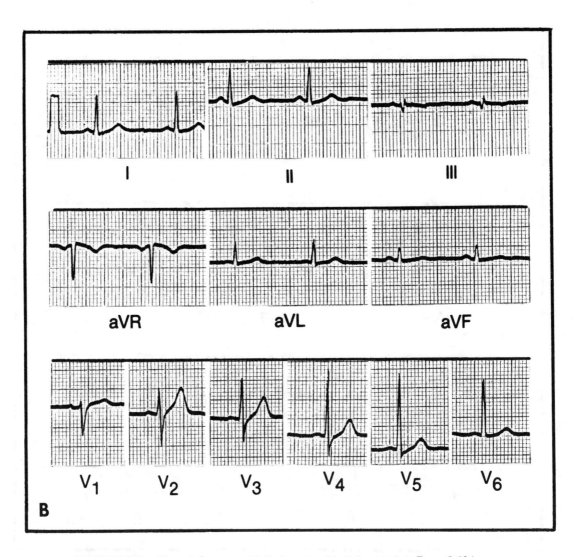

FIGURE 3-10B.   Normal. Compare with the hypertrophied left ventricle in Figure 3-10A.

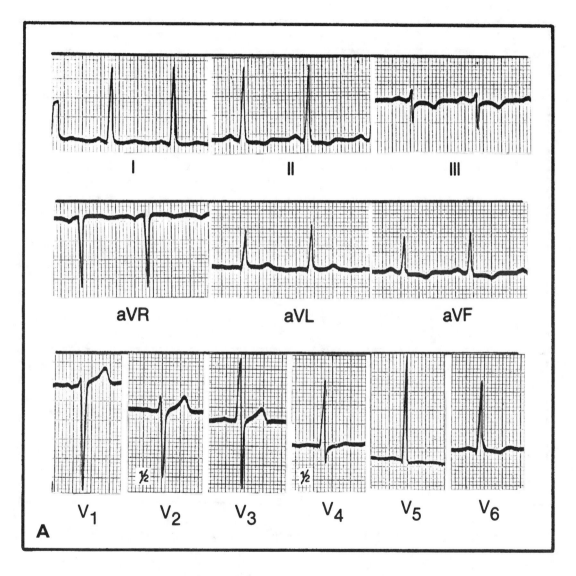

FIGURE 3-11A. Left ventricular hypertrophy in an elderly patient with aortic valve disease. The chest leads V_2 and V_4 are on half standard; remember therefore to double the size of these leads in making your "magnitude" calculations.

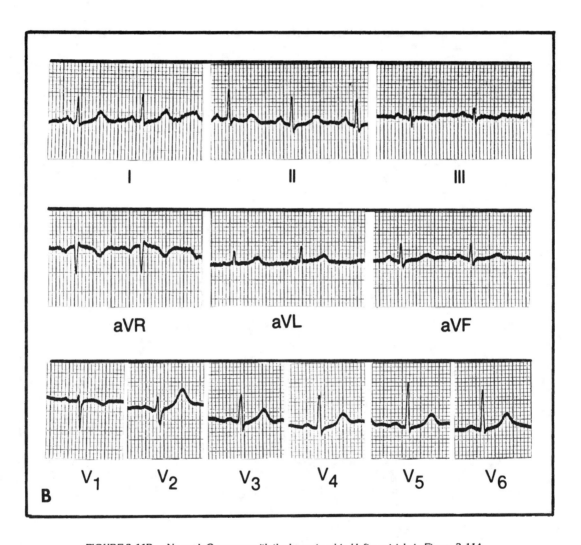

FIGURE 3-11B. Normal. Compare with the hypertrophied left ventricle in Figure 3-11A.

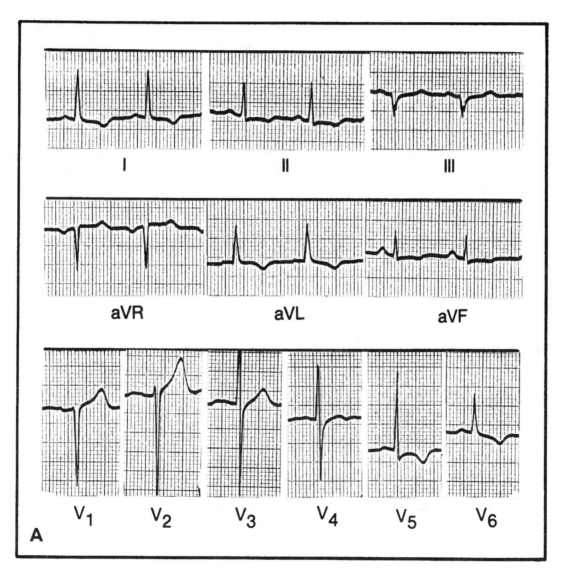

FIGURE 3-12A.   *Hypertrophied left ventricle in an adult with hypertension.*

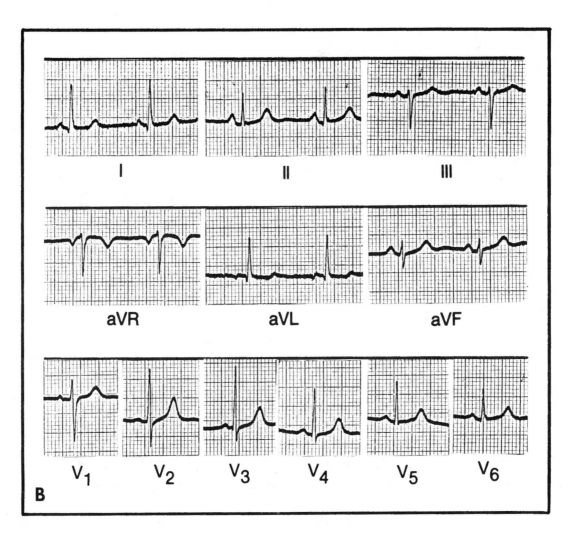

FIGURE 3-12B. Normal. Compare with the hypertrophied left ventricle in Figure 3-12A.

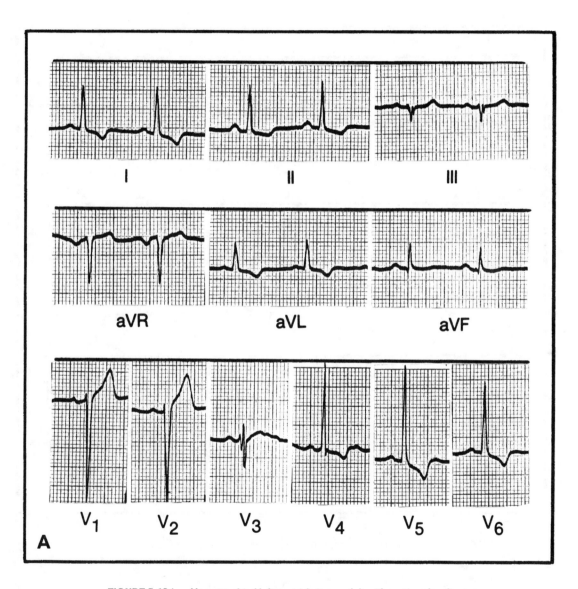

FIGURE 3-13A. Hypertrophied left ventricle in an adult with aortic valve disease.

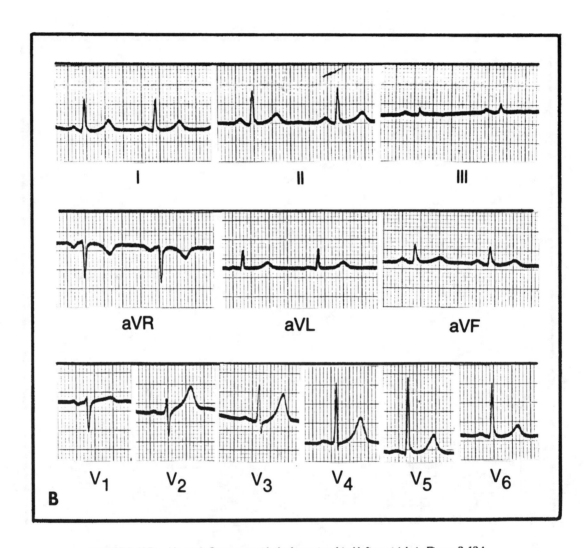

FIGURE 3-13B.   Normal. Compare with the hypertrophied left ventricle in Figure 3-13A.

Electrocardiograms 3-14 to 3-25 are examples of left ventricular hypertrophy. Practice analyzing them by detailing all the criteria for left ventricular hypertrophy, including (a) increased magnitude of the mean QRS vector, (b) repolarization abnormalities, and (c) left axis deviation.

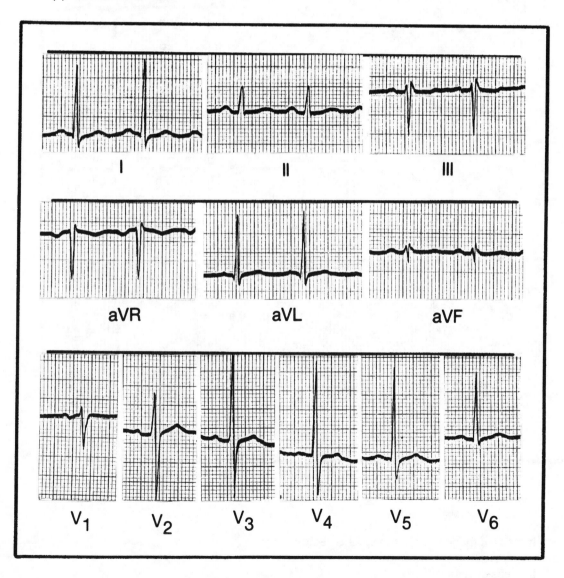

FIGURE 3-14.   *Left ventricular hypertrophy in an adult with hypertension.*

Analysis:

a.   increased magnitude of mean QRS vector:

b.   repolarization abnormalities:

c.   left axis deviation:

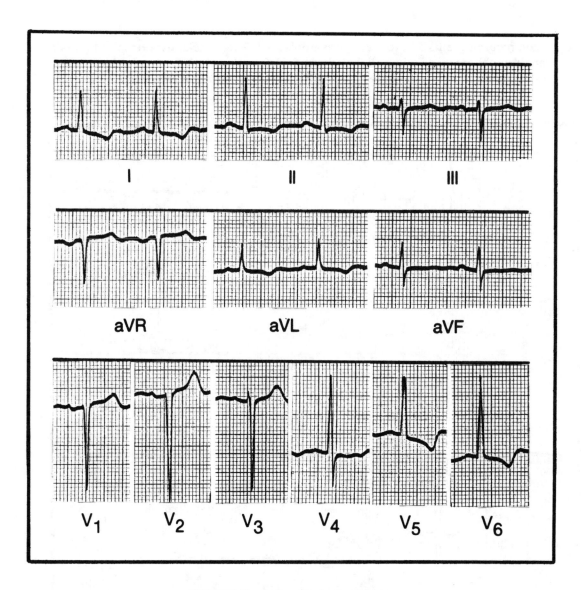

FIGURE 3-15.   Left ventricular hypertrophy.

Analysis:
a. increased magnitude of mean QRS vector:
b. repolarization abnormalities:
c. left axis deviation:

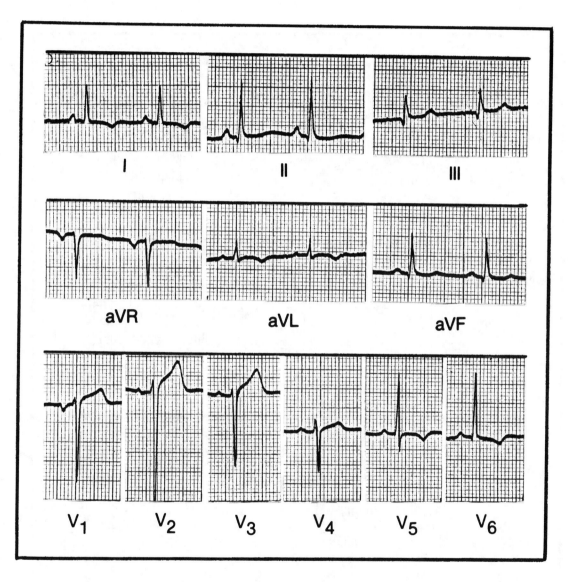

FIGURE 3-16.   Left ventricular hypertrophy.

Analysis:

a.   increased magnitude of mean QRS vector:

b.   repolarization abnormalities:

c.   left axis deviation:

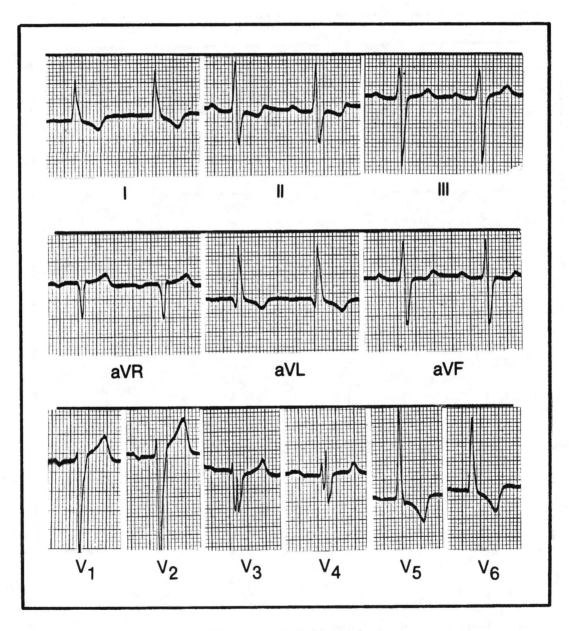

FIGURE 3-17. Left ventricular hypertrophy.

Analysis:
a. increased magnitude of mean QRS vector:
b. repolarization abnormalities:
c. left axis deviation:

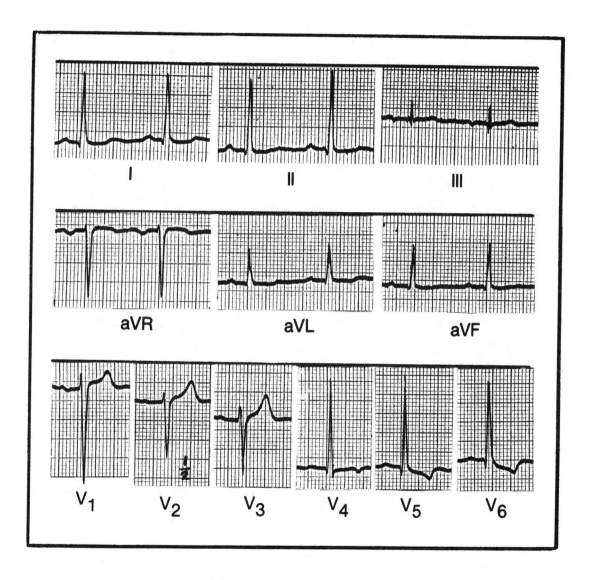

FIGURE 3-18.   Left ventricular hypertrophy.

Analysis:
a. increased magnitude of mean QRS vector:
b. repolarization abnormalities:
c. left axis deviation:

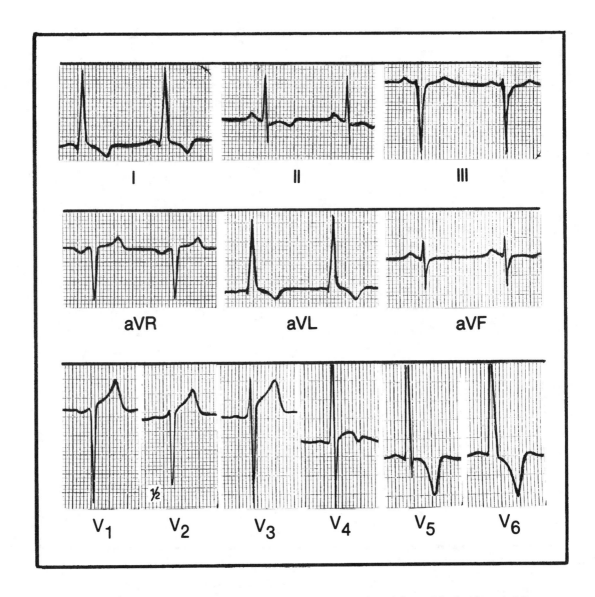

FIGURE 3-19. *Left ventricular hypertrophy. Although this patient had a large left ventricle, the characteristic shape of the markedly inverted T waves in leads V_5 and V_6 represent primary repolarization abnormalities of myocardial ischemia. These primary abnormalities are added to the secondary repolarization abnormalities of hypertrophy. The term "ischemia" should not be applied to the secondary repolarization abnormalities of hypertrophy. This will again be studied in Chapter 4.*

Analysis:

a. increased magnitude of mean QRS vector:

b. repolarization abnormalities:

c. left axis deviation:

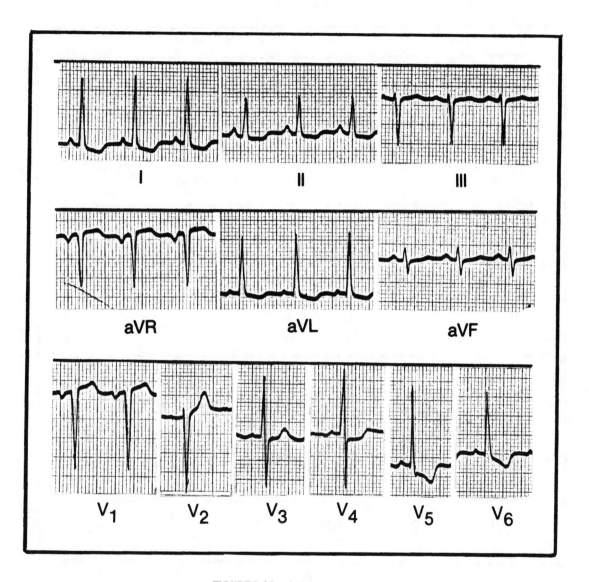

FIGURE 3-20.   Left ventricular hypertrophy.

Analysis:
a. increased magnitude of mean QRS vector:
b. repolarization abnormalities:
c. left axis deviation:

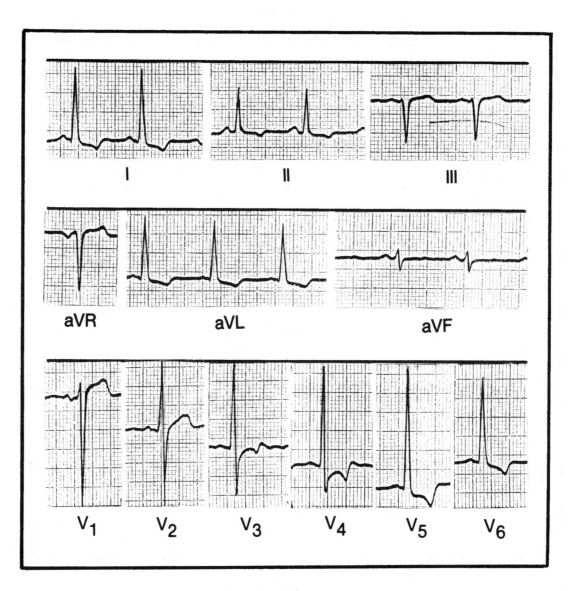

FIGURE 3-21. *Left ventricular hypertrophy.*

Analysis:
a. increased magnitude of mean QRS vector:
b. repolarization abnormalities:
c. left axis deviation:

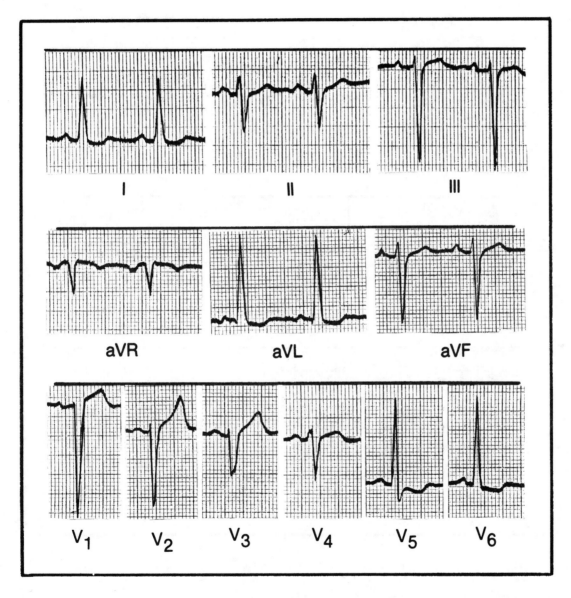

FIGURE 3-22.   *Left ventricular hypertrophy.*

Analysis:
a. increased magnitude of mean QRS vector:
b. repolarization abnormalities:
c. left axis deviation:

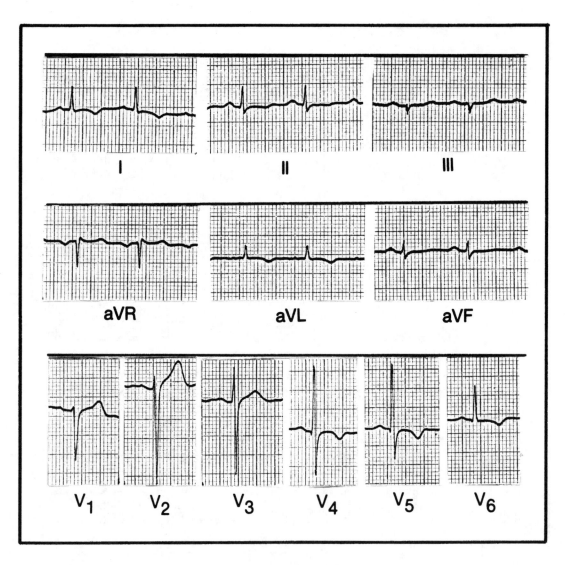

FIGURE 3-23.   Left ventricular hypertrophy.

Analysis:
a. increased magnitude of mean QRS vector:
b. repolarization abnormalities:
c. left axis deviation:

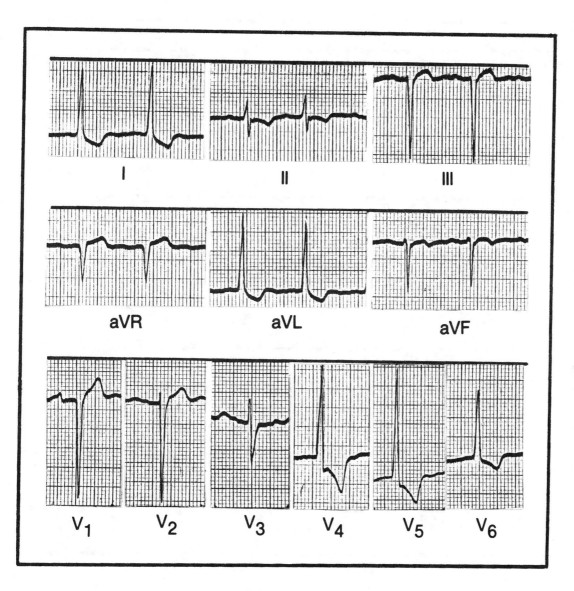

FIGURE 3-24.   Left ventricular hypertrophy.

Analysis:
a.   increased magnitude of mean QRS vector:
b.   repolarization abnormalities:
c.   left axis deviation:

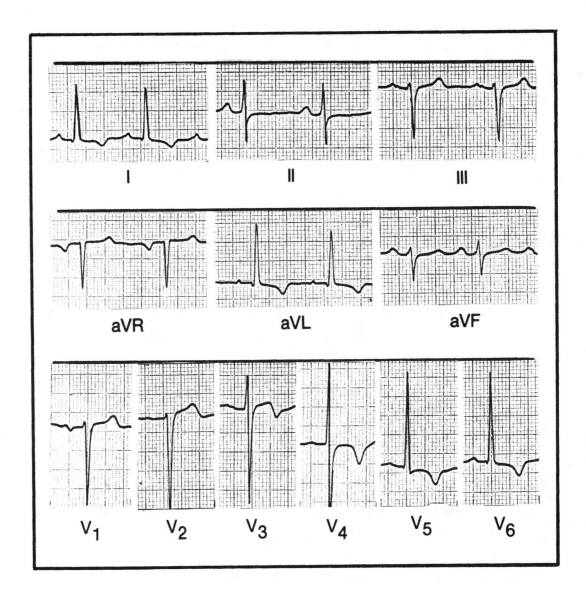

FIGURE 3-25.   Left ventricular hypertrophy.

Analysis:
a.   increased magnitude of mean QRS vector:
b.   repolarization abnormalities:
c.   left axis deviation:

> After completing the analyses proceed to the post-test on the next page.

DIRECTIONS. Supply the information requested in each of the following.

1. What is the major electrocardiographic criterion of left ventricular hypertrophy?

2. When you studied electrocardiographic diagnosis of right ventricular hypertrophy, you learned the importance of a rightward shift of the mean QRS vector. Is a leftward QRS vectorial shift as important in the diagnosis of left ventricular hypertrophy?

3. What is an "ischemia" pattern on the electrocardiogram? Explain the "strain" pattern. Should these terms be used?

4. What is abnormal left axis deviation of the mean QRS vector?

5. Is left axis deviation ever found in the absence of left ventricular hypertrophy? Is left ventricular hypertrophy ever found in the absence of left axis deviation?

6. When can you securely make the diagnosis of left ventricular hypertrophy only on the basis of repolarization abnormalities?

7. List the three criteria for making the diagnosis of left ventricular hypertrophy electrocardiographically.

8. Under what circumstances may magnitude criteria be seen in the horizontal plane but not in the frontal plane in left ventricular hypertrophy?

9. List the magnitude criteria for electrocardiographic diagnosis of left ventricular hypertrophy in the frontal and horizontal plane leads.

10. What are the lower limits of the magnitude criteria in the normal electrocardiogram?

> Check your responses on the following pages.

ANSWERS TO
POST-TEST

1. The major electrocardiographic criterion in the determination of left ventricular hypertrophy is *magnitude* of the mean QRS vector.

2. No. The *normal left ventricle,* having a wall several times as thick as the normal right ventricle, is the dominant ventricle; therefore, the normal mean QRS vector, reflecting this dominance, is to the *left, inferior,* and *posterior.* In contrast to right ventricular hypertrophy, left ventricular hypertrophy is often accompanied by an *accentuation of the normal vector.*

3. The wide QRS-T angle has been referred to as an "ischemia" pattern and S-T segment abnormalities, together with a wide QRS-T angle, in the hypertrophied ventricle, as a "strain" pattern. These terms are not proper terms since these repolarization abnormalities are *secondary* and not *primary* abnormalities. These repolarization abnormalities are expected with hypertrophy.

4. Abnormal left axis deviation refers to a mean QRS vector from -30 to $-90°$.

5. The answer to both questions is yes. At one time it was thought that left axis deviation was strongly suggestive of left ventricular hypertrophy; it is now, however, considered to be a conduction disturbance. Left axis deviation may occur without left ventricular hypertrophy and left ventricular hypertrophy may occur without left axis deviation.

6. You *should not* make the diagnosis of left ventricular hypertrophy solely on the basis of repolarization abnormalities; you should also have magnitude criteria in at least some of the leads.

7. The three criteria for making the diagnosis of left ventricular hypertrophy are:

   a. increase in the magnitude of the mean QRS vector.

   b. repolarization abnormalities (abnormalities of the S-T segment and T wave).

   c. left axis deviation.

8. In a markedly posterior (common in the enlarged left ventricle) mean QRS vector, the QRS deflections in the horizontal plane reflect the vector more in its fuller length. The deflections in the frontal plane reflect the vector more on-end. The very same, large mean QRS vectorial force may therefore seem to be large in some leads and small in others; you must examine all the leads.

9. The magnitude criteria for the electrocardiographic diagnosis of left ventricular hypertrophy are as follows:

    Frontal Plane Leads: I, II, III, aVR, aVL, and aVF.

    $R_I + S_{III}$ and/or $R_{aVL} + S_{aVF} \geq 35$ mm. (in association with left axis deviation)

    $R_{aVL} \geq 12$ mm. (especially in presence of a *normally oriented* mean QRS vector)

    Horizontal Plane Leads: V_1 to V_6
    (QRS magnitude criteria in an adult over the age of 30 years, of normal height and weight).

    S_{V_1} or $S_{V_2} + R_{V_5}$ or $R_{V_6} \geq 35$ mm.

    S_{V_1} or $S_{V_2} \geq 25$ mm.

    R_{V_3} or $R_{V_6} \geq 25$ mm. (especially if $R_{V_6} \geq R_{V_3}$).

10. The lower limits of the magnitude criteria in the normal electrocardiogram are

    Frontal plane (leads I, II, III, aVR, aVL, and aVF)

        at least 5 mm. in any lead

    Horizontal plane (leads V_1 to V_6)

        at least 10 mm. in any lead

NOTES AND REFERENCES

From Pages 209–210 (Table 3-1)

The many criteria recommended as evidence of left ventricular hypertrophy (LVH) attest to the fact that none have both the desired sensitivity and specificity. As in right ventricular hypertrophy, most have much greater specificity than sensitivity. Sensitivity and specificity are defined on page 192. These criteria attempt to identify the enlarged mean QRS vector of LVH. The concept of the increased vectorial magnitude will remain although the numbers may change with new information.

Frontal plane criteria are generally less reliable than horizontal plane criteria. The reason for this is illustrated on page 214 (Figure 3-5B). Furthermore, various factors, including thin chests in young patients, obesity and bulk of intervening lung, affect the size of the QRS complex in addition to the myocardial mass. Feldman and associates [3-1] recorded a $41 \pm 8\%$ increase in R wave amplitude in leads V_5 and V_6 in the change from the supine to the left lateral position. The study concluded that both the size and the distance of the left ventricle to leads V_5 and V_6 are major determinants of R wave amplitude.

Additional electrocardiographic evidence of LVH is cited below under the name or names of the investigators. Owing to the large number of studies relating to all aspects of the electrocardiographic identification of LVH, these references will be restricted to QRS amplitude criteria except for the point score system of Romhilt and Estes.

Sokolow and Lyon[3-2]

$S_{V_1} + R_{V_5} > 35$ mm.

R_{V_5} or $R_{V_6} > 26$ mm.

Schamroth[3-3]

S_{V_1} or $R_{V_6} \geq 20$ mm.

$S_{V_1} > 15$ mm. is a "pointer to potential diagnosis of LVH"

Griep[3-4]

Holt and Spodick[3-5]

$R_{V_6} > R_{V_5}$

Generally the R wave in lead V_5 is taller than the R wave in lead V_6. These studies indicate that if, in addition to increased QRS voltage, the R wave in lead V_6 is taller than the R wave in lead V_5, additional evidence for LVH is present. This is seen in Figures 3-15 and 3-22.

Roberts and Day[3-6]

Total QRS amplitude in all 12 electrocardiographic leads > 175 mm.

Casale and associates[3-7]

$$R_{aVL} + S_{V_3} > 28 \text{ mm. in men}$$

$$> 20 \text{ mm. in women}$$

Romhilt and Estes[3-8]

Romhilt and Estes developed a point score system for the electrocardiographic diagnosis of left ventricular hypertrophy as follows:

		Points
1.	Amplitude	3
	Any limb lead R or S $\geq$ 20 mm.	
	or S_{V_1} or S_{V_2} or $\geq$ 30 mm.	
	or R_{V_5} or $R_{V_6} \geq$ 30 mm.	
2.	ST-T abnormalities typical of LVH	
	Without digitalis	3
	With digitalis	(1)
3.	Left atrial involvement	3
	Terminal negativity of P_{V_1} is $\geq$ 1 mm. in depth with duration $\geq$ 0.04 sec.	
4.	Left axis deviation	2
	$\geq$ $-30°$ in the frontal plane.	
5.	QRS duration $\geq$ 0.09 sec.	1
6.	Intrinsicoid deflection in V_5 or $V_6 \geq$ 0.05 sec.	1
	Maximum total	13

5 points signifies LVH
4 points signifies probable LVH

From Pages 217–218 (Figure 3-8A)

Heretofore we have been describing left ventricular hypertrophy due to *systolic overload* as found in systemic hypertension, aortic stenosis, hypertrophic cardiomyopathy, and coarctation of the aorta. *Systolic overload* is *pressure* overload with resistance to left ventricular systolic outflow. We see characteristic QRS voltage criteria in addition to a wide QRS-T angle and S-T segment abnormalities.

In Figure 3-8A we have an example of left ventricular hypertrophy due to *diastolic overload* in aortic insufficiency. It also may occur with mitral insufficiency, patent ductus arteriosus, and ventricular septal defect. Diastolic overload refers to *volume overload* with diastolic overfilling of the left ventricle. In Figure 3-8A we see the characteristic QRS voltage criteria of left ventricular hypertrophy, but the QRS-T angle is not wide; this is common in diastolic overload. Often Q waves are prominent in leads V_5 and V_6. After the aortic valve was replaced in this patient with coronary artery disease and systemic hypertension the systolic overload pattern became apparent (Figure 3-8B). The patient, in spite of coexistent disease, was much improved clinically following surgery.

Biventricular Hypertrophy (RVH + LVH)

During the study of right ventricular hypertrophy, Figure 2-20, pages 172 and 194, it was stated that biventricular hypertrophy would be discussed following the study of left ventricular hypertrophy. Biventricular hypertrophy is suggested by the P wave of left atrial abnormality (large left atrium as a criterion of LVH) in addition to any of the following criteria of RVH according to Murphy and associates[3-9]:

1.   R/S ratio in lead V_5 or $V_6 \leq 1$

2. S_{V_5} or $S_{V_6} \geq 7$ mm. or

3.   RAD of the QRS $> + 90°$

Figure 2-20 satisfies 1 and 2 above.

References

3-1. Feldman, T., et al.: Relation of electrocardiographic R-wave amplitude to changes in left ventricular chamber size and position in normal subjects. Am. J. Cardiol., *55*:1168, 1985.

3-2. Sokolow, M., and Lyon, T.P.: The ventricular complex in left ventricular hypertrophy as obtained by unipolar precordial and limb leads. Am. Heart J., *37*:161, 1949.

3-3. Schamroth, L.: The 12 Lead Electrocardiogram. Oxford, Blackwell Scientific Publications, 1989, p. 34.

3-4. Griep, A.H.: Pitfalls in electrocardiographic diagnosis of left ventricular hypertrophy: a correlative study of 200 autopsied patients. Circulation, *20*: 30, 1959.

3-5. Holt, D.H., and Spodick, D.H.: The R_{V_6}:R_{V_5} voltage ratio in left ventricular hypertrophy. Am. Heart J., *63*:65, 1962.

3-6. Roberts, W.C., and Day, P.J.: Electrocardiographic observations in clinically isolated, pure, chronic severe aortic regurgitation: analysis of 30 necropsy patients aged 19 to 65 years. Am. J. Cardiol., *55*:431, 1985.

3-7. Casale, P.N., et al.: Improved sex-specific criteria of left ventricular hypertrophy for clinical and computer interpretation of electrocardiograms: validation with autopsy findings. Circulation, *75*:565, 1987.

3-8. Romhilt, D.W., and Estes, E.H.: A point-score system for the ECG diagnosis of left ventricular hypertrophy. Am. Heart J., *6*:752, 1968.

3-9. Murphy, M.L., et al.: Reevaluation of electrocardiographic criteria for left, right and combined cardiac ventricular hypertrophy. Am. J. Cardiol., *53*:1140, 1984.

4

**REPOLARIZATION
(S-T SEGMENT AND T WAVE)
ALTERATIONS**

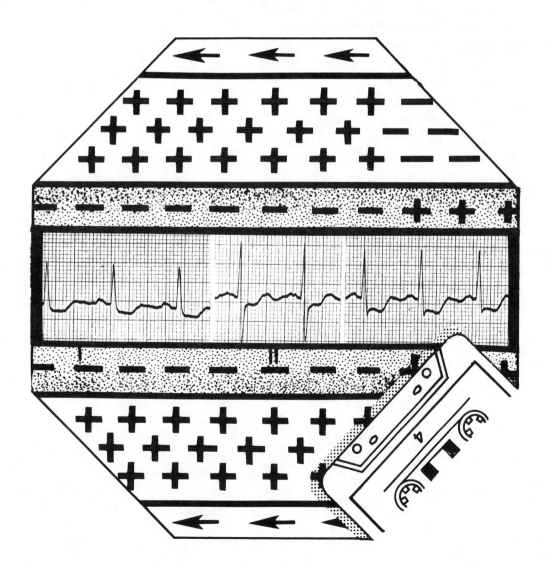

CHAPTER 4
CONTENTS

INTRODUCTION

The lability of the ventricular repolarization phase (S-T segment and T wave) is emphasized, and reference is made to atrial repolarization alterations. Repolarization, in contrast to depolarization, is the energy-consuming phase, and as such, is much more prone to abnormality under a variety of circumstances. On the other hand, not every S-T segment or T wave which appears abnormal at first is actually abnormal. This will be seen in the "early repolarization" and "juvenile" patterns.

There are many causes of repolarization alterations, some of which are beyond the scope of this course, and more will be described in the future. Prototypes, therefore, are used. For example, digitalis serves as the prototype of drug-induced repolarization changes. The repolarization abnormalities resulting from myocardial infarction have been bypassed, except for an example of ventricular aneurysm, since Chapter 5 is entirely devoted to myocardial infarction. It should be remembered, however, that myocardial infarction is responsible for significant repolarization abnormalities.

OBJECTIVES

Upon completion of this chapter, you should be able to:

1. Recognize the difference between primary and secondary repolarization abnormalities.

2. Acknowledge the rotation of the mean T vector from youth to old age.

3. Recognize the "juvenile" pattern.

4. Recognize the electrocardiographic manifestations of digitalis "effects."

5. Evaluate electrocardiographic alterations which may be due to coronary heart disease.

6. Recognize "early repolarization" and differentiate it from more ominous causes of S-T segment displacement.

7. Recognize the electrocardiographic manifestations of ventricular aneurysm.

8. Identify the repolarization abnormalities in a patient with pericarditis.

9. Recognize electrocardiographic evidence of electrolyte imbalance.

10. Recognize abnormalities in atrial repolarization.

P R E T E S T

DIRECTIONS. This pretest consists of five electrocardiograms. Write a brief analysis of each in the space provided.

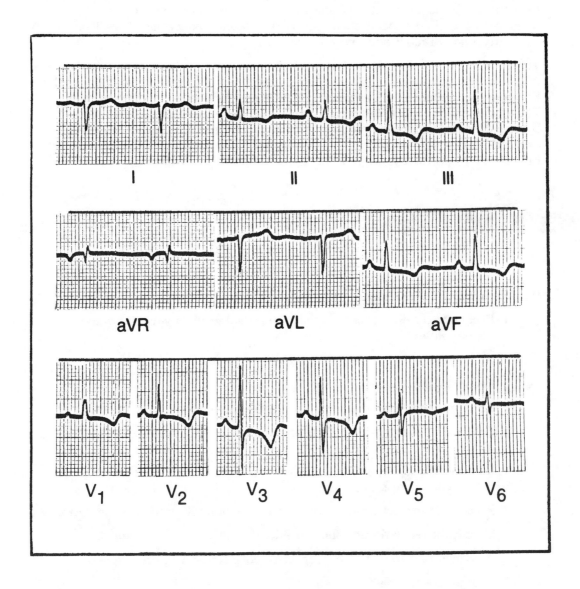

FIGURE 4-2.

1. Analysis:

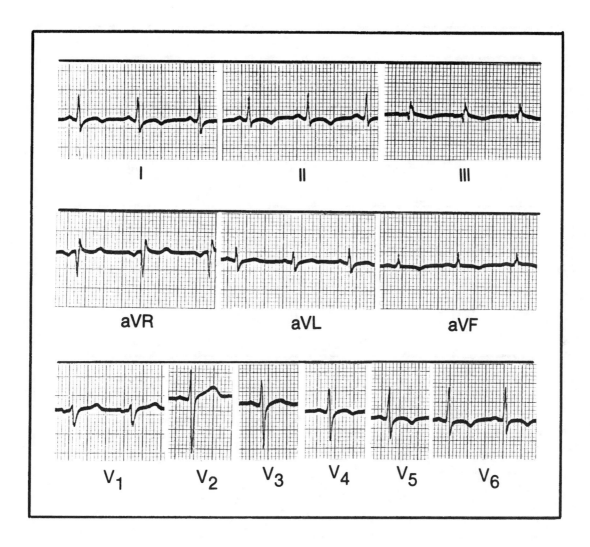

FIGURE 4-7.

2. Analysis:

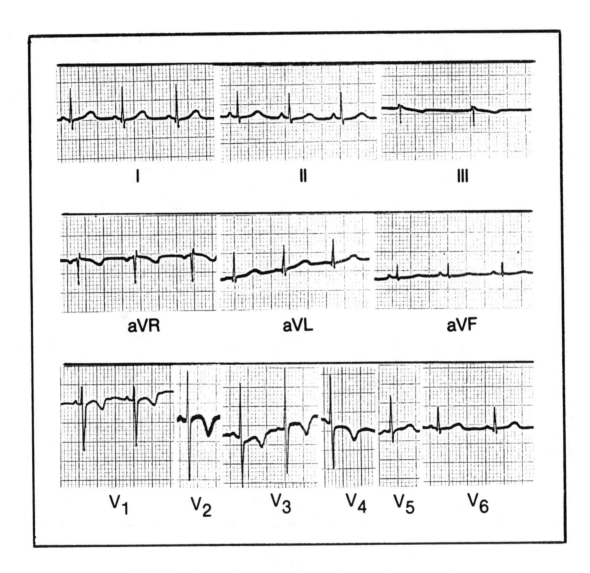

FIGURE 4-8. Analyze this electrocardiogram from a healthy young patient.

3. Analysis:

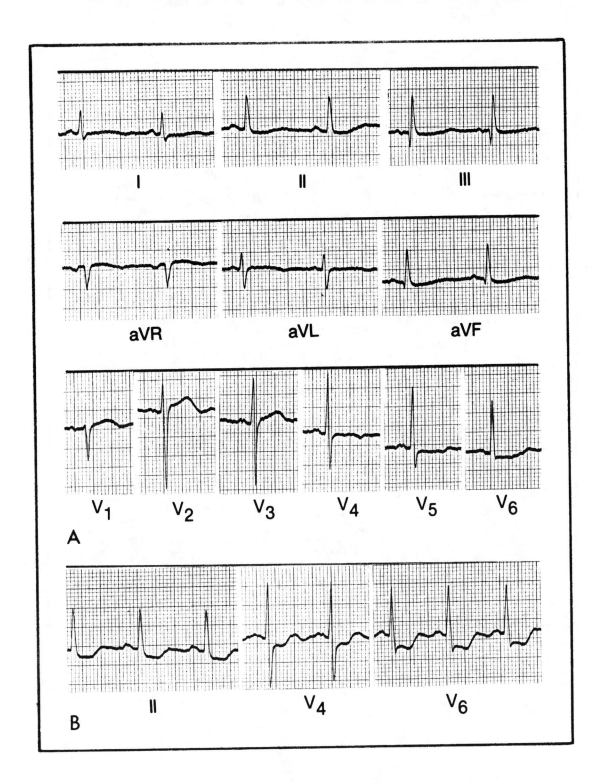

FIGURE 4-19.   A, At rest. B, After exercise.

4.   Analysis:

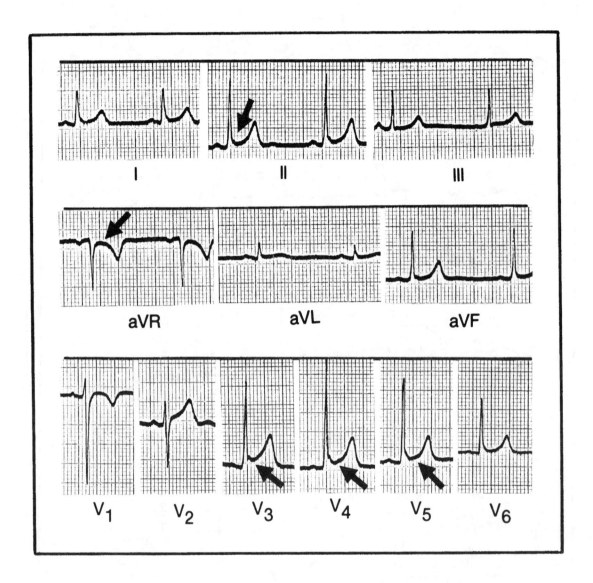

FIGURE 4-22.   Analyze this electrocardiogram from a normal young patient.

5.   Analysis:

> Solutions to the pretest will be indicated later in this chapter.

> When you have completed the pretest start Cassette Side 9 and continue on the next page.

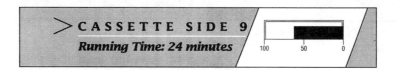

CASSETTE SIDE 9
Running Time: 24 minutes
100   50   0

NORMAL REPOLARIZATION AND REPOLARIZATION ALTERATIONS

A. Normal Repolarization

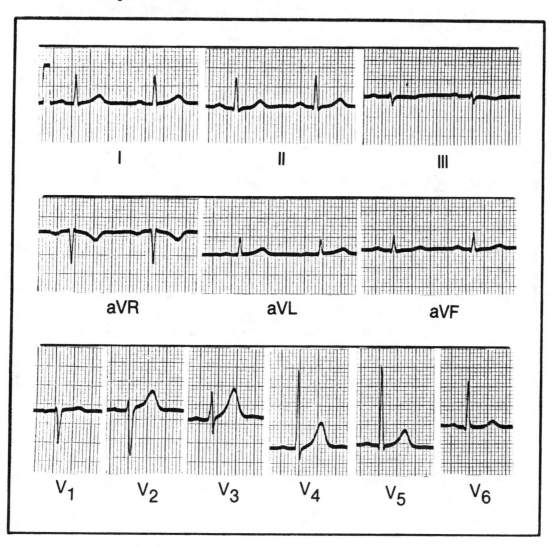

FIGURE 4-1.   Normal electrocardiogram. Depolarization of the ventricles is represented by the QRS complexes; repolarization is represented by the S-T segments and T waves.

You have actually been studying repolarization throughout the course. In the study of the normal electrocardiogram (Chapter 1) you learned that repolarization is studied in its relationship to depolarization (QRS-T angle). In the study of the hypertrophied right ventricle (Chapter 2) and the hypertrophied left ventricle (Chapter 3), you noted abnormalities in repolarization, abnormal QRS-T angles, and abnormal S-T segments. Review all the features which make the electrocardiogram in Figure 4-1 a normal one. Describe the P waves, P-R intervals, rhythm, QRS complexes, QRS-T angle, and S-T segments.

B. Ventricular Repolarization Alterations

There are numerous causes of ventricular repolarization abnormalities. Examples are given below.

1. Right Ventricular Hypertrophy

Figure 4-2 reveals the principal findings of right ventricular hypertrophy in the adult. There is marked right axis deviation (+120°) of the mean QRS vector, which is also anterior (the R wave is the main ventricular deflection in lead V_1). Repolarization abnormalities are striking, with a very wide QRS-T angle.

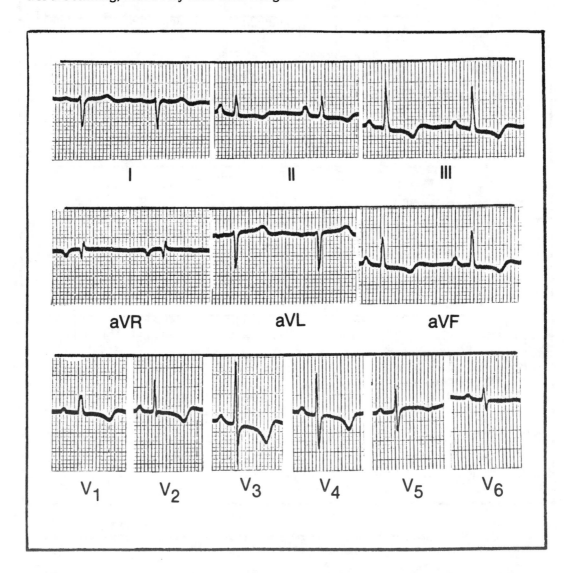

FIGURE 4-2. *Right ventricular hypertrophy. Calculate the mean QRS vector and QRS-T angle and describe the S-T segments. Compare with the normal electrocardiogram in Figure 4-1. If you have any questions as to the characteristics of the hypertrophied right ventricle, especially repolarization abnormalities, take the time to review Chapter 2.*

> The analysis of Figure 4-2 in the text and on the tape is the solution to item 1 on the pretest.

2. *Left Ventricular Hypertrophy*

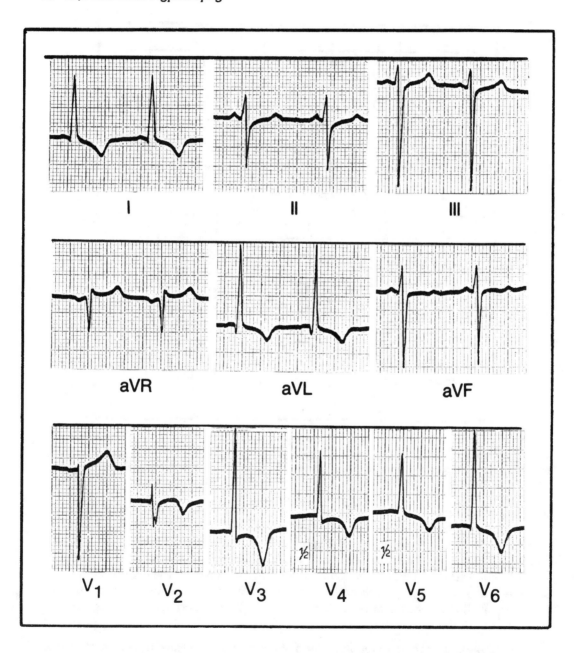

FIGURE 4-3.   *Left ventricular hypertrophy. Review all the criteria for left ventricular hypertrophy (Chapter 3), especially the repolarization abnormalities. If you have reviewed and understand the electrocardiograms in Figures 4-1, 4-2, and 4-3, you have actually reviewed all that we have studied in Chapters 1, 2, and 3.*

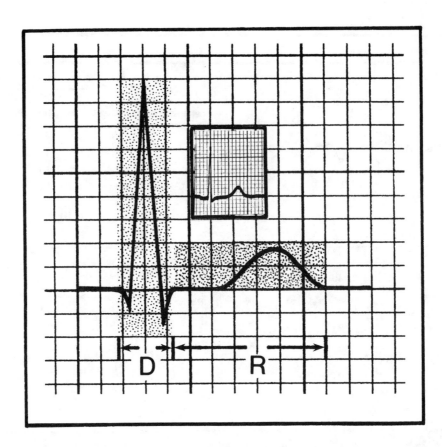

FIGURE 4-4. Electrocardiographic manifestations of ventricular depolarization and repolarization (D and R, respectively). Since repolarization is a much longer process than depolarization and consumes relatively more energy, it is more prone to abnormality; hence the multiple causes of S-T segment and T wave abnormalities.

Repolarization abnormalities may be primary, secondary, or both. Figure 4-5A illustrates repolarization abnormalities resulting from *abnormal depolarization*. Note the abnormally wide QRS complexes (representing left bundle branch block, to be studied in Chapter 6). When repolarization is abnormal because depolarization is abnormal, the repolarization abnormalities are *secondary*. How do we know that the abnormalities are *secondary* and not *primary* in this patient? Figure 4-5B is from the same patient during intermittent *normal* ventricular conduction; the QRS-T angle and S-T segments are normal.

Since patients with *secondary* repolarization abnormalities may also have *primary* repolarization abnormalities (abnormalities of repolarization *not due* to abnormalities of depolarization), how do you distinguish between *secondary* and *primary* abnormalities of repolarization in the presence of abnormal depolarization? Serial electrocardiographic tracings yield important information in the careful follow-up of a patient.

3. Secondary Repolarization Abnormalities

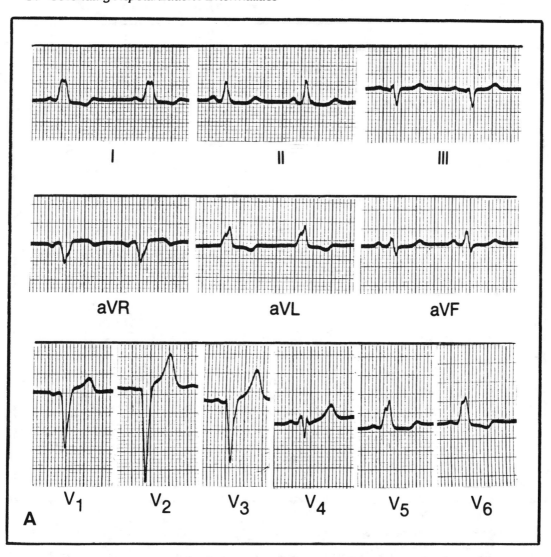

FIGURE 4-5A. *This electrocardiogram represents a ventricular conduction disturbance (left bundle branch block), which will be studied later in the course. For the present, note the abnormal width of the QRS complexes and repolarization abnormalities (S-T segment and T wave abnormalities). When repolarization abnormalities are caused by abnormal depolarization, they are known as secondary repolarization abnormalities (secondary S-T segment and T wave abnormalities). Figure 4-5B is from the same patient during normal conduction.*

The repolarization abnormalities accompanying ventricular hypertrophy are also *secondary,* as noted in Chapters 2 and 3.

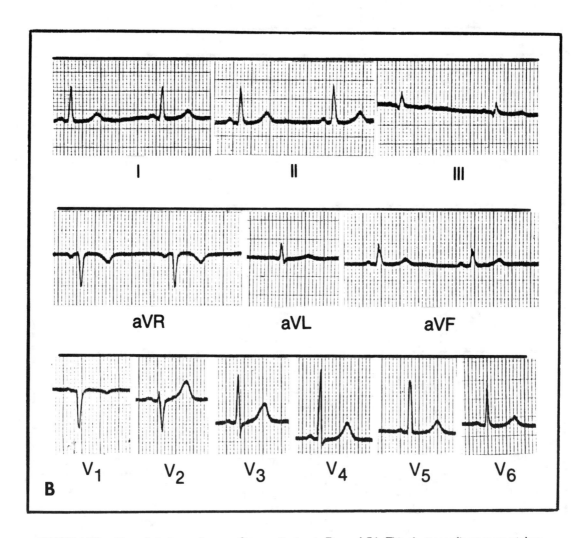

FIGURE 4-5B.   Normal electrocardiogram. Same patient as in Figure 4-5A. This electrocardiogram was taken
during normal ventricular conduction (normal depolarization with normal QRS complexes), which alternated
with abnormal conduction at a critical rate. During this normal depolarization, the repolarization was completely
normal; therefore, the repolarization abnormalities seen in Figure 4-5A, following abnormal depolarization, are
strictly secondary repolarization abnormalities.

4. Primary Repolarization Abnormalities

When repolarization abnormalities are seen with normal depolarization, they are *primary* (abnormalities due to intrinsic problems in the repolarization phase and not secondary to abnormal depolarization). As previously learned, the phase of repolarization requires more energy, relative to depolarization, and is therefore more prone to abnormality. There are numerous causes of repolarization abnormalities, including a host of metabolic derangements and drug states, coronary heart disease, as well as variants of normal. Repolarization abnormalities have been recorded with posture change, cold drinks, anxiety, hyperventilation, smoking, and eating.

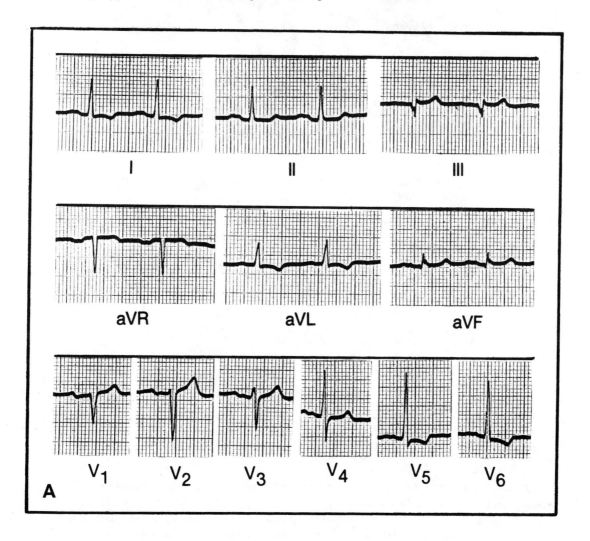

FIGURE 4-6A. Primary *repolarization (S-T segment and T wave) abnormalities.*

5. Rotation of Mean T Vector from Youth to Old Age

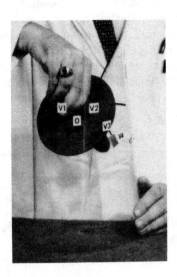 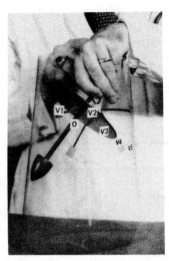

Youth   Old Age

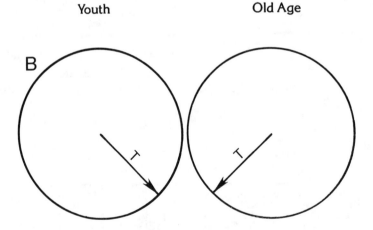

FIGURE 4-6B.   Rotation of mean T wave vector from youth to old age. The mean T wave vector in youth is frequently found to be the left, inferior, and posterior, inscribing a T wave across the chest (see vector model above) as follows: leads V_1, V_2, and V_3 negative, V_4, V_5, and V_6 positive. The T wave may be negative as far as lead V_4. This "juvenile" pattern is illustrated in Figure 4-8.

With increasing age, the mean T vector rotates *rightward* and *anteriorly*, inscribing a T wave across the chest as follows: leads V_1, V_2, V_3, and V_4 positive, V_5 and V_6 negative (see vector model above). This does not always happen; not every elderly patient has negative T waves in V_5 and V_6, nor is it considered normal to have negative T waves in these leads. Many an asymptomatic elderly patient, however, upon being told by an unwary physician that his heart is "ischemic" or "straining" has been prodded into symptoms. You must always treat the patient, not the electrocardiogram detached from the patient.

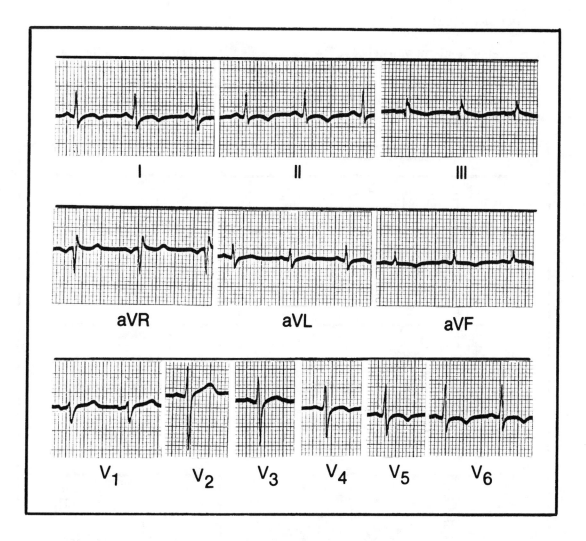

FIGURE 4-7.   *Wide QRS-T angle.*

The QRS-T angle is abnormally wide. This patient, with primary repolarization abnormalities, had symptoms of myocardial ischemia. If you read this electrocardiogram without knowing the patient, however, you might call these "non-specific" repolarization abnormalities. In the variations from normal there are numerous false positives and false negatives, emphasizing the importance of knowing your patient.

The analysis of Figure 4-7 in the text and on the tape is the solution to item 2 on the pretest.

6. "Juvenile" Pattern

The "juvenile" pattern, with negative T waves in leads V_1 to V_4 is not infrequently seen in normal, healthy young patients well into the third decade of life. It is not abnormal. This emphasizes once again that the electrocardiogram should not be detached from the patient and should not be read without knowing the age of the patient or without knowledge of pertinent clinical information. 4-1, 4-2

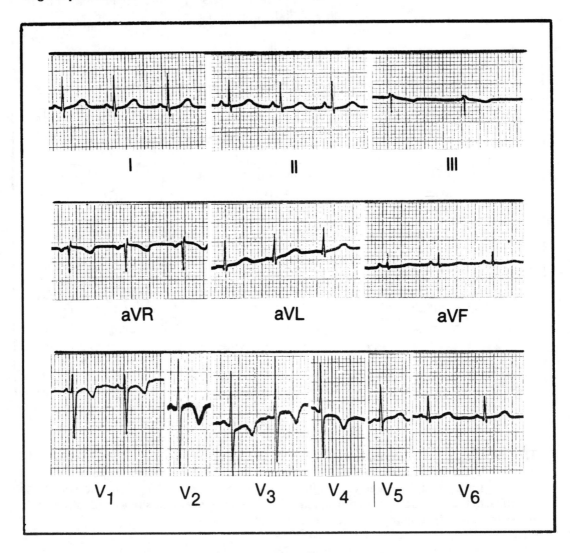

FIGURE 4-8. "Juvenile" pattern in a healthy young patient (refer to the discussion in Figure 4-6B). Describe the mean T vector and contrast with the many normals already seen.

> The analysis of Figure 4-8 in the text and on the tape is the solution to item 3 on the pretest.

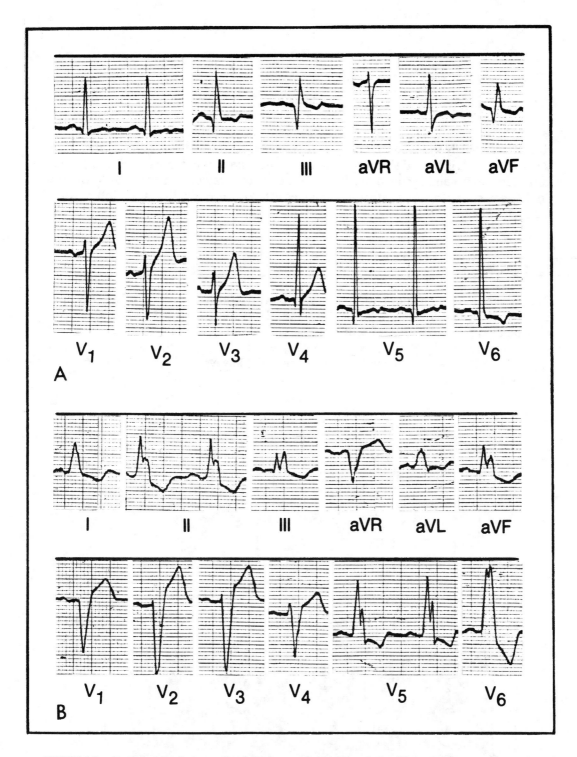

FIGURE 4-9.   *Patient with inferior myocardial infarction before (A) and after (B) the development of a conduction disturbance (left bundle branch block, LBBB).*

Figure 4-9A is from a patient with an inferior myocardial infarction (this subject will be studied in Chapter 5). For the present, describe the repolarization abnormalities (abnormal S-T segments and T waves). This patient also had left ventricular hypertrophy. Figure 4-9B is from the same patient following the development of a ventricular conduction disturbance (left bundle branch block, LBBB, to be studied in Chapter 6).

Note the markedly widened QRS complexes and the diminution or disappearance of the Q waves in leads II, III, and aVF. Note also the further changes in repolarization. The repolarization abnormalities due to LBBB were added to the previously abnormal repolarization. The best way to appreciate these changes is to know your patients and follow with serial electrocardiograms.

---

7. *Digitalis*

Digitalis has long been known for its effects on ventricular repolarization. The "classic" changes of digitalis are described as a "fist-like" depression of the S-T segment (as if you were placing your fist in the S-T segment and depressing it), or "paint-brush" inscription (as if you were painting the S-T segment with gradual widening of the paintbrush as you approach the S-T segment from the downslope of the R wave), or "scooping" of the S-T segment.

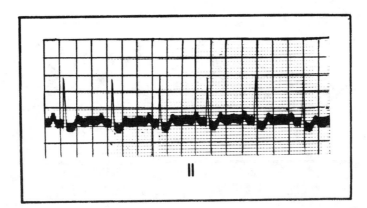

II

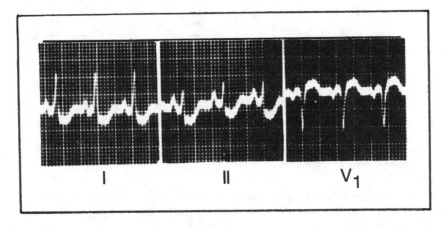

I   II   V₁

FIGURE 4-10.   "Classic" changes on the S-T segments caused by digitalis in two patients. (Electrocardiograms reduced in size.)

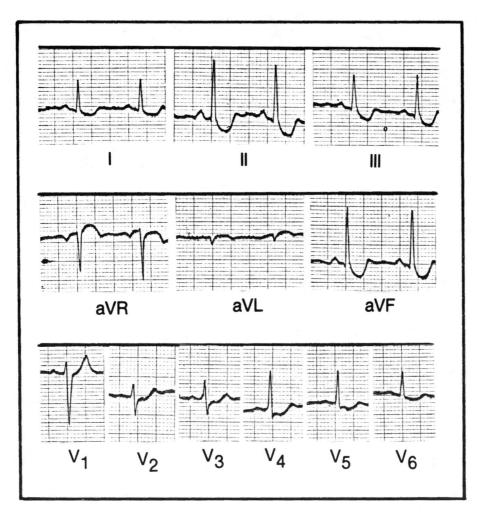

FIGURE 4-11.   Review the effects of digitalis on ventricular repolarization.

It has been repeatedly emphasized in this course that it is best to read the electrocardiograms of your patients. If you do not know the patient, an electrocardiographic pattern as seen above may represent myocardial ischemia or digitalis effects or both. The repolarization findings are therefore *nonspecific*.

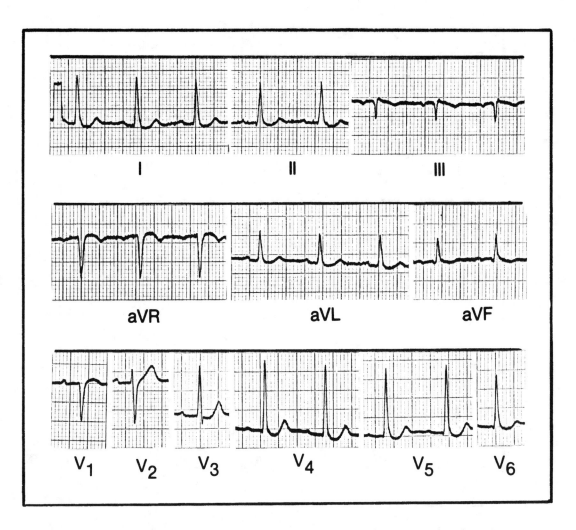

FIGURE 4-12.   Patient receiving digitalis. Describe the "classic" changes in the early part of repolarization caused by digitalis and known as "digitalis effects."

Figures 4-13 to 4-16 are from studies of digitalis effects on repolarization. In spite of the well-accepted "classic" changes on early repolarization (S-T segment), the effects on later repolarization (T wave) were just as dramatic. In a substantial number of patients it was not possible to predict which part, or whether the entire phase, of repolarization would be affected (both the S-T segment and the T wave). This again emphasizes the need to follow each patient closely without relying on "predictable" changes.

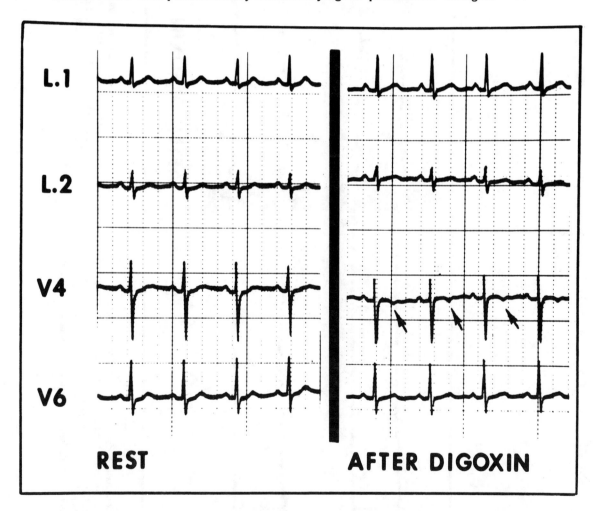

FIGURE 4-13.   *Repolarization changes due to a digitalis preparation (digoxin). In spite of the "classic" changes ascribed to digitalis on the early part of repolarization (S-T segment) note the effect of a subdigitalizing dose of digoxin on late repolarization (T wave). (Electrocardiogram reduced in size.)*

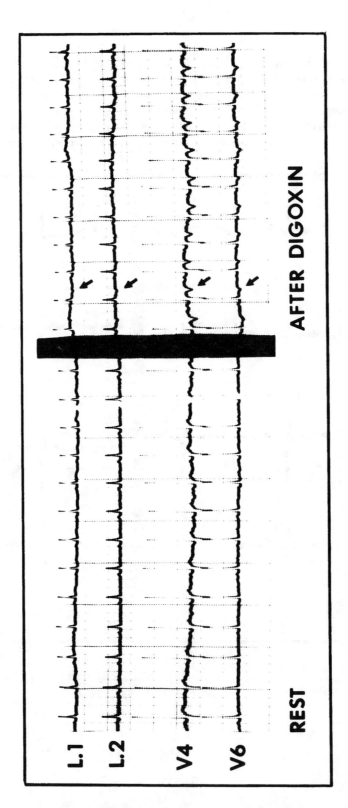

REST

AFTER DIGOXIN

L.1

L.2

V4

V6

FIGURE 4.14. *Repolarization changes due to digitalis. A dramatic effect is seen in late repolarization (T wave) due to a small dose of the digitalis preparation digoxin. There was no other intervention here; the thick black line in the center is where the recording machine was stopped for one hour following the administration of digoxin. It cannot, therefore, be said dogmatically that digitalis affects only the early part of repolarization; the effect on the T waves may be much more marked than the effect on the S-T segments. Repolarization should be dealt with as a unit; the S-T segments and T waves should not be categorically separated. Digitalis may affect one, the other, or both. (Electrocardiogram reduced in size.)*

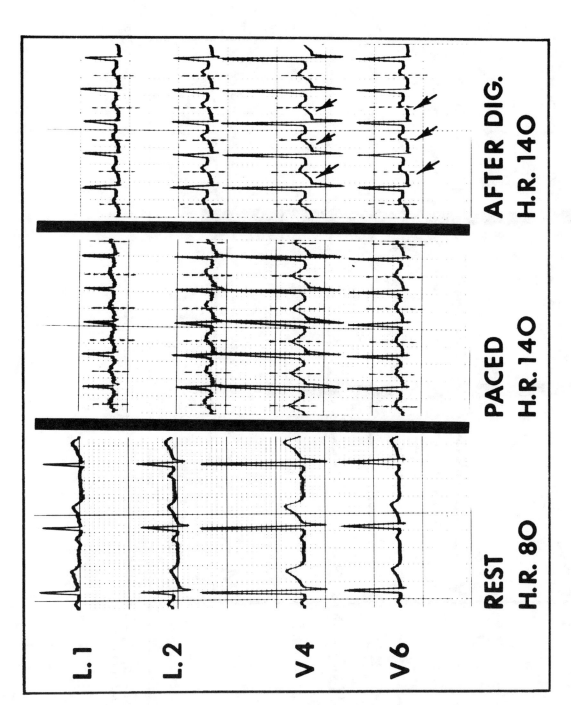

FIGURE 4.15.　Repolarization changes due to digitalis. The arrows point to the effects of digitalis on the S-T segments at a given paced heart rate, compared with the same paced heart rate without digitalis. (Electrocardiogram reduced in size.)

CASSETTE SIDE 10
Running Time: 25 minutes

100   50   0

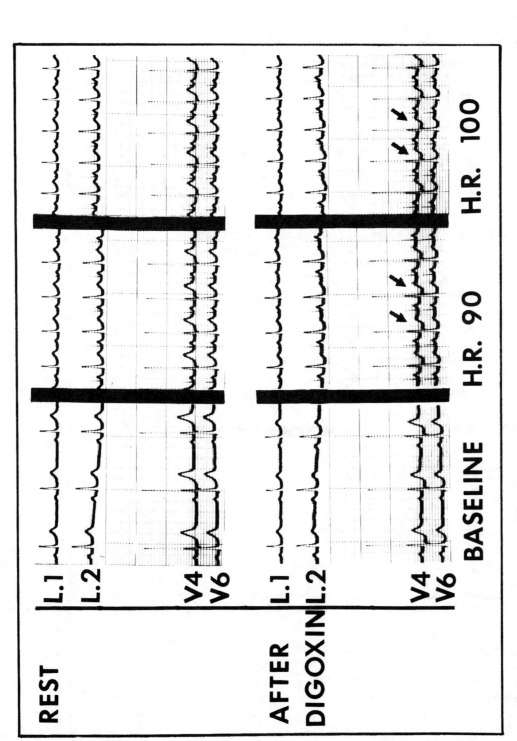

REST

L.1
L.2

V4
V6

AFTER DIGOXIN

L.1
L.2

V4
V6

BASELINE   H.R. 90   H.R. 100

FIGURE 4-16.   Digitalis effects on repolarization. Compare the effects of digitalis on each of the paired heart rates, baseline, 90 per minute, and 100 per minute. (Electrocardiogram reduced in size.)

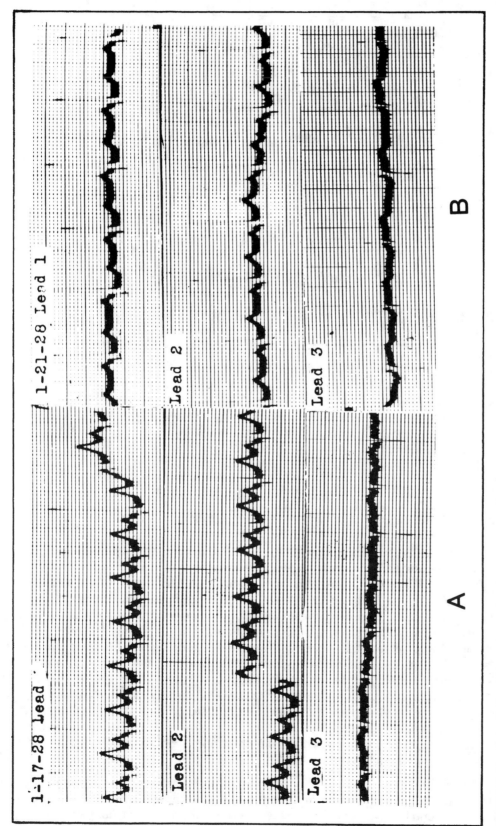

FIGURE 4.17.   Before (A) and after (B) "digitalization." Describe the changes which have occurred during ventricular repolarization (both S-T segment and T wave). That digitalis could affect the entire phase of repolarization was recognized years ago.

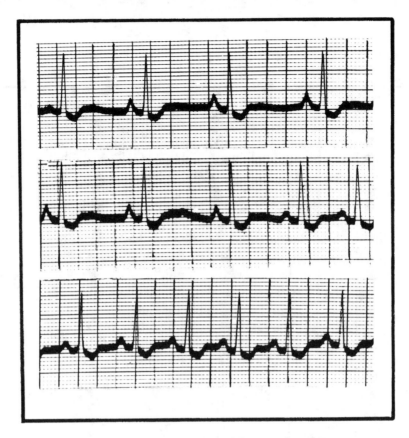

FIGURE 4-18.   Repolarization and changes in heart rate.

Often you will hear that an increase in heart rate will cause a change in repolarization. You have already seen that the effects of digitalis on repolarization were more pronounced at the higher rates (Figures 4-15 and 4-16). Always evaluate critically; repolarization is not readily predictable. In Figure 4-18 there is no marked change in repolarization in spite of an increased heart rate.

8.   Coronary Heart Disease

Coronary heart disease, or as others prefer, the broader term ischemic heart disease, is a major cause of ventricular repolarization abnormalities. Figure 4-19 shows the effects of activity (Figure 4-19B) on the already abnormal repolarization (Figure 4-19A) in a patient with angina pectoris. The S-T segment in lead V_6 (Figure 4-19B), depressed and downsloping, is commonly seen in patients with myocardial ischemia. Many a patient with a typical history of angina pectoris will have an electrocardiogram with normal ventricular repolarization at rest; this is seen in Figure 4-20A and was seen in multiple resting electrocardiograms. The electrocardiogram of the same patient following a walk from her room to the electrocardiography office is seen in Figure 4-20B. Activity (utilizing the patient's normal activity, such as taking a walk), rather than provocative testing, will often yield important information in the *initial* evaluation. This activity did not produce pain, yet the effect on ventricular repolarization is obvious. In Figure 4-21B we see the striking S-T segment elevations (lead II), during an episode of chest pain in a patient with a history of angina pectoris at rest.

Some patients with "classic" angina pectoris have been found to have normal-appearing coronary arteries by arteriography. Of great interest are the patients with clinical myocardial infarction found to have normal-appearing coronary arteries. Much has yet to be learned in this field.

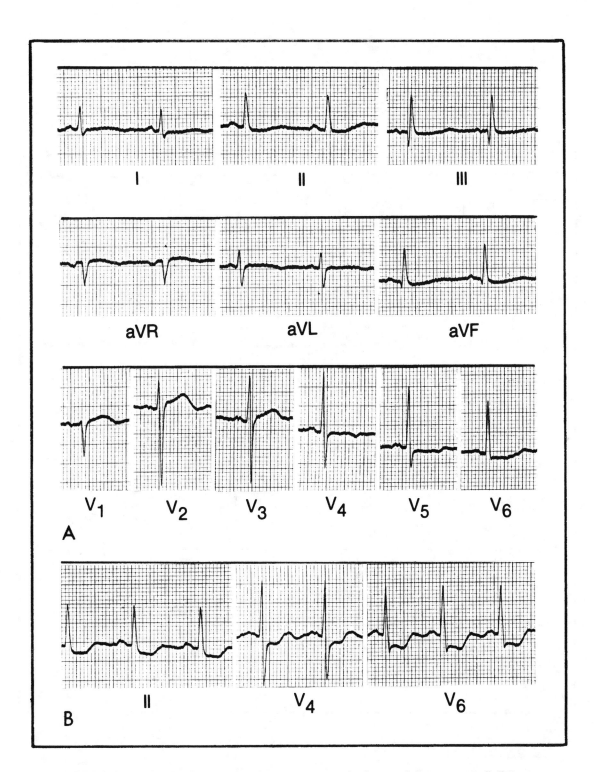

FIGURE 4-19.   A, Repolarization abnormalities in a patient with a history of angina pectoris. B, Following activity, repolarization abnormalities became quite pronounced with a typical picture of myocardial ischemia. Note the depression and downsloping of the S-T segment.

> The analysis of Figure 4-19 in the text and on the tape is the solution to item 4 on the pretest.

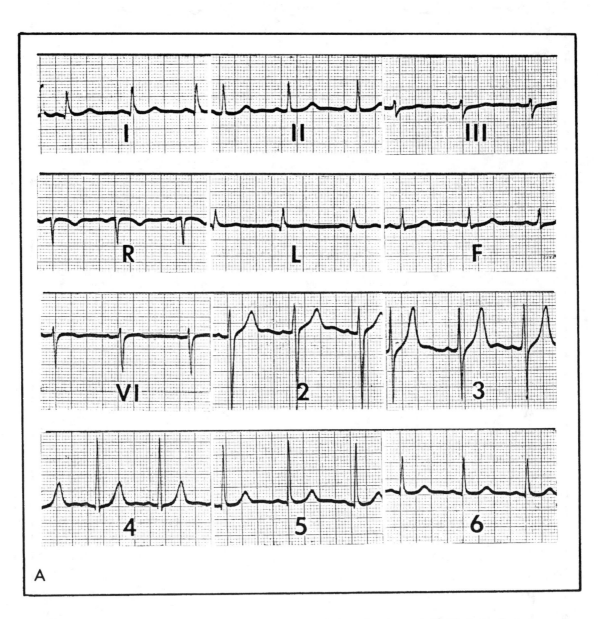

FIGURE 4-20A.   Resting electrocardiogram of a patient with a history of angina pectoris. (Electrocardiogram reduced in size.)

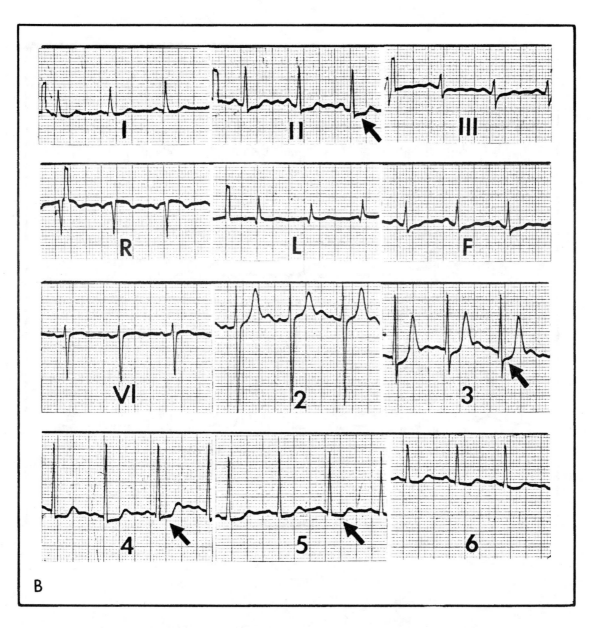

FIGURE 4-20B.   Electrocardiogram of same patient as in Figure 4-20A following a walk from her room to the electrocardiography office. The treadmill is most commonly used for exercise or stress testing.[43] Activity utilizing the patient's normal activity, such as taking a walk, rather than provocative testing, will often yield important information. (Electrocardiogram reduced in size.)

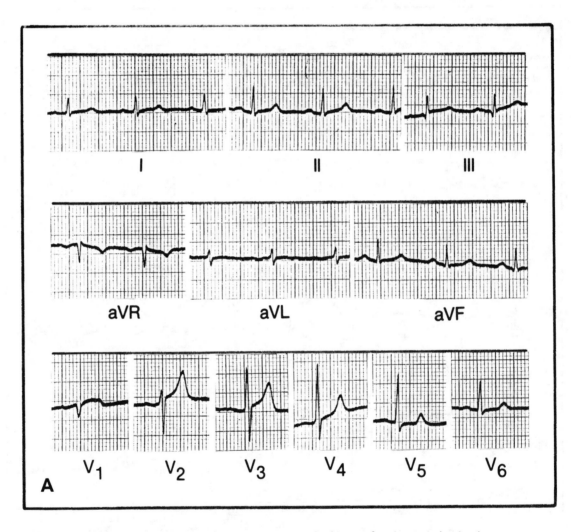

FIGURE 4-21A.   *Electrocardiogram of a patient with a history of angina pectoris, at rest.*

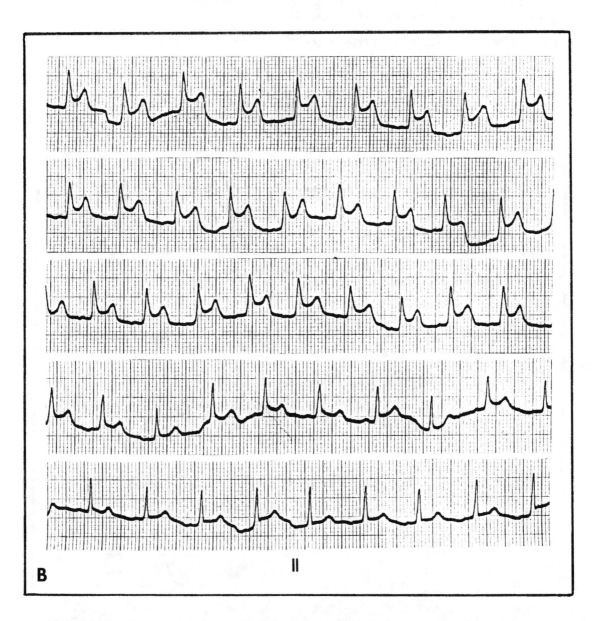

FIGURE 4-21B.   The electrocardiogram of the same patient as in Figure 4-21A during an episode of chest pain at rest, showing a continuous lead II with return of the S-T segments toward normal on subsidence of chest pain. This was described by Prinzmetal and associates as a variant form of angina pectoris.[4,4,4,5] How do these S-T segments differ from the S-T segments in previous electrocardiograms of patients with angina pectoris? There is nothing categorically explicit about what will be found on the electrocardiogram among a group of patients with the same symptoms. Each patient must be closely followed and any change carefully evaluated.

9. Early Repolarization

This pattern is not infrequently seen in young asymptomatic patients.[4.6,4.7] The S-T segment is elevated (leads II and V_3 to V_5) and depressed (lead aVR) following the orientation of the T wave. The QRS–S-T junction is also displaced. Of importance is the need to distinguish "early repolarization" from the more ominous causes of S-T segment displacement such as pericarditis and myocardial infarction.

Distinguishing features of "early repolarization" include:
1. Clinical correlation: the patient is young and well.
2. The S-T segment displacement is associated with increased T wave magnitude.
3. Normal QRS-T angle.
4. The mean S-T and T vectors are similarly oriented. The S-T segment is elevated with tall T waves and depressed with deep T waves.

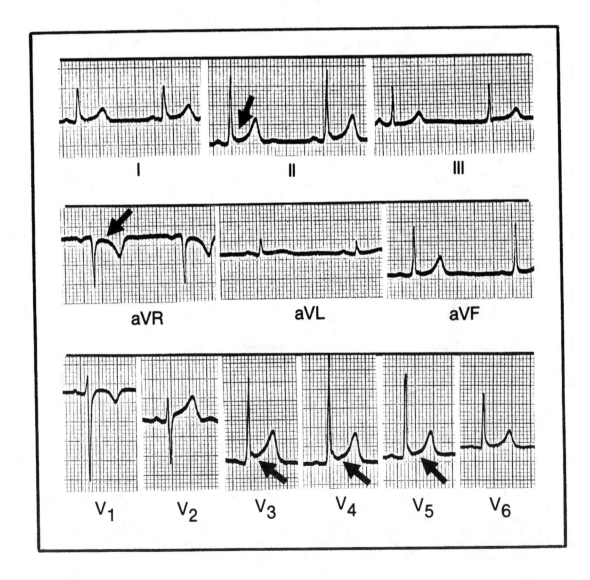

The analysis of Figure 4-22 in the text and on the tape is the solution to item 5 on the pretest.

10. Ventricular Aneurysm

Figure 4-23, from a patient with a ventricular aneurysm years after a myocardial infarction, illustrates one of the effects of myocardial infarction on ventricular repolarization. The persistent elevation of the S-T segment, described as a persistent "monophasic" curve of injury, represents a ventricular aneurysm, an outpouching of a section of scarred ventricular myocardium. The subject of myocardial infarction will be discussed in Chapter 5.

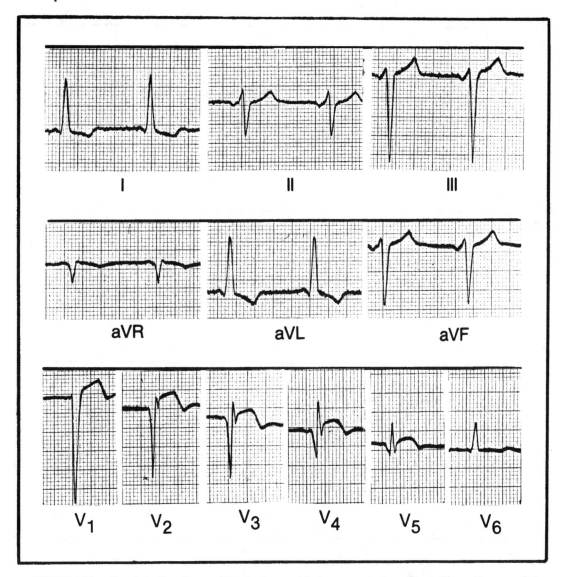

FIGURE 4-23. Repolarization abnormalities due to a ventricular aneurysm in a patient with an old myocardial infarction. This patient also had a large left ventricle. Note that the rhythm is not sinus.

11. Pericarditis

Repolarization abnormalities in a patient with pericarditis are seen in Figure 4-24. Since the early part (S-T segment) of repolarization is affected, we should expect the abnormality, anatomically, to be in the epicardial area of the heart, nearest the pericardium. Often, in the evolutionary serial electrocardiographic tracings the T wave (later repolarization) is also affected. Do not confuse this abnormal, changing, evolving pattern with "early repolarization" (Figure 4-22), found in many normal, healthy young patients.[48-410] Clinical correlation must again be emphasized since the pattern seen in Figure 4-24 may not be distinguishable from that of a patient with an acute myocardial infarction.

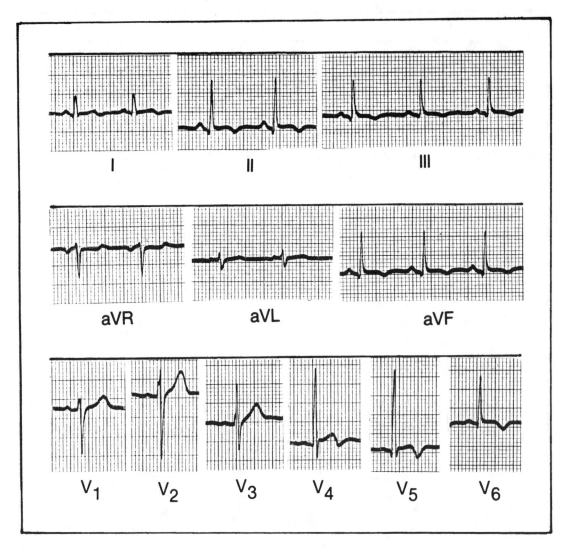

FIGURE 4-24.   Repolarization abnormalities in a young patient with pericarditis.

> After completing the study of Figure 4-24, stop the tape and analyze Figures 4-25B, 4-27, and 4-28, electrocardiograms from patients with electrolyte imbalance.

---

12. Electrolyte Imbalance

Electrolyte imbalance is another common cause of ventricular repolarization abnormalities. If the imbalance is severe, *atrioventricular conduction* as well as *ventricular depolarization* may also be affected, as seen in Figure 4-25B. This elderly patient with borderline renal function, whose baseline abnormal electrocardiogram is seen in Figure 4-25A, became *hyperkalemic*. In comparing Figures 4-25B with 4-25A note the changes in the:

1. QRS complex (ventricular depolarization).
2. S-T segment and T wave (ventricular repolarization).
3. P-R interval (atrioventricular conduction). The P waves are seen clearly in leads II, III, and aVF in Figure 4-25B.

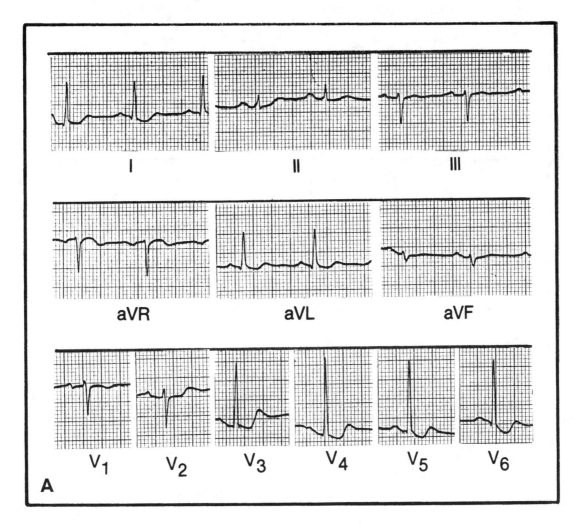

FIGURE 4-25A. Describe the abnormal repolarization.

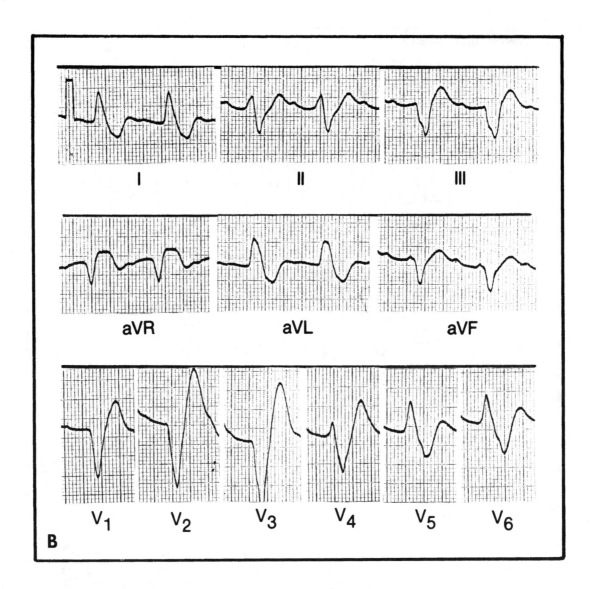

FIGURE 4-25B.   Hyperkalemic state in patient whose prior electrocardiogram was seen in Figure 4-25A. Describe the additional abnormalities seen here during repolarization, as well as during depolarization and atrioventricular conduction.

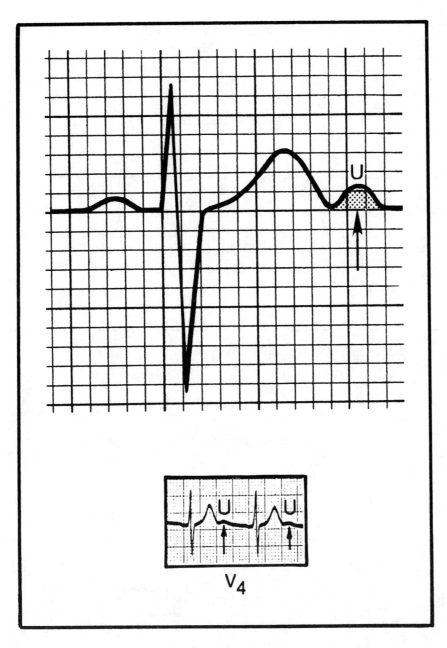

FIGURE 4-26. The U Wave.

Hypokalemia may produce striking electrocardiographic abnormalities, such as depression of the S-T segment, lowering and flattening of the T wave, and appearance of a prominent *U wave*. The U wave follows the T wave and has been associated with hypokalemia, although it may be found normally, as above. The normal small U wave, when present, is seen best in the midprecordial leads. In Figure 4-27 there appears to be a prolonged Q-T interval in leads II, 'II, aVR, and aVF. The Q-T interval should be 0.28 sec., not 0.36 sec. at the rate of 125 beats per minute. Lead V₂, however, reveals the hypokalemic U wave on the descending limb of the T wave.

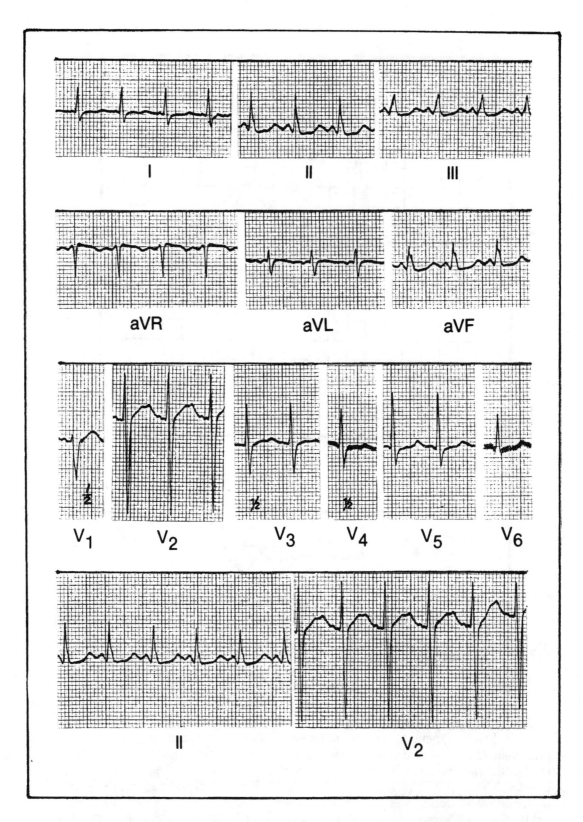

FIGURE 4-27. *Hypokalemia in a patient with sinus tachycardia. Leads V_1, V_3, and V_4 are one half standard.*

Figure 4-28 reveals the marked *prolongation of the Q-T interval* in a patient with long-standing *hypocalcemia*. The heart rate of the patient is 84 beats per minute. At this rate the Q-T interval should be 0.34 sec., rather than 0.48 sec., as seen here. Refer to Chapter 1 for the relationship between the Q-T interval and the heart rate. *Hypercalcemia* is often represented electrocardiographically by a short Q-T interval (see p. 311). There is an inverse relationship between the Q-T interval and the level of serum calcium.

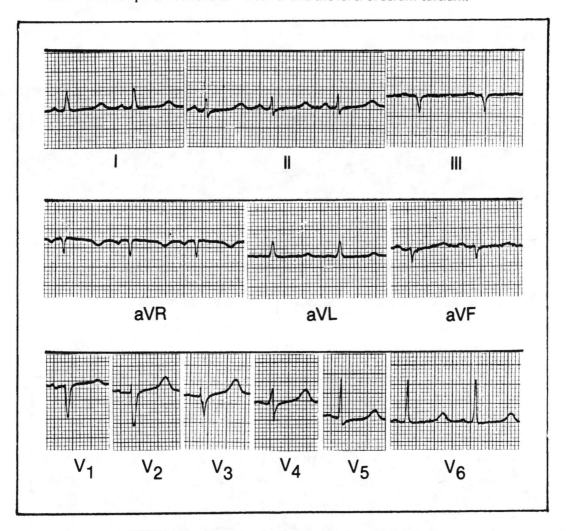

FIGURE 4-28.   Hypocalcemia of longstanding in an elderly patient.

After completing your analyses, restart the tape and also refer to pages 308–311 for explanations and additional illustrations of the electrocardiographic manifestations of electrolyte imbalance.

C. Atrial Repolarization Alterations

Although the subject of this chapter is repolarization of the ventricles, atrial repolarization must not be neglected. This is usually not evident on the clinical electrocardiogram because the P wave itself is relatively small and is quickly followed by the prominent QRS complex. Under special circumstances, parts of the atrial repolarization phase may be seen as in Figures 4-29 and 4-30.

1. Atrial Enlargement

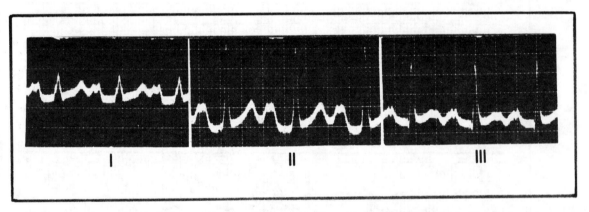

FIGURE 4-29.   Left and right atrial enlargement and first degree atrioventricular block in a patient with mitral stenosis. Note the size of the P waves in lead II. The prolonged P-R interval of the atrioventricular block gives us the opportunity to see an abnormally depressed P-R segment. Normal atrial repolarization does not produce P-R segment depression of this magnitude, best seen in lead II. (Electrocardiogram enlarged.)

2. Myocardial Infarction

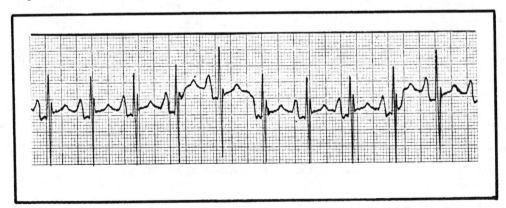

FIGURE 4-30.   Abnormal atrial repolarization in a patient with myocardial infarction involving the atria. Always look for abnormalities in atrial repolarization; you may find clues not seen anywhere else in the electrocardiogram. This precordial lead is from a patient with myocardial infarction involving the atria. Note the depression of the P-R segment. Among the causes of abnormal atrial repolarization are atrial enlargement, pericarditis involving the atria, myocardial infarction involving the atria, manipulation, and injury to the atria during open heart surgery. (Electrocardiogram reduced in size.)

"MARCH OF THE ARROWS" CONCEPT

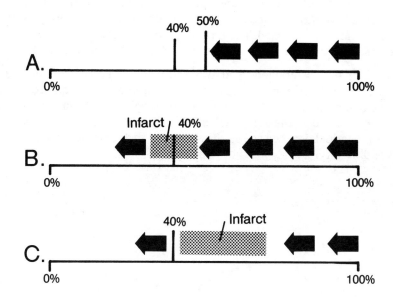

FIGURE 4-31. The "march of the arrows" concept in coronary heart disease. See below.

The emphasis in this course has always been on the concept rather than on memorized patterns and normal values. Since the study of ventricular repolarization is so closely related to coronary heart disease, the "march of the arrows" concept (Figure 4-31) will be introduced at this point, prior to the actual study of myocardial infarction. The natural history of coronary heart disease may be considered according to this concept. The assumption is made that at least 40% of functioning myocardium is needed for asymptomatic, full activity (this is only an assumption; it may or may not be accurate). The 100% starting point represents birth. As a person matures and ages, the arrows continue to march inexorably toward the 0 point.

1. *Figure 4-31A.* A man had reached the age of 95 years with 50% of his myocardium fibrosed. He had been asymptomatic, that is, with no chest pain nor shortness of breath. He did not run around a football field but did whatever a 95-year-old man wished to do. At postmortem examination his heart was small and the coronary arteries were markedly narrowed, but not occluded. Many were amazed that he had been able to function so well with so much myocardial destruction.

2. *Figure 4-31B.* A 50-year-old man was asymptomatic until he suffered a myocardial infarction a year ago. He never recovered fully and has continued to have both angina pectoris and shortness of breath on effort. There was enough myocardial destruction resulting from the infarct to cross the bar at 40%. The arrows have continued to march with time and symptoms have been progressive.

3. *Figure 4-31C.*   A 60-year-old man had had a massive myocardial infarction at age 58. He recovered fully and was asymptomatic for about 1 year. During the following year he began to experience both chest pain and shortness of breath. This panel shows that the infarction caused substantial myocardial destruction, but the bar at 40% had still not been crossed. The crossing took place at a later date coinciding with the onset of symptoms. The infarction hastened the process.

The concept, which may be applied to other organ systems, and which permits you to see change in an orderly fashion, may appear oversimplified; it is. The process is far more complex, and hidden within it are the secrets of aging. There are those who stand at a podium and give you all the answers; I am merely raising some of the questions. Why does one individual proceed so rapidly along the path to disaster while another has relatively little difficulty?

> A number of entities affecting repolarization have been discussed; you will learn many more as you continue with electrocardiography. Based on the material learned to date you should be able to analyze Figures 4-32 to 4-40.

REVIEW
ELECTROCARDIOGRAMS

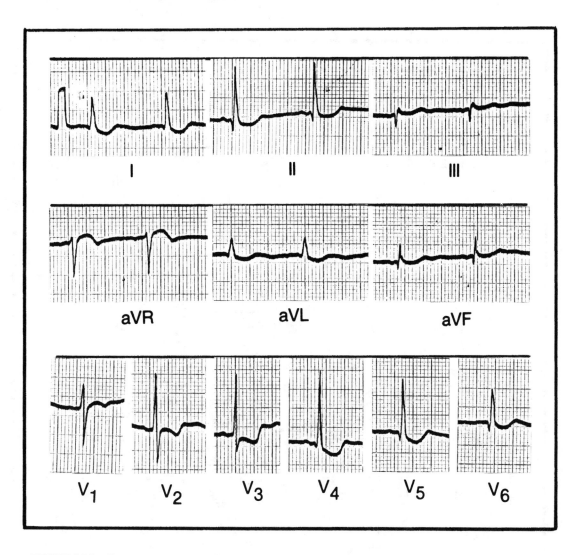

FIGURE 4-32. Describe the repolarization abnormalities. Can you state with absolute certainty, from this one electrocardiogram, that all the repolarization abnormalities are due to digitalis?

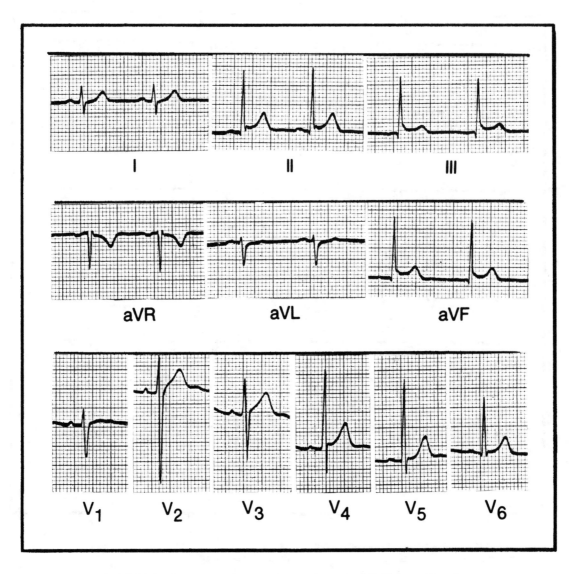

FIGURE 4-33. Analyze this electrocardiogram from a healthy 18-year-old student.

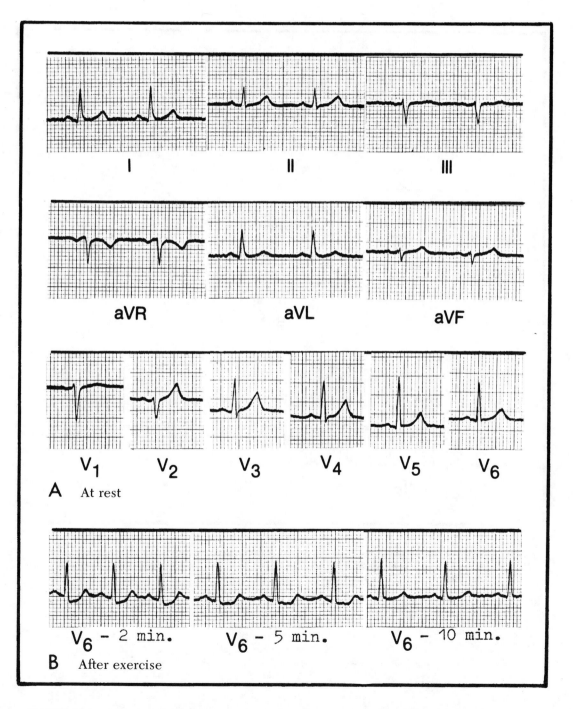

FIGURE 4-34. A, At rest. B, After exercise. What changes have occurred in repolarization after exercise in this patient with a history of angina pectoris?

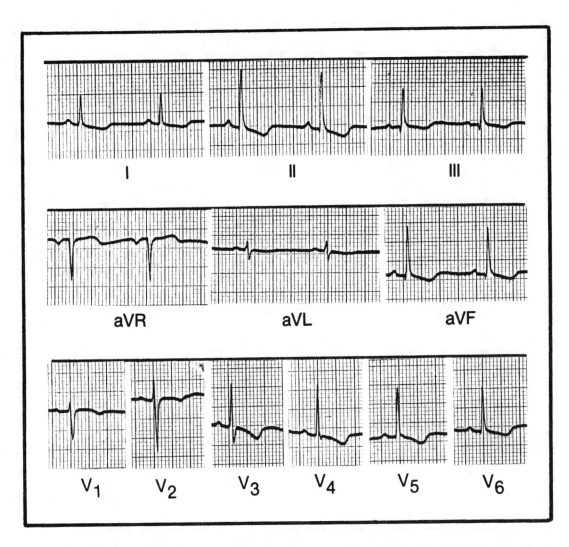

FIGURE 4-35.   *Abnormal repolarization (nonspecific) in a middle-aged, asymptomatic patient with a normal-sized heart. This patient may have coronary heart disease; the diagnosis, however, should not be made from the electrocardiogram alone.*

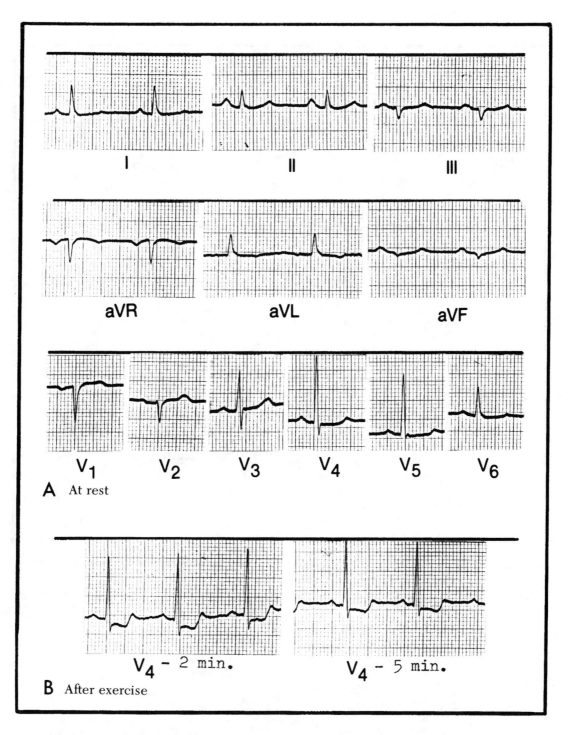

FIGURE 4-36.   A, At rest. B, After exercise. What changes have occurred following activity in this patient with a history of coronary heart disease?

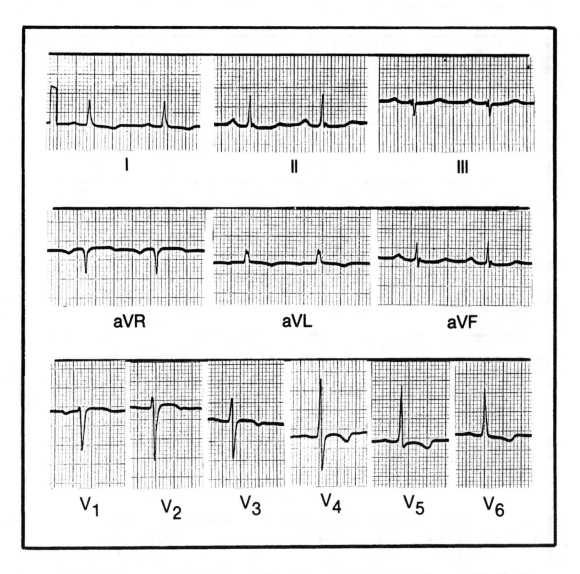

FIGURE 4-37.   Abnormal repolarization in a middle-aged, asymptomatic patient with a normal-sized heart.

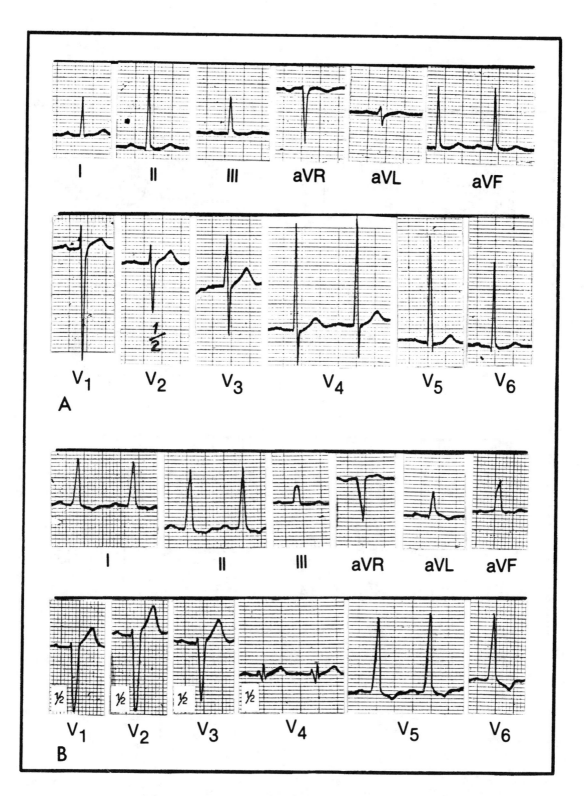

FIGURE 4-38. *What changes are seen as this patient alternates between "normal" conduction and left bundle branch block (a ventricular conduction disturbance)? Are the S-T segment and T wave abnormalities in B primary or secondary?*

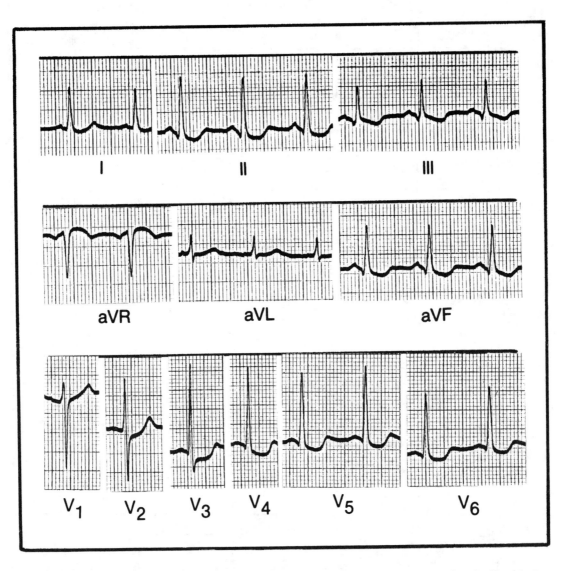

FIGURE 4-39.   Repolarization abnormalities in a patient on digitalis. Even before receiving digitalis this patient had repolarization abnormalities.

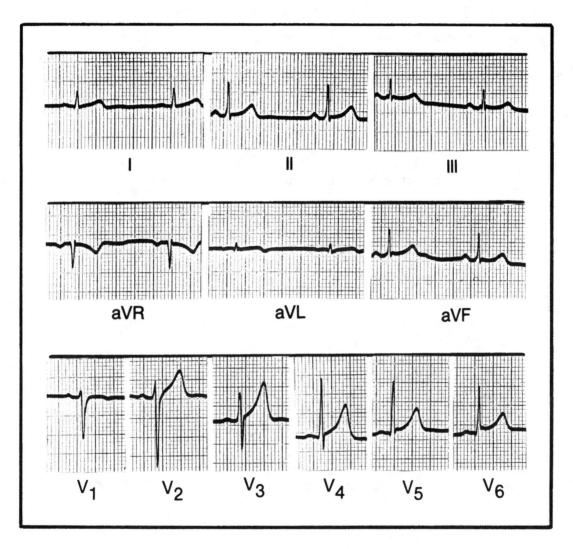

FIGURE 4-40.   *"Early repolarization" in a normal young man.*

POST·TEST A

DIRECTIONS.   Supply the information requested in each of the following.

1. Describe the electrocardiographic "juvenile" pattern.

2. Describe the rotation of the mean T vector from youth to old age.

3. Differentiate between primary and secondary abnormalities of ventricular repolarization.

4. Describe the common electrocardiographic alterations found in many patients with coronary heart disease.

5. Is "early repolarization" a normal phenomenon? If so, state the distinguishing features.

6. Describe the electrocardiographic alterations of hypocalcemia.

7. How may hypercalcemia be detected electrocardiographically?

8. Describe the electrocardiographic features of hypokalemia.

9. Describe the "classic" electrocardiographic alterations due to digitalis.

10. Discuss the differences between ventricular depolarization and ventricular repolarization. Include in your discussion differences in duration and energy consumption.

> Check your responses on the following pages.

ANSWERS TO
POST-TEST A

1. In the young, the mean T vector is found to be to the left, inferior, and posterior, inscribing negative T waves as far as lead V_4, but positive in V_5 and V_6. When this pattern persists it is called a "juvenile" pattern (see Figure 4-6B).

2. The mean T wave vector in youth is frequently found to be to the left, inferior, and posterior, inscribing a T wave across the chest (see vector model, page 264) as follows: leads V_1, V_2, and V_3 negative, V_4, V_5, and V_6 positive. The T wave may be negative as far as lead V_4. This "juvenile" pattern is illustrated in Figure 4-8.

   With increasing age, the mean T vector rotates *rightward* and *anteriorly*, inscribing a T wave across the chest as follows: leads V_1, V_2, V_3, and V_4 positive, V_5 and V_6 negative. This does not always happen; not every elderly patient has negative T waves in V_5 and V_6, nor is it considered normal to have negative T waves in these leads. Many an asymptomatic elderly patient, however, upon being told by an unwary physician that his heart is "ischemic" or "straining," has been prodded into symptoms. You must always treat the patient, not the electrocardiogram detached from the patient. See Figure 4-6B.

3. Repolarization abnormalities may be primary, secondary, or both. When repolarization abnormalities follow abnormalities in depolarization, the abnormalities are *secondary*. When abnormalities of repolarization are not due to abnormalities in depolarization, they are *primary*. Since patients with secondary abnormalities are not immune to primary abnormalities, serial electrocardiograms are often needed to make the distinction.

4. Coronary heart disease is a major cause of ventricular repolarization abnormalities. Figure 4-19 shows the effects of activity (Figure 4-19B) on the already abnormal repolarization (Figure 4-19A), in a patient with a history of angina pectoris. Many a patient with a typical history of angina pectoris will have an electrocardiogram with normal ventricular repolarization at rest; this is seen in Figure 4-20A and was seen in multiple resting electrocardiograms. The electrocardiogram of the same patient following a walk from her room to the electrocardiography office is seen in Figure 4-20B. Activity (utilizing the patient's normal activity, such as taking a walk), rather than provocative testing, will often yield important information in the *initial* evaluation. This activity did not produce pain, yet the effect on ventricular repolarization is obvious. In Figure 4-21B we see the striking S-T segment elevations (lead II), during an episode of chest pain in a patient with a history of angina pectoris at rest. There is nothing categorically explicit about what will be found on the electrocardiogram among a group of patients with the same symptoms. Each patient must be closely followed and any change carefully evaluated. This must be continually emphasized. Some patients with "classic" angina pectoris have been found to have normal-

appearing coronary arteries (by arteriography). Of even greater interest are the patients with clinical myocardial infarction found to have normal-appearing coronary arteries. Much has yet to be learned in this field.

5. A common repolarization variant seen in normal young adults is S-T segment displacement usually associated with tall or deep T waves. This pattern (Figure 4-22) has been known as "early repolarization" and is not considered abnormal. As mentioned earlier, repolarization actually begins before the end of the QRS complex and is reflected in the patients with "early repolarization" by the frequent occurrence of QRS–S-T junction displacement. In these normal patients the mean T and S-T vectors are generally parallel. In Figure 4-22 the S-T segment is elevated (leads II and V_3 to V_5 and depressed (lead aVR) following the orientation of the T wave. Note the displacement of the QRS–S-T junction.

Of importance is the need to distinguish "early repolarization" from the more ominous causes of S-T segment displacement such as pericarditis and myocardial infarction. Distinguishing features of "early repolarization" include:

   a. Clinical correlation: the patient is young and well.

   b. The S-T segment displacement is associated with increased T wave magnitude.

   c. Normal QRS-T angle.

   d. The mean T and S-T vectors are generally parallel. The S-T segment is elevated with tall T waves and depressed with deep T waves.

6. Hypocalcemia may result in marked prolongation of the Q-T interval. This is seen in Figure 4-28, in a patient with longstanding hypocalcemia. The heart rate of the patient is 84 beats per minute. At this rate the Q-T interval should be 0.35 sec., rather than 0.48 sec., as seen here. Refer back to Chapter 1 for the relationship between the Q-T interval and the heart rate.

7. Hypercalcemia is often represented electrocardiographically by a short Q-T interval. There is an inverse relationship between the Q-T interval and the blood level of calcium.

8. Hypokalemia may produce striking electrocardiographic abnormalities, such as depression of the S-T segment, lowering and flattening of the T wave and appearance of a U wave (Figure 4-26). See also Figure 4-27.

9. The "classic" changes of digitalis are described as a "fist-like" depression of the S-T segment (as if you were placing your fist in the S-T segment and depressing it), or "paintbrush" inscription (as if you were painting the S-T segment with gradual widening of the paintbrush as you approach the S-T segment from the downslope of the R wave), or "scooping" of the S-T segment. See Figures 4-10 to 4-12.

10. Depolarization of the ventricles (QRS complex) proceeds from endocardium to epicardium, from the inner areas of the ventricular muscle to the outer areas, and repolarization (S-T segment and T wave) proceeds in the reverse direction, from epicardium to endocardium.

   a. Depolarization (QRS complex) is a relatively short process.

   b. Repolarization (S-T segment and T wave) is a much longer process.

   c. Depolarization consumes relatively little energy.

   d. Repolarization consumes more energy.

   Since repolarization is the energy-consuming phase, it is more prone to abnormality; hence the multiple causes of S-T segment and T wave abnormalities.

N O T E S

From Page 286 (Figure 4-25B):
Hyperkalemia

The appearance of *a tall, peaked T wave* is often a manifestation of hyperkalemia (high blood level of potassium). With increasingly high levels of potassium the P-R interval may become prolonged, with a widening QRS interval. In more extreme cases of hyperkalemia the P waves become flatter and the QRS complexes continue to widen, as seen in Figure 4-25B. Ventricular fibrillation may then ensue if the level of potassium continues to rise.

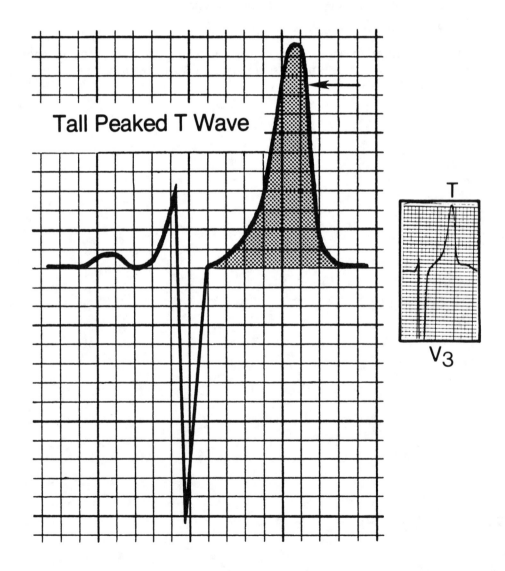

From Page 288 (Figure 4-27):
Hypokalemia

Hypokalemia may produce striking electrocardiographic abnormalities, such as depression of the S-T segment, lowering and flattening of the T wave, and appearance of a prominent U wave. The U wave follows the T wave and has been associated with hypokalemia, although it may be found normally (Figure 4-26). The normal small U wave, when present, is seen best in the midprecordial leads. In Figure 4-27 there appears to be a prolonged Q-T interval in leads II, III, aVR, and aVF. The Q-T interval should be 0.28 sec., not 0.36 sec. at the rate of 125 beats per minute. Lead V_2, however, reveals the hypokalemic U wave on the descending limb of the T wave. During treatment of the hypokalemia, electrocardiographic monitoring revealed a T wave that gradually became taller and a U wave that gradually disappeared. The events described in Figure 4-27 are graphically illustrated below. A represents the normal control with the true Q-T interval between the vertical lines. B represents lead II; the prominent U wave, if read as a T wave would lead to the wrong interpretation as a prolonged Q-T interval. C reveals both T and U waves in lead V_2.

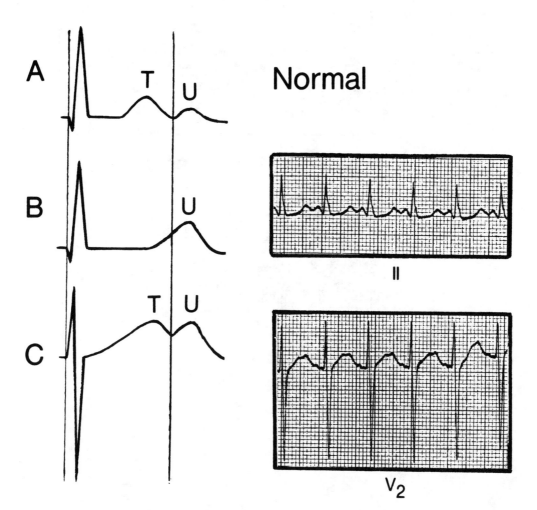

From Page 289: Hypocalcemia

Figure 4-28 reveals the striking *prolongation of the Q-T interval* in a patient with long-standing *hypocalcemia* (low blood level of calcium). Refer to Chapter 1 for the relationship between the Q-T interval and the heart rate.

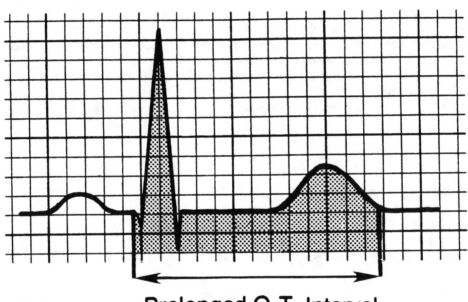

Prolonged Q-T Interval

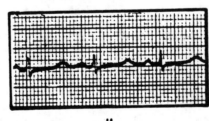

II

From Page 289: Hypercalcemia

Hypercalcemia is often represented electrocardiographically by a *short Q-T interval.*
There is an inverse relationship between the Q-T interval and the level of serum calcium.

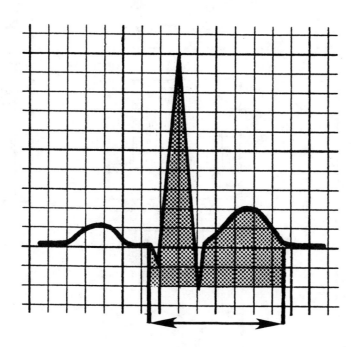

Shortened Q-T
Interval

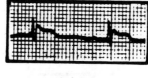

V₂

> After completing your review, proceed to Post-Test B on the next page.

POST·TEST B

DIRECTIONS.   Identify the etiology of each of the following repolarization abnormalities.

1.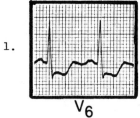
V_6

6.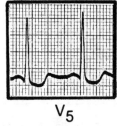
V_5

11.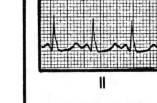
II

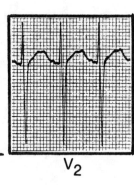
V_2

2.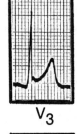
V_3

7.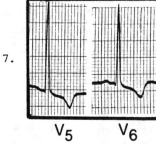
V_5 V_6

3.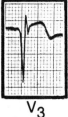
V_3

8.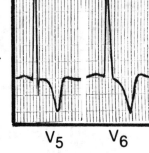
V_5 V_6

12.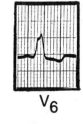
V_6

4.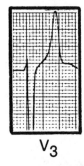
V_3

9.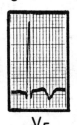
V_5

5.
II

10.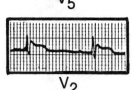
V_2

1._____
2._____
3._____
4._____
5._____
6._____
7._____
8._____
9._____
10._____
11._____
12._____

> Check your responses on the following pages.

ANSWERS TO
POST-TEST B

1. Ischemia. The flat or downsloping S-T segment is frequently seen as a result of myocardial ischemia in a patient with coronary heart disease. If it is not seen at rest it may be seen with activity, as in Figure 4-19B (p. 277).

2. Early repolarization. This pattern is not infrequently seen in young asymptomatic patients (p. 282, Figure 4-22).

3. Injury. This elevated S-T segment has been described as a "monophasic" curve of injury. It may be found in a patient with a recent myocardial infarction, or it could represent, as in this case, a ventricular aneurysm, years after the infarction (p. 283, Figure 4-23).

4. Hyperkalemia. The appearance of a *tall, peaked T wave* is a manifestation of hyperkalemia. With increasingly high blood levels of potassium, the P-R interval may become prolonged, with a widening QRS interval. In more extreme cases of hyperkalemia, the P waves become flatter and the QRS complexes continue to widen. Ventricular fibrillation may then ensue if the level of potassium continues to rise (pp. 285-286, Figure 4-25A and B; p. 308).

5. Hypocalcemia. The Q-T interval may be *markedly prolonged* in a patient with hypocalcemia (p. 289, Figure 4-28; p. 310).

6. Digitalis effects or nonspecific repolarization abnormalities. These abnormalities may be due to digitalis effects or to ischemia or both. If you do not know the patient these abnormalities may be termed nonspecific (p. 300, Figure 4-39).

7. Left ventricular hypertrophy. These repolarization abnormalities, consisting of S-T segment depression and asymmetric inversion of the T wave in the lateral precordial leads, are the secondary repolarization abnormalities of left ventricular hypertrophy (pp. 206-261).

8. Ischemia. As seen in Figure 3-19, although this patient had a large left ventricle, the characteristic shape of the markedly inverted T waves in leads V_5 and V_6 represents *primary* repolarization abnormalities of mycardial ischemia. These primary abnormalities are added to the *secondary* repolarization abnormalities of hypertrophy (p. 234, Figure 3-19). T wave inversion of this magnitude may be seen with myocardial infarction, with or without Q waves (this will be studied in the next chapter).

9. Pericarditis. Ventricular repolarization abnormalities are common in patients with pericarditis. Often both the S-T segment and the T wave are involved. Do not confuse this abnormal, changing, evolving pattern with "early repolarization" (Figure 4-22) found in many normal, healthy young patients. Clinical correlation must again be emphasized since the pattern seen in Figure 4-24 may not be distinguishable from that of a patient with an acute myocardial infarction (p. 284, Figure 4-24).

10. Hypercalcemia. Hypercalcemia is often represented electrocardiographically by a short Q-T interval. There is an inverse relationship between the Q-T interval and the level of serum calcium (p. 311).

11. Hypokalemia. In lead II there appears to be a prolonged Q-T interval. Lead V_2, however, reveals that hypokalemic U wave on the descending limb of the T wave (p. 288, Figure 4-27; p. 309).

12. Left bundle branch block. When the repolarization abnormalities are due to abnormalities in depolarization, as occurs in left bundle branch block, the repolarization abnormalities are *secondary* (pp. 261-262, Figure 4-5A and B).

R E F E R E N C E S

4-1. Wasserburger, R.H.: Obervations on the "juvenile pattern" of adult Negro males. Am. J. Med., *18:*428, 1955.

4-2. Reiley, M.A., et al.: Racial and sexual differences in the standard electrocardiogram of black vs white adolescents. Chest, *75:*474, 1979.

4-3. Amsterdam, E.A., et al.: Toward improved interpretation of the exercise test. Cardiology, *66:*236, 1980.

4-4. Prinzmetal, M., et al.: Angina pectoris. I. A variant form of angina pectoris. Am. J. Med., *27:*375, 1959.

4-5. Prinzmetal, M., et al.: Variant form of angina pectoris, previously undelineated syndrome. JAMA, *174:*1794, 1960.

4-6. Kambara, H., and Phillips, J.: Long-term evaluation of early repolarization syndrome (normal variant RS-T segment elevation). Am. J. Cardiol., *38:*157, 1976.

4-7. Mirvis, D.: Evaluation of normal variations in S-T segment patterns by body surface isopotential mapping: S-T segment elevation in absence of heart disease. Am. J. Cardiol., *50:*122, 1982.

4-8. Spodick, D.H.: Differential characteristics of the electrocardiogram in early repolarization and acute pericarditis. N. Engl. J. Med., *295:*523, 1976.

4-9. Spodick, D.H.: Pathogenesis and clinical correlations of the electrocardiographic abnormalities of pericardial disease. Cardiovasc. Clin., *8:*201, 1977.

4-10. Ginzton, L.E., and Laks, M.M.: The differential diagnosis of acute percarditis from the normal variant: new electrocardiographic criteria. Circulation, *65:*1004, 1982.

5

MYOCARDIAL INFARCTION

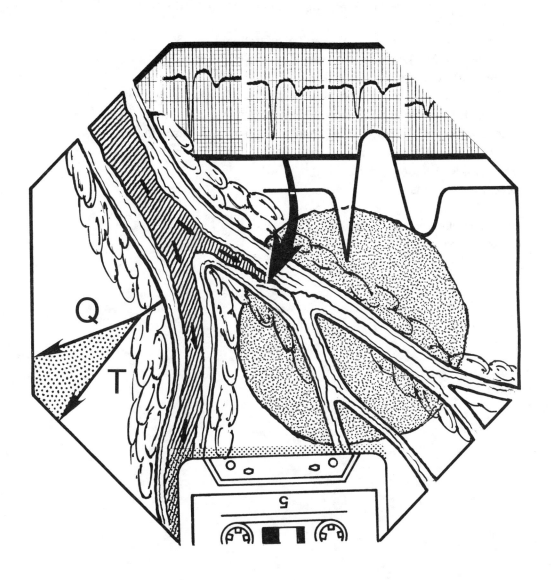

CHAPTER 5
CONTENTS

INTRODUCTION

Nowhere in the entire study of electrocardiography should the failings of the clinical electrocardiogram be emphasized more than in the study of myocardial infarction. Nowhere have diagnoses been made with such erudition and such explicitness, only to be shown to be completely wrong on examination of the heart. Myocardial infarction, from the smallest infarct to the most extensively scarred heart, may be manifest on the clinical electrocardiogram by:

1. No abnormalities.
2. "Nonspecific" abnormalities.
3. "Classic" abnormalities.

Especially does this problem arise in the case of multiple infarctions. Which came before which and where are they located? Conceivably, the balance of vectorial forces resulting from multiple infarctions may deceptively "normalize" the electrocardiogram.

There are three "nevers" that must always be kept in mind.

1. Never finalize the age of an infarct from a single electrocardiogram.

2. Never prognosticate as to the outcome of the myocardial infarction from a single electrocardiogram. So many patients with normal electrocardiograms are ill, while others with the most striking electrocardiographic abnormalities are well clinically. The electrocardiogram, in a state of flux, such as occurs with infarction of the heart, should be studied sequentially. Always ask for serial electrocardiograms.

3. Never allow the electrocardiogram to be anything more than an adjunct to the practice of medicine, as has already been stressed. It can never replace clinical acumen.

O B J E C T I V E S

Upon completion of this chapter, you should be able to:

1. Identify the electrocardiographic manifestations of: (a) inferior (diaphragmatic) myocardial infarction; (b) anterolateral myocardial infarction; (c) apical myocardial infarction; (d) anterior or anteroseptal myocardial infarction; (e) true posterior myocardial infarction; (f) subendocardial myocardial infarction; and (g) ventricular aneurysm.

2. Explain the formation of Q waves in myocardial infarction.

3. Explain the significance of Q waves in lead III only, varying with respiration.

4. State the importance of repolarization (S-T segment and T wave) alterations in the recognition of myocardial infarction.

5. Recognize the evolutionary electrocardiographic changes following acute myocardial infarction.

6. State the differential diagnosis of a predominant R wave in lead V_1.

7. Recognize the importance of serial electrocardiograms in the evaluation of electrocardiographic manifestations of myocardial infarction.

P R E T E S T

DIRECTIONS.   This pretest consists of four electrocardiograms. Write a brief analysis of each in the space provided.

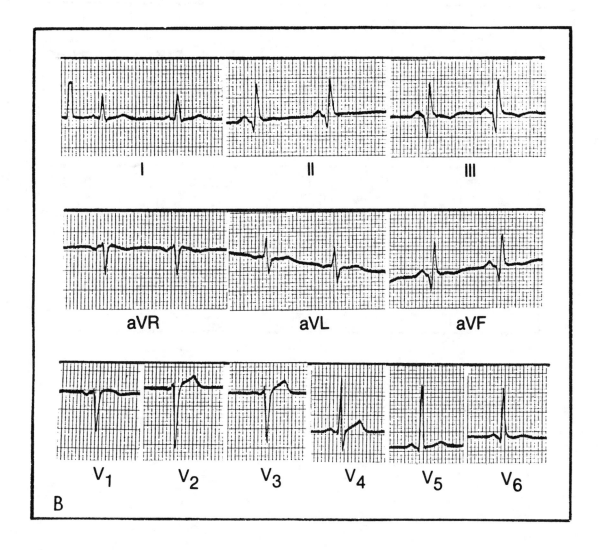

FIGURE 5-6B.

1.   Analysis:

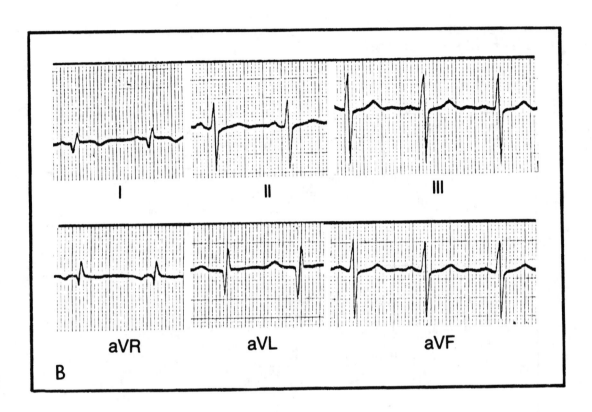

FIGURE 5-7B.

2. Analysis:

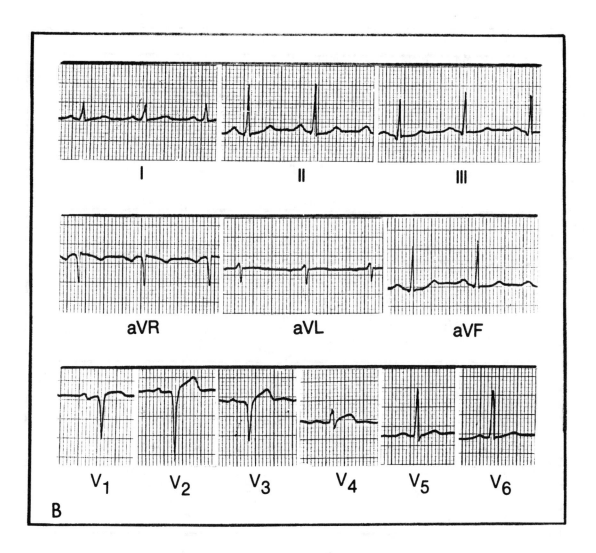

FIGURE 5-9B.

3. Analysis:

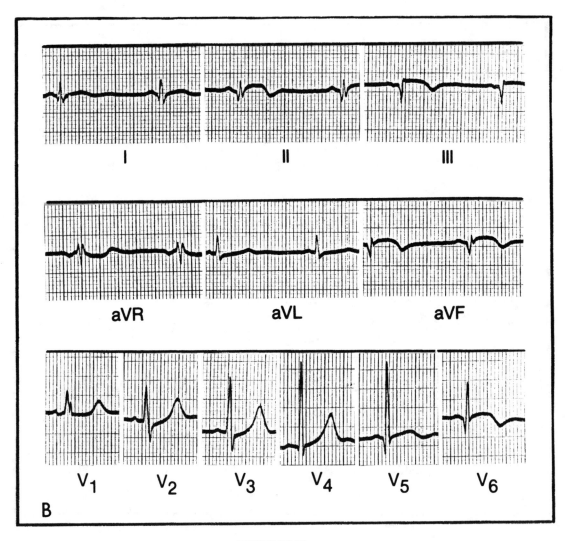

FIGURE 5-10B.

4. Analysis:

> Solutions to the pretest will be indicated later in this chapter.

> When you have completed your analyses start Cassette Side 11 and continue on
the next page.

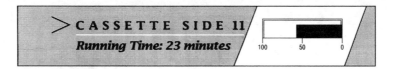

ELECTROCARDIOGRAPHIC MANIFESTATIONS OF MYOCARDIAL INFARCTION

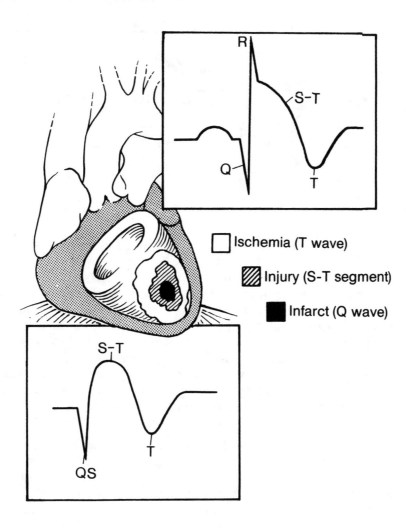

FIGURE 5-1.   *"Classic" electrocardiographic patterns of myocardial infarction.*

The early electrocardiographers illustrated the electrocardiographic patterns associated with infarction of the heart as follows: the *Q wave; elevated S-T segment;* and *inverted T wave.* The Q wave (or QS complex, if there was no R wave) represented infarction, the elevated S-T segment signified injury, and the inverted T wave, ischemia. The accompanying diagram would show a dead zone surrounded by zones of injury and ischemia.

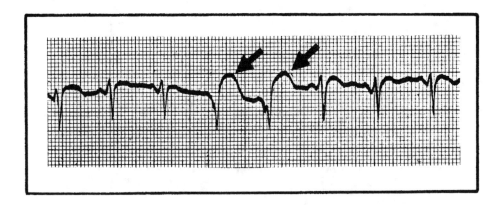

FIGURE 5-2. Electrocardiogram during pericardiocentesis.

A myocardial infarction is not, however, needed to show all the "classic" findings of infarction. The electrocardiographic tracing in Figure 5-2 was recorded during an electrocardiographically monitored therapeutic pericardiocentesis. The arrows point to the two complexes recorded when the tip of the needle "touched" the epicardium. Here it did not represent myocardial infarction, although all the features described were present. As soon as the needle was withdrawn a minute distance, the normal processes ensued. We are using this example in spite of the fact that it could be argued that we are dealing with a different process. Depolarization and repolarization were altered because of epicardial "touching" of the heart. This example is offered merely to show that a myocardial infarction is not needed to produce all the "classic" electrocardiographic manifestations.

Benchimol and associates found that the electrocardiographic configuration of the premature ventricular beat might offer a clue to the presence of myocardial infarction not seen in the sinus beat.[5-1] Wahl and associates,[5-2] however, concluded that although the Q waves of premature ventricular beats indicated the presence of myocardial infarction in 67% of patients, they yielded little or no diagnostic information to that obtained from the sinus beats.

On a vectorial basis, infarction of the heart may be studied as follows:

1.   Initial QRS vector abnormalities—the formation of the Q wave.

2.   Repolarization abnormalities (abnormalities of the S-T segment and T wave).

3.   Terminal QRS vector abnormalities.

Before beginning the study of initial QRS vector abnormalities, and the formation of the Q wave, study Figure 5-3.

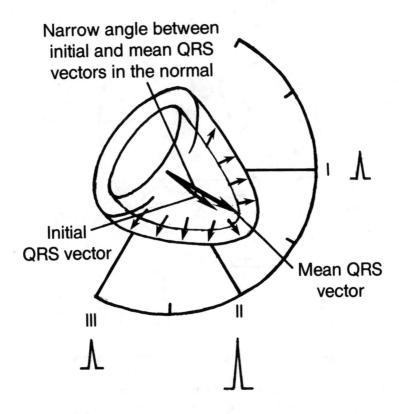

FIGURE 5-3.   *Narrow angle between the initial QRS vector (initial 0.04-sec. vector) and mean QRS vector (the entire 0.08-sec. vector) in the normal.*

This illustration, of the left ventricle, shows the relationship between the initial QRS vector (the first 0.04-sec. vector) and the mean QRS vector (the mean vector of the entire QRS complex, the 0.08-sec. vector) in the *normal*. The mean QRS vector in the normal is to the left and inferior (Chapter 1) and depolarization of the ventricles, as already seen, proceeds from endocardium to epicardium. If we study the initial QRS vector, the first 0.04-sec. vector of the QRS (the first part of the QRS, written within one small box on the electrocardiogram), we find that the angle between it and the mean QRS vector is *narrow*.

A. Initial QRS Vector Abnormalities: The Formation of the Q Wave in Myocardial Infarction

Although an area of left ventricular myocardium is infarcted (Figure 5-4, shaded area), the *mean QRS vector* may not be changed. Compare Figures 5-3 and 5-4. Owing to the interference with early depolarization caused by the infarct, there is a shift of the *initial* vector. The small arrows in Figure 5-4, representing the initial vector, tend to summate *away* from the area of infarction.

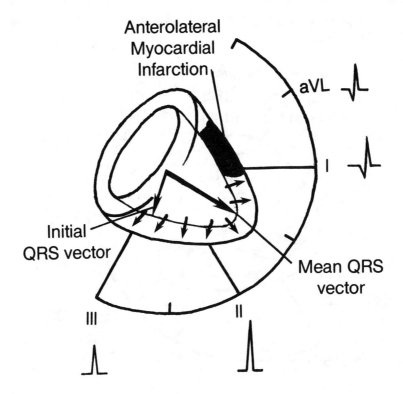

FIGURE 5-4. Disturbance of the initial QRS vector as a result of myocardial infarction.

This example shows an infarct which is on the anterolateral surface of the heart; the initial vector faces *away* from lead I, hence the Q wave.

The Q wave *does not* represent a "hole" in the heart; it represents initial vectorial forces going away from the electrode at the point of recording. The Q wave of significance is frequently at least 0.04 sec. in duration (one small box) and from one fourth to one third the size of the QRS complex.

Note: The diagram in Figure 5-4 (as well as the diagrams in other chapters) is presented to explain a concept and may not represent strict anatomic accuracy. Of importance is the concept; once you learn the concept you can incorporate new information with greater ease.

> The significant Q wave is illustrated on page 397.

Figure 5-5 shows the five regions of the left ventricle, designated by Grant, where infarction may occur.

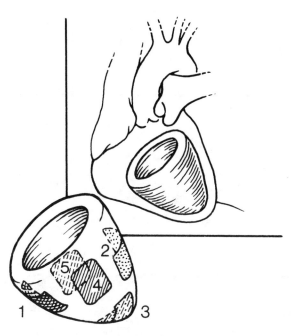

FIGURE 5-5.   *Divisions of the left ventricle according to Grant (see text).* *(Redrawn from Beckwith, J.R.: Grant's Clinical Electrocardiography, 2nd Ed. New York, McGraw-Hill, 1970.)*

Grant divided the left ventricle into five regions as follows:

1. Inferior or diaphragmatic.
2. Anterolateral.
3. Apical.
4. Strictly anterior or anteroseptal.
5. Strictly (true) posterior.

Although we are studying infarction of the left ventricle, where infarction commonly occurs, it should be noted that infarction of the right ventricle as well as infarction of the atria may occur. Infarction of the right ventricle should be considered when, in addition to the findings of inferior wall infarction, there is S-T segment elevation in one (lead V_1) or more of the right precordial leads.[53] Erhardt and associates,[54] studying patients with inferior myocardial infarction, found that S-T segment elevation of more than 1 mm. in lead V_4R (same place as lead V_4 *but on the right side of the chest*) strongly indicated extension of the infarct to the right ventricle. Atrial infarction was seen in Figure 4-30, with significant depression of the P-R segment.

> An example of right ventricular infarction is illustrated on page 398.

1. *Inferior or Diaphragmatic Myocardial Infarction*

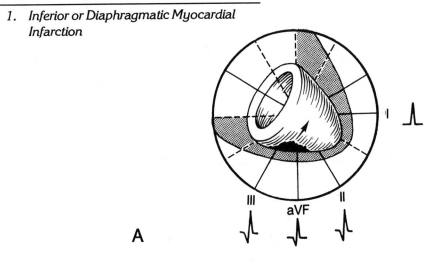

A

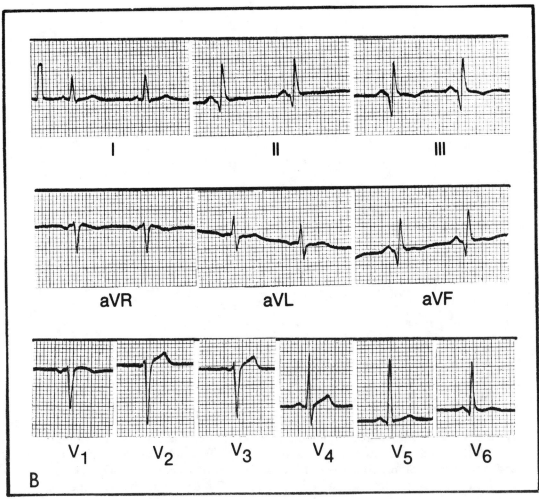

FIGURE 5-6. Inferior (diaphragmatic) myocardial infarction. As seen in Figure 5-6A, the initial vector of depolarization (arrow) faces away from the inferior surface of the left ventricle. This is reflected on the electrocardiogram (Figure 5-6B) by the initial negative or Q waves in leads II, aVF, and III, since the initial vector of depolarization faces away from these leads.

> The analysis of Figure 5-6 in the text and on the tape is the solution to item 1 on the pretest.

2. *Anterolateral Myocardial Infarction*

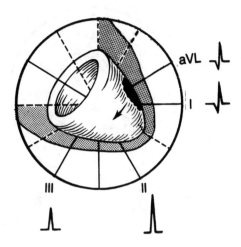

A

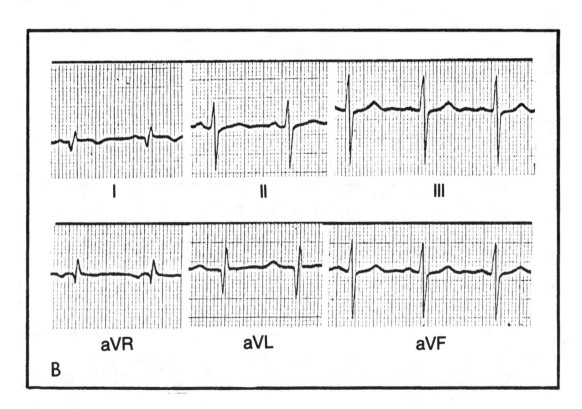

B

FIGURE 5-7.   *Anterolateral myocardial infarction. The initial QRS vector, pointing away from the anterolateral myocardial infarction, produces Q waves in leads I and aVL and sometimes, depending on the vectorial direction, in leads V_5 and V_6.*

> The analysis of Figure 5-7 in the text and on the tape is the solution to item 2 on the pretest.

3. *Apical Myocardial Infarction*

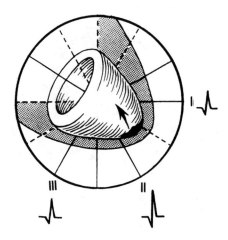

A

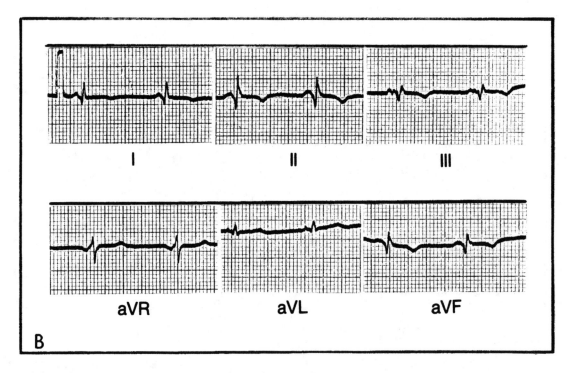

B

FIGURE 5-8.   A and B, Apical myocardial infarction. The initial QRS vector, pointing away from the apical myocardial infarction and from leads I, II and III, produces Q waves in all three leads. The question arises: did one myocardial infarction produce these abnormalities, or are they the result of more than one infarction at different times? See Figure 5-8C.

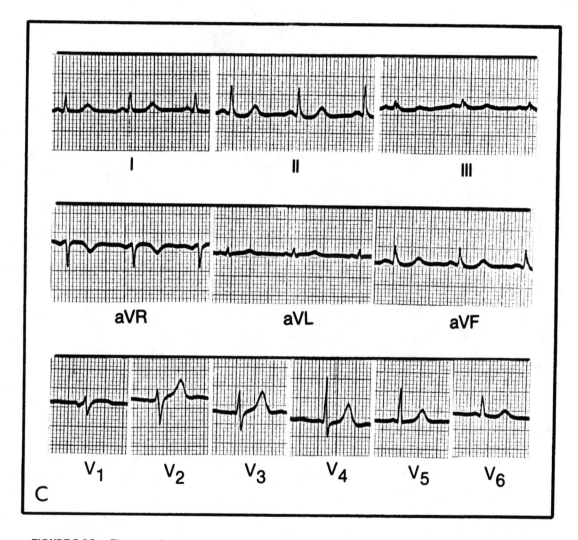

FIGURE 5-8C. Electrocardiogram just prior to the infarction which brought about the changes seen in Figure 5-8B. The only way to answer the question posed in Figure 5-8B is to follow the patient clinically and have serial electrocardiograms.

Apical myocardial infarction has not been as clearly defined electrocardiographically as the other areas of myocardial infarction. The concept, as suggested by Grant,[5-5] is here emphasized.

4. *Strictly Anterior or Anteroseptal*
   Myocardial Infarction

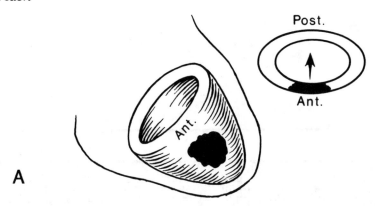

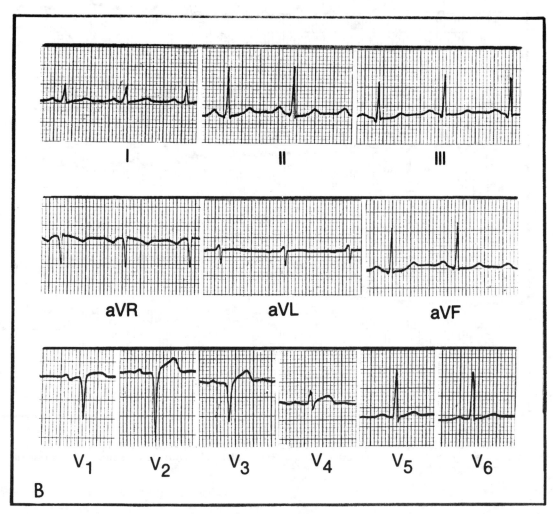

FIGURE 5-9.   Strictly anterior or anteroseptal myocardial infarction. The initial vector of depolarization (arrow in Figure 5-9A), the initial QRS vector, facing away from the anterior area, points posteriorly, inscribing Q waves or QS complexes in the precordial leads. When these are limited to leads V_1 to V_3, the infarct is generally termed "anteroseptal." If these extend beyond lead V_3 the infarct is termed "anterior" and if they extend as far as leads V_5 and V_6 the term "lateral" is added. Depending on the orientation of this initial vector, the frontal plane leads may also be affected.

> The analysis of Figure 5-9 in the text and on the tape is the solution to item 3 on the pretest.

5. Strictly (True) Posterior Myocardial Infarction

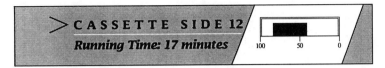

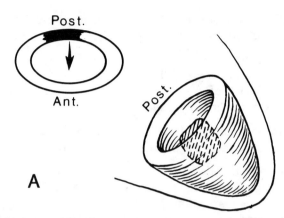

A

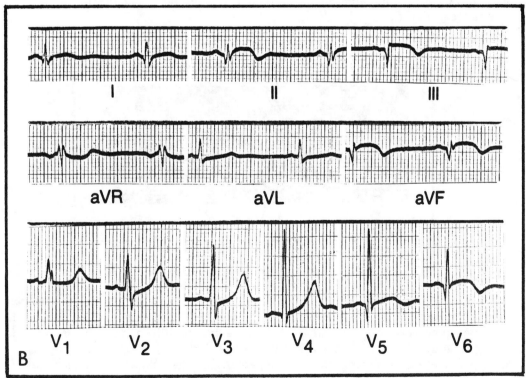

FIGURE 5-10.   Old true posterior and more recent inferior (diaphragmatic)-lateral myocardial infarction. In the true posterior myocardial infarction the initial QRS vector is anteriorly oriented (arrow in Figure 5-10A), away from the posterior area of the heart. This initial vector, facing anteriorly, produces a prominent R wave in lead V_1 (Figure 5-10B). More recently, the patient suffered an inferior (diaphragmatic)-lateral myocardial infarction. This is seen with Q waves or QS complexes in leads II, II, aVF, V_5, and V_6, with elevation of the S-T segments in the form of monophasic curves of injury and inversion of the T waves, reflecting the evolutionary changes of a recent myocardial infarction.

As noted in Figure 5-10B, the R wave in lead V_1 is the main ventricular deflection. The differential diagnosis of such an R wave includes:

1. Right ventricular hypertrophy.
2. Strictly, or true, posterior wall myocardial infarction.
3. Right bundle branch block (RSR').
4. Pre-excitation (Wolff-Parkinson-White) syndrome.

The term "true" posterior myocardial infarction is used since the old terminology identified inferior (diaphragmatic) myocardial infarction as "posterior."

Figure 5-11 is from a patient with strictly anterior or anteroseptal myocardial infarction, a diagnosis made decades ago. Much credit is due the early electrocardiographers who recognized the Q wave and repolarization abnormalities as signs of myocardial infarction. They carefully correlated clinical-pathologic findings and made the most of what they had to work with.

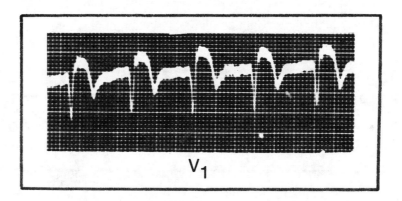

FIGURE 5-11.   Anterior or anteroseptal myocardial infarction.

The findings on the clinical electrocardiogram are the result of the balancing of vectorial forces. Much depends on the forces prior to infarction, often unknown in a given patient. It also becomes more and more difficult to localize the site with each ensuing infarct. It is so vital to study each problem carefully with serial electrocardiograms, observing changes as they occur. You must know your patients and their clinical histories since Q waves may be found in conditions other than myocardial infarction, as in cardiomyopathy, ventricular hypertrophy, left bundle branch block, the Wolff-Parkinson-White syndrome, and the hemiblocks. Fulton and Marriott reported a case of acute pancreatitis electrocardiographically simulating myocardial infarction.[5,6] In addition, Figure 5-16 illustrates Q waves in a normal patient.

B. *Ventricular Repolarization (S-T Segment and T Wave) Abnormalities*

The S-T segment and T wave represent the early to late repolarization phase of the ventricles (epicardium to endocardium) and are sensitive indicators of the state of myocardium.

The altered state of early (S-T segment) repolarization in acute myocardial infarction, the current of injury, is reflected in a mean S-T vector oriented *toward* the site of infarction, opposite the initial QRS vector (Q wave). Late repolarization results in a mean T vector of the same orientation as the initial QRS vector. In summary, in acute myocardial infarction, the Q wave and T wave are of the same orientation and opposite the S-T segment. This is seen in Figure 5-12.

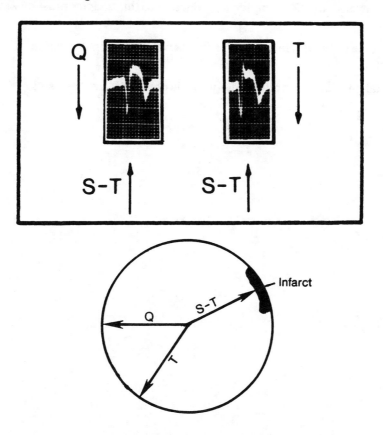

FIGURE 5-12.   Acute anterior myocardial infarction (lead V₁) showing the abnormal depolarization and repolarization.

These changes (Q wave, elevated S-T segment, and inverted T wave), occurring with myocardial infarction, indicate the location of the infarction. The changes in the leads on the opposite surface of the heart, away from the area of infarction are known as reciprocal changes. An example of reciprocal changes is illustrated on page 399.

As a review of A (Initial QRS Vector Abnormalities) and B (Ventricular Repolarization Abnormalities), three sets of serial electrocardiograms will be presented—Figures 5-13A to E, 5-14A to D, and 5-15A to C.

1. All three patients are alive and *well,* two of the three more than 5 years after the myocardial infarction.

2. The electrocardiographic "extent" of the infarct varies. The patient whose electrocardiograms appear the most foreboding (Figure 5-13, page 339) is the most active of the three.

3. The three "nevers" mentioned in the introduction to this chapter must be kept in mind.

4. The evolutionary changes in depolarization (Q wave) and repolarization (S-T and T) are illustrated.

5. The importance of serial electrocardiograms is obvious from these sets.

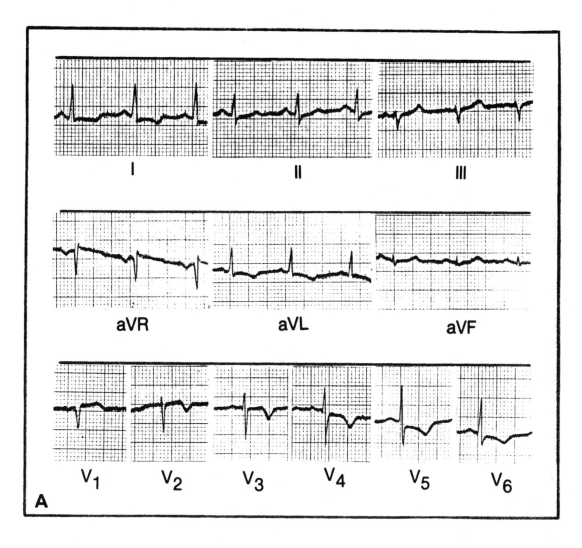

FIGURE 5-13A.   Onset of chest pain in a previously asymptomatic patient. Describe the abnormalities noted here.

A number of terms have been used to describe the evolutionary electrocardiographic changes associated with myocardial infarction—hyperacute (minutes to hours), acute (hours to days to weeks), subacute or recent (weeks to months), and old (stabilized, months to years after infarction). As you can readily see, there is much overlap and these terms can be misleading. A good way to time an infarct is to carefully follow your patients clinically and with serial electrocardiograms. To reemphasize the importance of serial tracings these sets are presented.

> Evolutionary electrocardiographic changes following blood flow obstruction are illustrated on page 400.

> The hyperacute phase of anterior myocardial infarction is also illustrated in Chapter 6, Figure 6-33B.

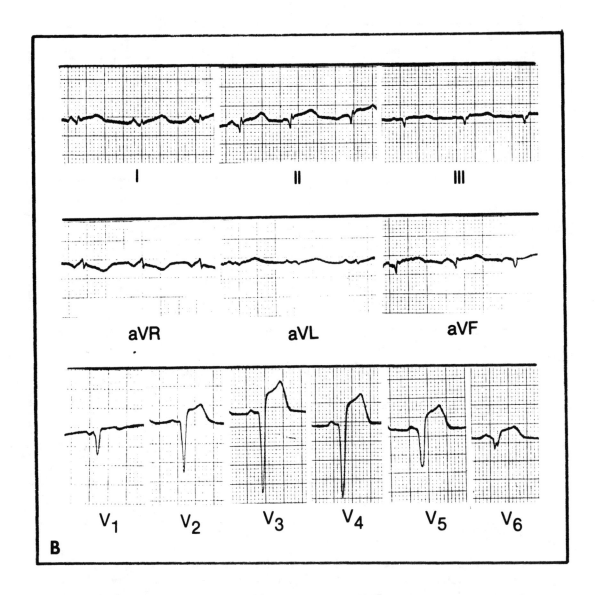

FIGURE 5-13B. *Following onset of "crushing" chest pain in the same patient. Blood enzymes became abnormal at this time. Describe the depolarization (Q wave) and repolarization (S-T segment and T wave) abnormalities.*

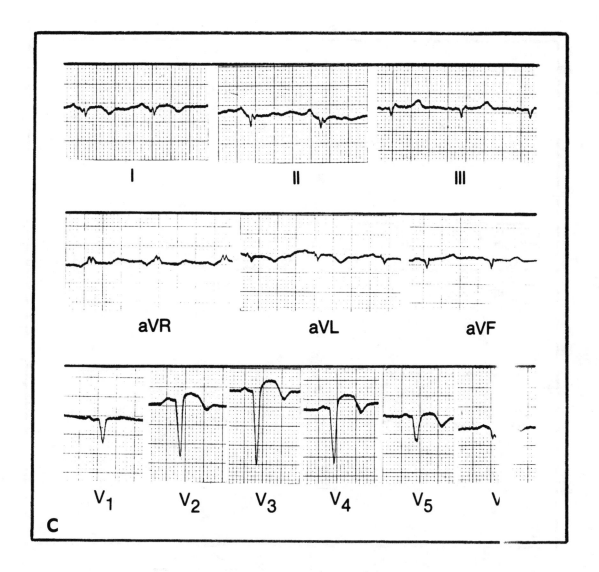

FIGURE 5-13C.   Evolutionary changes in acute myocardial infarction (1 week after Figure 5-13B). The chest pain had subsided. Compare each lead with those in the previous electrocardiograms and describe the serial evolutionary changes.

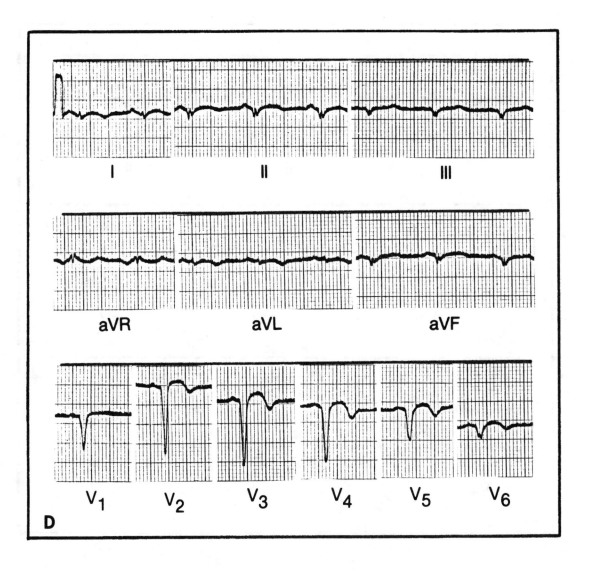

FIGURE 5-13D.   Evolutionary changes in acute myocardial infarction (3 days after Figure 5-13C).

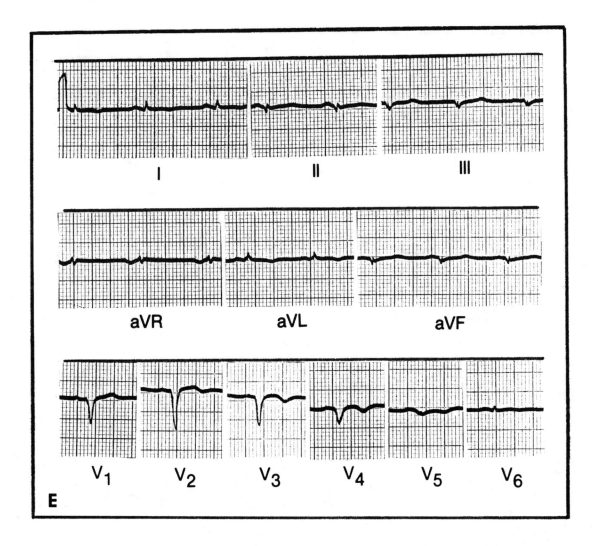

FIGURE 5-13E. Stabilized electrocardiogram obtained a year and a half after Figure 5-13D. The patient is currently asymptomatic and active in business. Review and carefully analyze this entire series. Could you predict an asymptomatic, active patient from these "terrible-looking" electrocardiograms, indicating an "extensive infarction, covering a large area of myocardium?" Remember the dictum that the patient is to be treated, not the electrocardiogram.

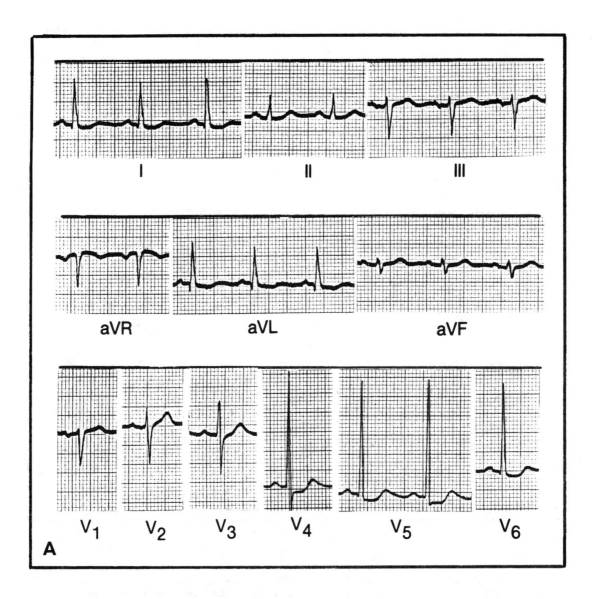

FIGURE 5-14A.   Onset of intermittent chest pain in a previously asymptomatic patient. Describe the repolarization abnormalities. Are there any significant Q waves? Are there any criteria for left ventricular hypertrophy?

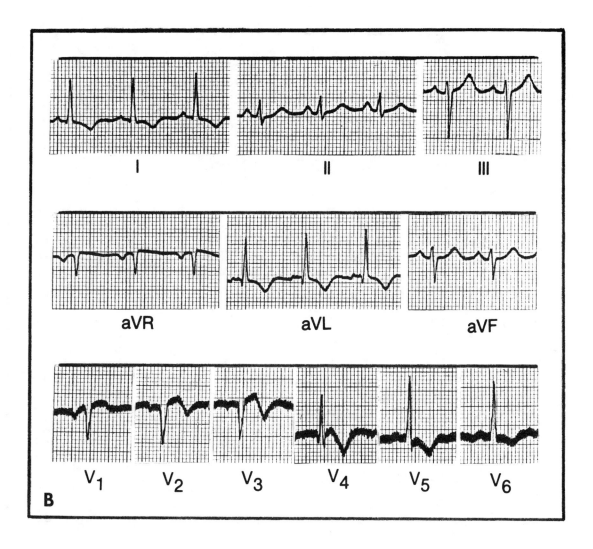

FIGURE 5-14B. *Electrocardiogram 1 week after Figure 5-14A. The patient experienced "crushing" chest pain and blood enzymes became abnormal. Describe the abnormalities in depolarization (Q waves) and repolarization (S-T segments and T waves).*

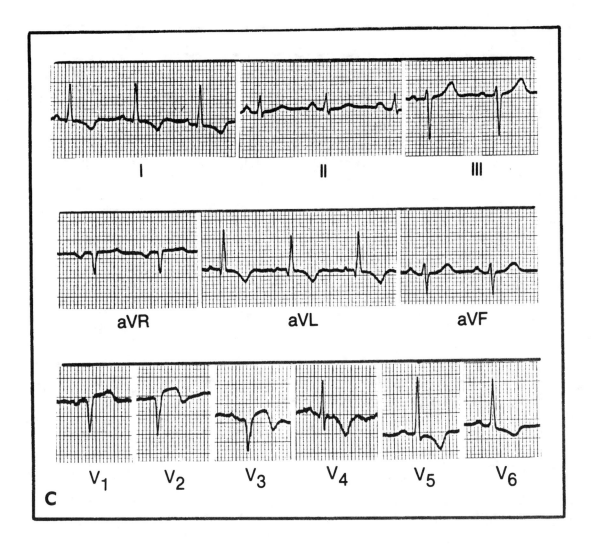

FIGURE 5-14C.   *Evolutionary changes in strictly anterior or anteroseptal infarction 1 week after Figure 5-14B. Describe.*

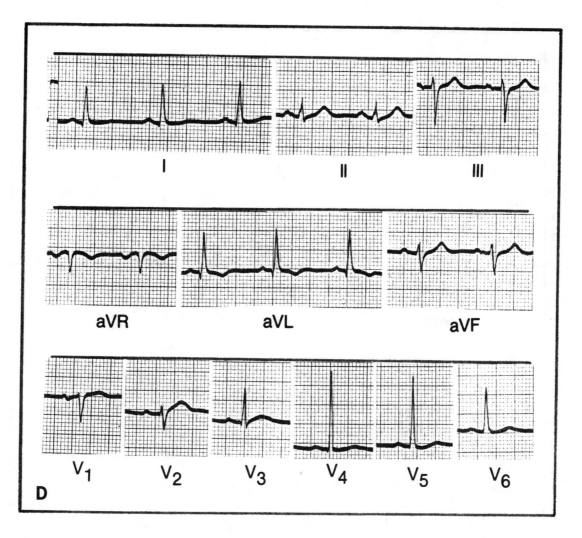

FIGURE 5-14D.   Electrocardiogram 3 years after Figure 5-14C. Any sign of the infarct? Are you surprised? Could you make the diagnosis of anteroseptal myocardial infarction if you did not have the serial electrocardiograms?

Wasserman and associates,[57] in a study of 4524 participants who were followed for 3 years, found that 14.2% lost documented significant Q waves.

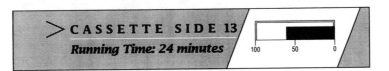

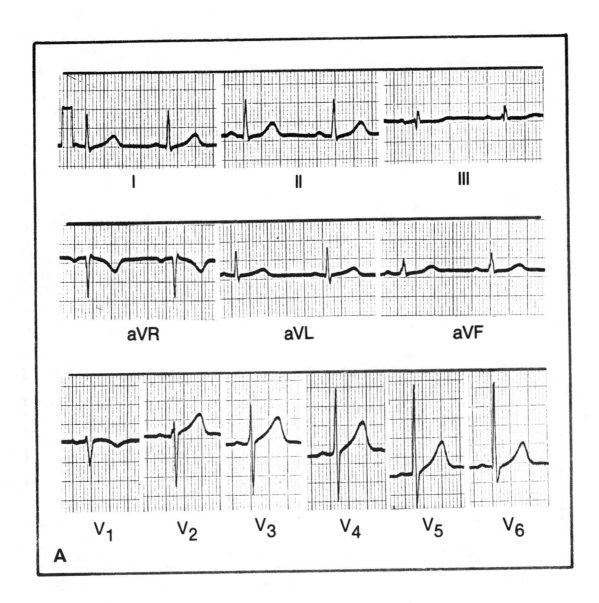

FIGURE 5-15A. Baseline electrocardiogram in a patient who subsequently developed a myocardial infarction (Figures 5-15B and C).

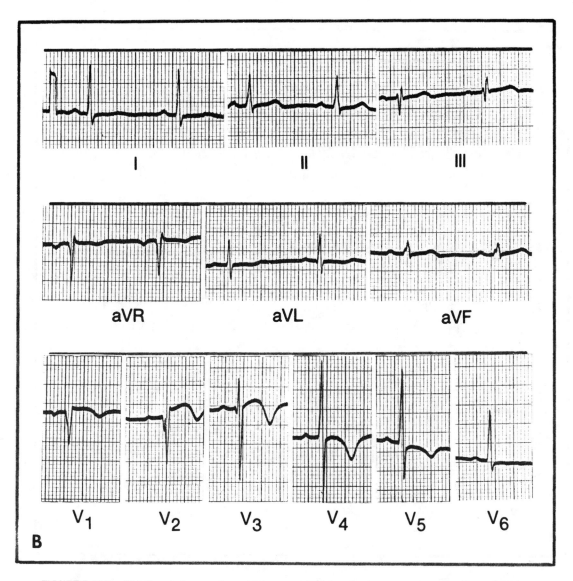

FIGURE 5-15B.   Strictly anterior or anteroseptal myocardial infarction in same patient as in Figure 5-15A. Describe abnormalities.

The significant Q wave (described on page 328 and illustrated on page 397) is at least 0.04 sec. in duration (one small box wide) and at least one quarter to one third the size of the QRS complex. However, there is one major exception. In the precordial leads, V_1 is predominantly negative as are leads V_2 and V_3 above. The transition has not been passed until we reach lead V_4. Prior to the transition even a small Q wave, as seen in lead V_3, is abnormal. This is known as the *pretransitional Q wave.* Sometimes the initial R wave is difficult to discern in lead V_1, but must be clearly seen in leads V_2 and V_3 if the transition has not been reached.

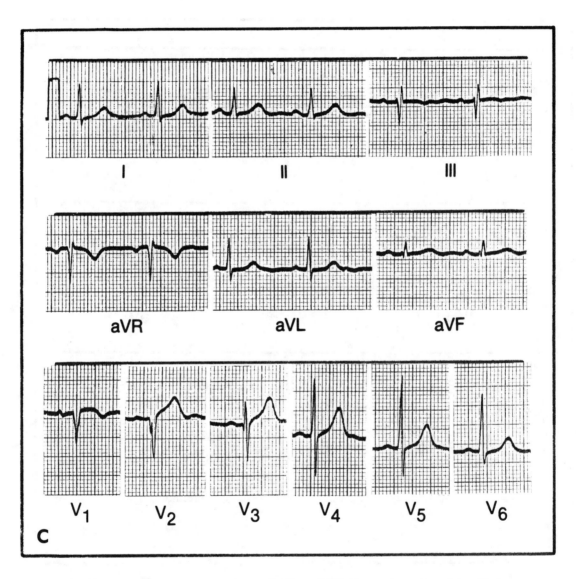

FIGURE 5-15C.　Stable electrocardiogram 1 year after Figure 5-15B. Review this series and describe the changes.

These cases (Figures 5-13, 5-14, and 5-15) emphasize the need for serial electrocardiograms. Few things of value will come to you accidentally. You must know what to look for; you must search to find.

Note again that in lead V_3 there is an initial Q wave in the presence of a predominantly *negative* QRS complex. This pretransitional Q wave is abnormal and represents the anteroseptal infarction.

Not all Q waves signify infarction of the heart, even though the Q wave is "significant." Figure 5-16 shows lead III in a normal patient. The Q wave in lead III may vary in size with respiration in a normal person due to slight vectorial shifts during respiration. This figure illustrates why it is not advisable to make the diagnosis of myocardial infarction from a single electrocardiogram with a "significant" Q wave in lead III. Conversely, this *does not* mean that a Q wave in lead III may not be the result of a myocardial infarction. How may serial electrocardiograms be of help?

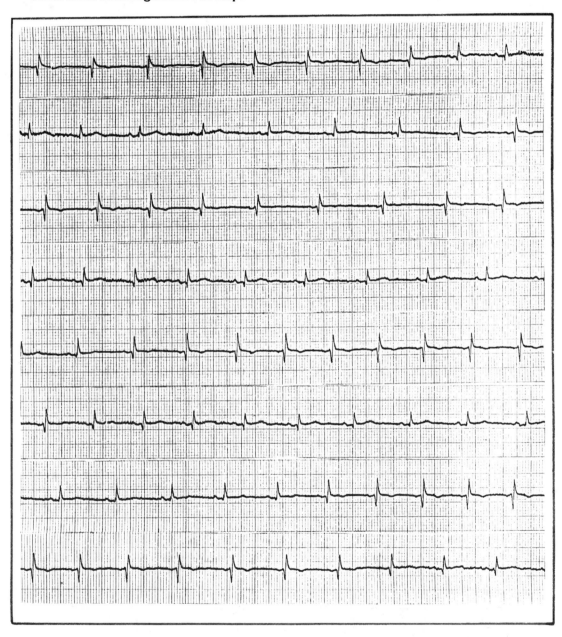

FIGURE 5-16.   Q waves in lead III in a normal patient. The Q wave in lead III may vary in size with respiration in a normal person, due to slight shifts in the vectorial forces during respiration. (Electrocardiogram reduced in size.)

> The vectorial illustration of Q wave formation in lead III in a normal patient is found on page 401.

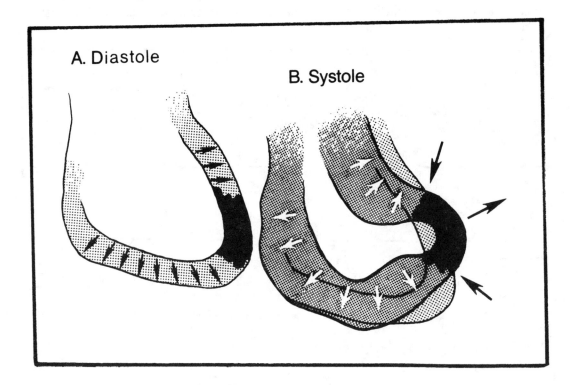

FIGURE 5-17.   Ventricular aneurysm. The scarred area of myocardium, following infarction, is not able to beat synchronously with the remainder of the ventricle. During systole, with ventricular contraction, this area bulges outward with "paradoxic" motion.

Figure 5-18 is from a patient with a ventricular aneurysm years after a myocardial infarction. The *persistent* elevation of the S-T segment, described as a persistent "monophasic" curve of injury, represents a ventricular aneurysm, an outpouching of a section of scarred ventricular myocardium, illustrated in Figure 5-17. During systole, with ventricular contraction, this area bulges outward with "paradoxic" motion. Paradoxic motion is also frequently seen during acute infarction. Paradoxic motion of the normal myocardium at the rim of the aneurysm may explain the elevated S-T segment in both acute myocardial infarction and ventricular aneurysm. A completely satisfactory explanation, however, has not been given. Only serial electrocardiograms will tell you the age of an elevated S-T segment. A favorite examination question is to show an "acute" myocardial infarction. Once you diagnose this "acute" infarction with certainty, the examiner will show you an identical electrocardiogram taken years before. Always ask for comparison electrocardiograms.

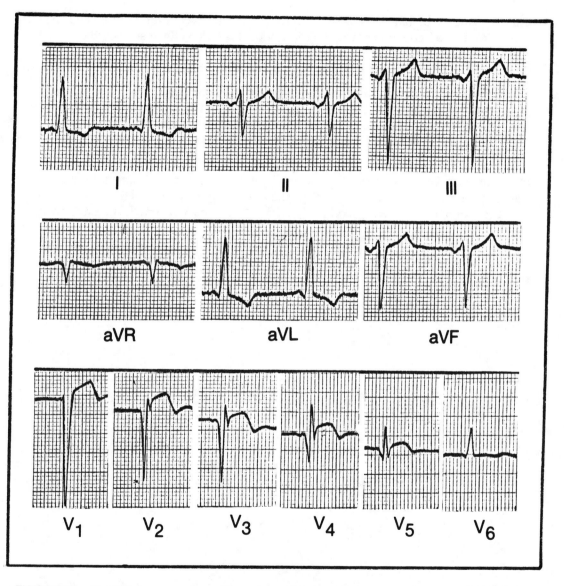

FIGURE 5-18. *Ventricular aneurysm in a patient with an old myocardial infarction. This patient also had a large left ventricle. Note that the rhythm is not sinus rhythm.*

"Subendocardial" Infarction

Clinical evidence of infarction of the heart (by history, physical examination, and enzyme abnormalities) is frequently encountered without Q waves on the electrocardiogram. It had been thought that when the subendocardium of the heart was infarcted the only electrocardiographic manifestations might be repolarization (S-T and T) abnormalities.

As noted earlier, there may not be exact electrical and anatomic correlation. Multiple combinations may be seen in spite of logical localizations and interpretations. The clinical picture of infarction should be quite clear before an electrocardiogram is labeled "subendocardial" infarction, since these repolarization abnormalities, although striking, may be nonspecific.

Although more common in transmural (involving the entire wall thickness) infarction, Q waves may be seen in both transmural and subendocardial (limited to the endocardium) infarction, or may be absent in both.[5-8] Spodick,[5-9] in an editorial, emphasizes the nonspecificity of electrocardiographic criteria for differentiating transmural and nontransmural lesions. Because of this problem it is common to refer to myocardial infarctions "with" or "without" Q waves. Of clinical significance, as noted by Schamroth,[5-10] is that the 1-year prognosis is similar in transmural and subendocardial infarction.

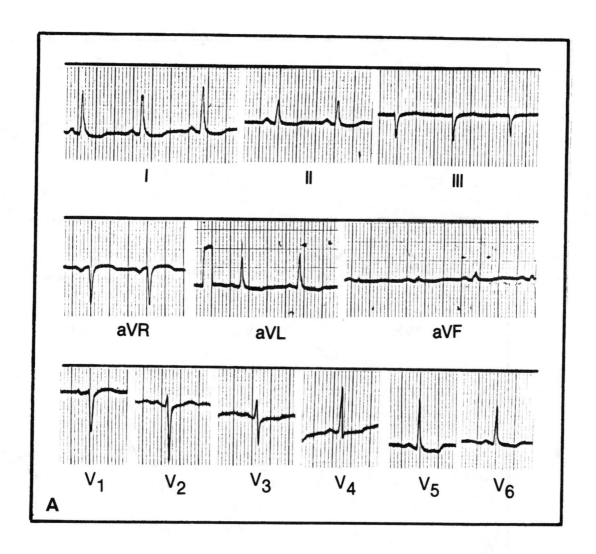

FIGURE 5-19A.   Baseline electrocardiogram prior to onset of subendocardial infarction. Is it normal?

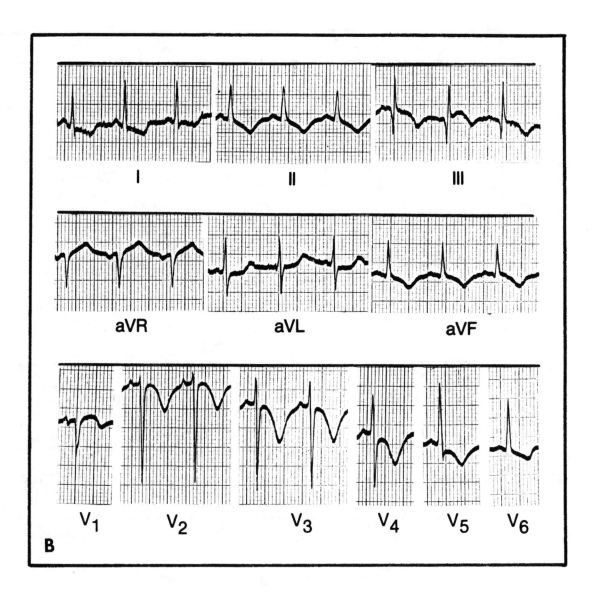

FIGURE 5-19B.   Electrocardiogram following onset of clinical evidence of myocardial infarction.

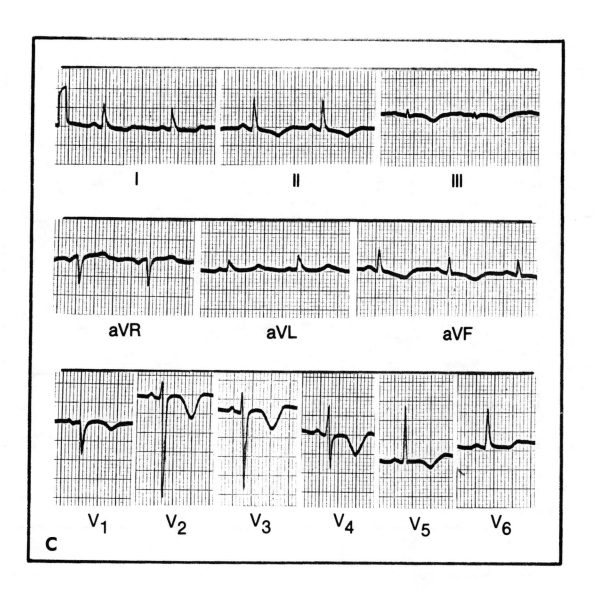

FIGURE 5-19C. Serial changes in subendocardial infarction. Are there any significant Q waves?

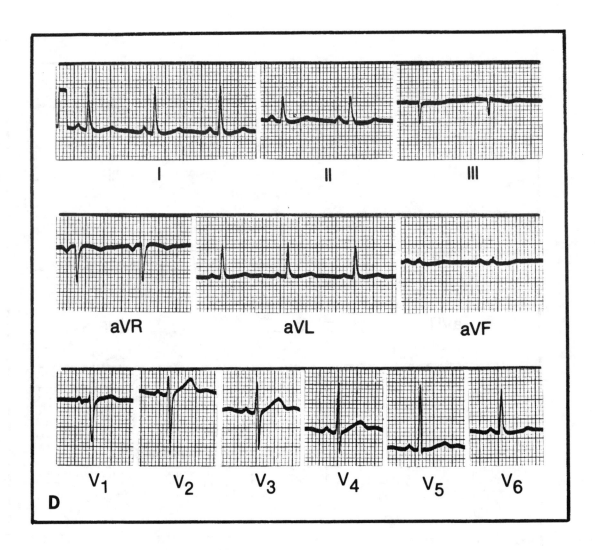

FIGURE 5-19D. Stable electrocardiogram 2¹/₂ years after Figure 5-19C. Compare with the original electrocardiogram (Figure 5-19A).

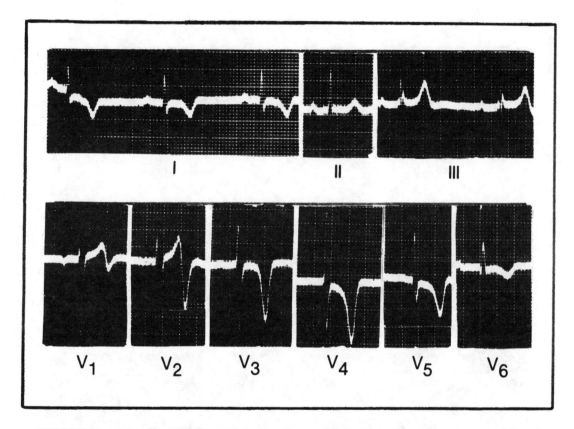

FIGURE 5-20.   Subendocardial (anterior) infarction. Myocardial infarction, without Q waves, was recognized many years ago. The biphasic T waves in leads V₁ and V₂, as well as the depth of T wave inversion, are highly suggestive of myocardial infarction.

De Zwaan, Bär, and Wellens observed that patients with the characteristic T wave pattern, shown above, have critical stenosis high in the left anterior descending coronary artery.[5-11] Prompt recognition and early treatment in patients with unstable angina who have this pattern may be lifesaving. Note that the mean T wave vector faces *away* from the infarction in the anterior wall.

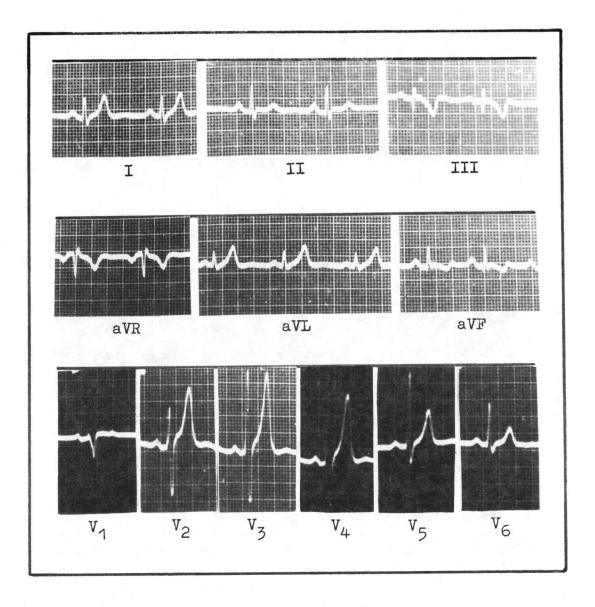

FIGURE 5-21. *Subendocardial (posterior) infarction. The mean T vector faces away from the infarction in the posterior wall.*[5-12] *Again, you must be certain that infarction is present clinically, since similar changes may be caused by electrolyte imbalance.*

C. Terminal QRS Vector Abnormalities

In examining for electrocardiographic alterations associated with myocardial infarction it has been customary to look for an abnormal initial QRS vector (Q wave) and abnormal repolarization (S-T and T abnormalities). Multiple examples have been seen in the preceding electrocardiograms. Terminal QRS vector abnormalities associated with myocardial infarction have received less attention, unfortunately; every electrocardiogram should be inspected for these changes. Figure 5-22 reveals the Q waves in lead I and aVL of an anterolateral infarction. Of great importance is also the fact that the terminal QRS vector shifted leftward as a result of the infarct, creating a wide angle between the initial and terminal QRS vectors. This had "classically" been called peri-infarction block due to anterolateral myocardial infarction.[513] Carefully inspect the electrocardiograms prior to infarction to be certain that the terminal vectorial abnormalities were not present *before* the infarct.

Figures 5-22 and 5-23 are presented to focus attention on terminal QRS vector abnormalities associated with myocardial infarction. Marriott notes that the left axis deviation resulting from anterolateral myocardial infarction most likely represents left anterior hemiblock.[514] The hemiblocks will be studied in Chapter 6.

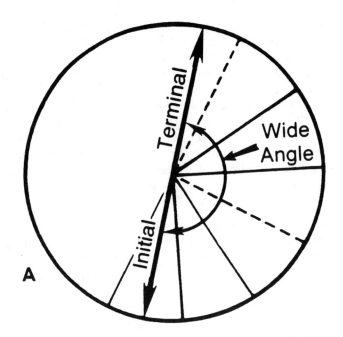

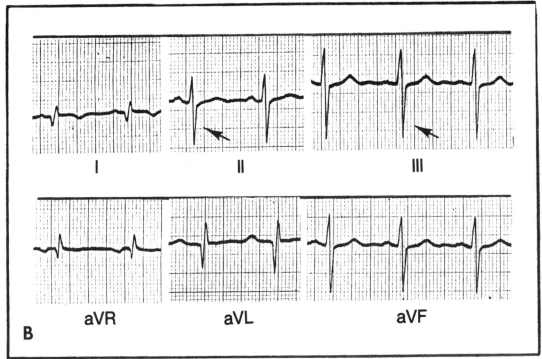

FIGURE 5-22.   Anterolateral myocardial infarction with leftward shift of the terminal QRS vector. The left axis deviation of the QRS vector will be discussed in the section on hemiblocks in Chapter 6. The arrows in leads II and III point to the deep S waves in leads II and III, signifying a terminal QRS vectorial shift to the left.

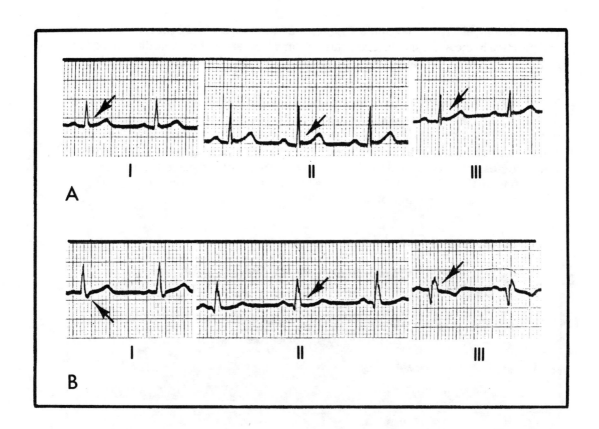

FIGURE 5-23.   A, Baseline electrocardiogram. B, Inferior myocardial infarction. In addition to the Q waves in leads II and III note the terminal QRS vectorial changes in all three leads (arrows). The terminal changes may represent the onset of right bundle branch block resulting from myocardial infarction, as above. The bundle branch blocks will be studied in Chapter 6.

REVIEW
ELECTROCARDIOGRAMS

The remaining electrocardiograms (Figures 5-24 through 5-48) are presented for continued practice in the analysis of electrocardiograms indicative of myocardial infarction. Included are several sets of serial electrocardiograms. Before proceeding, review the basic concepts of myocardial infarction.

Figure 5-25A and B is from a patient with dextrocardia, before and after anterior myocardial infarction. Review the mean P vector of dextrocardia in Chapter 1. Note that in the third panel of Figure 5-25A, marked V_1 to V_6, the R waves across the precordium are decreasing in size. This may be confused with "poor R wave progression" or "reversed R wave progression" (see page 379). However, when the leads are placed on the right side, rather than on the left side of the chest, the leads appear properly placed (fourth panel). Study this set; all the features of dextrocardia are illustrated.

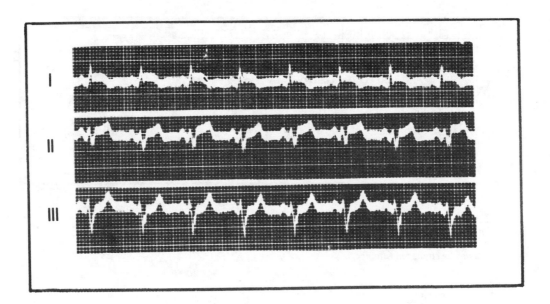

FIGURE 5-24. *Anterolateral myocardial infarction. This electrocardiogram was taken when the patient was experiencing chest pain, with clinical evidence of myocardial infarction. Describe. (Electrocardiogram reduced in size.)*

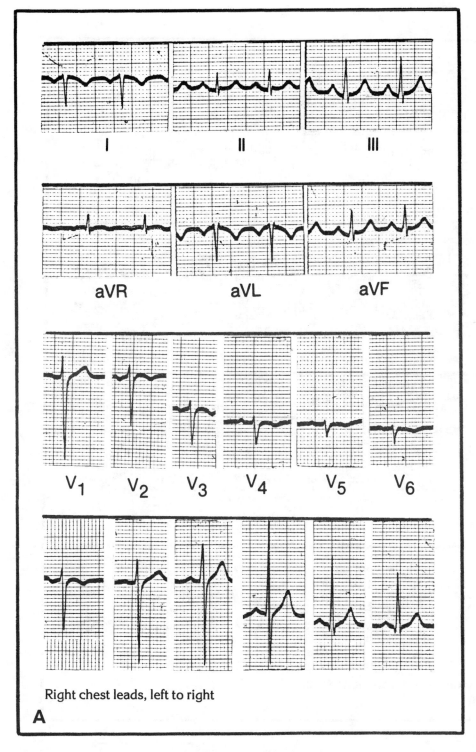

Right chest leads, left to right

A

FIGURE 5-25A.   Dextrocardia. This is the baseline electrocardiogram. Before proceeding to Figure 5-25B, review the mean P vector of dextrocardia in Chapter 1.

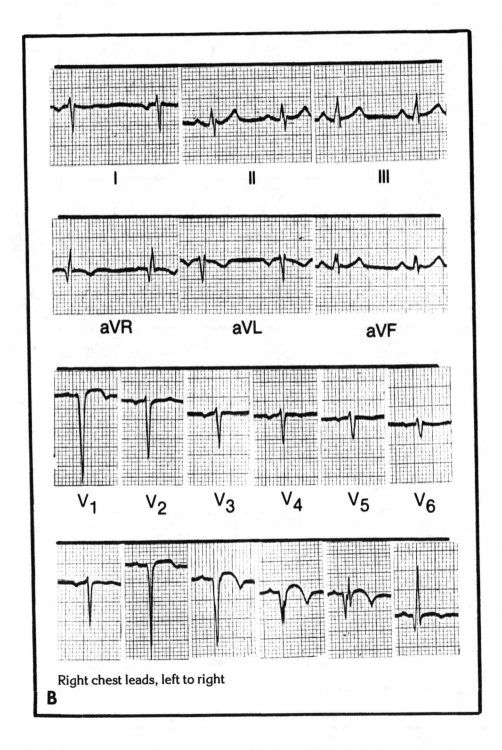

I II III

aVR aVL aVF

V₁ V₂ V₃ V₄ V₅ V₆

Right chest leads, left to right

B

FIGURE 5-25B.   Dextrocardia. This is the same patient as in Figure 5-25A following an anterior wall myocardial infarction. Explain the findings.

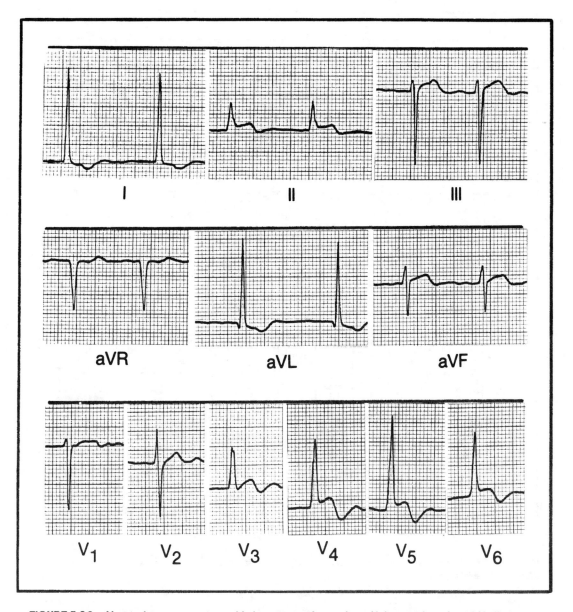

FIGURE 5-26.   *Ventricular aneurysm in an elderly patient with an enlarged left ventricle and atrial fibrillation. Could you make a diagnosis of myocardial infarction on the basis of Q waves? This pattern has been stable in this patient for about 5 years following acute myocardial infarction. How would you treat this patient if you did not know him and he walked into your office complaining of chest pain and exhibited this electrocardiogram?*

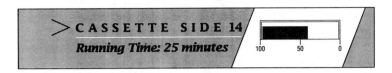

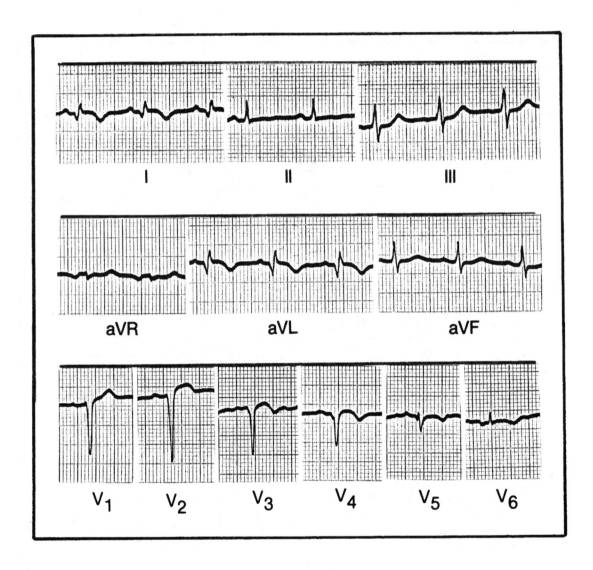

FIGURE 5-27.   Ventricular aneurysm following myocardial infarction. This is a stable pattern many months after the acute infarction.

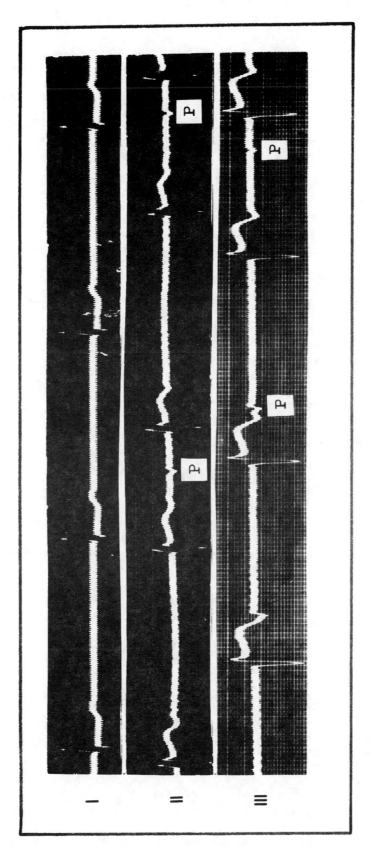

FIGURE 5-28. Inferior myocardial infarction. Why is the rhythm irregular? The P waves, where seen, are indicated in leads II and III. This electrocardiogram and Figure 5-30 are from patients with inferior myocardial infarction and disturbances of the conduction system of the heart. The answer is related to the structures supplied by the right coronary artery in most patients. This is not uncommon in myocardial infarction.

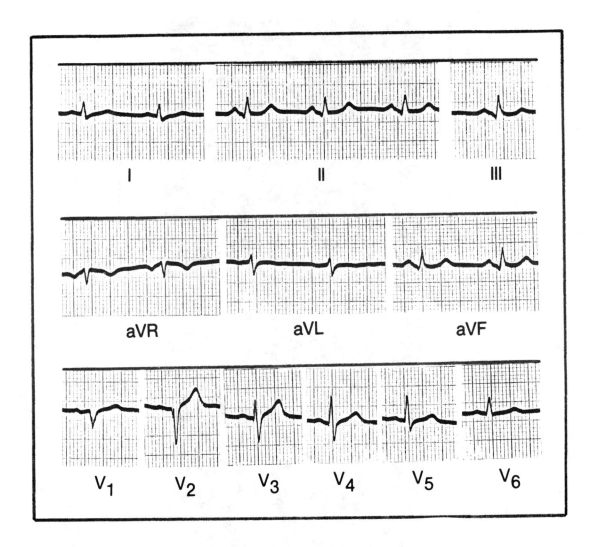

FIGURE 5-29. Anteroseptal myocardial infarction.

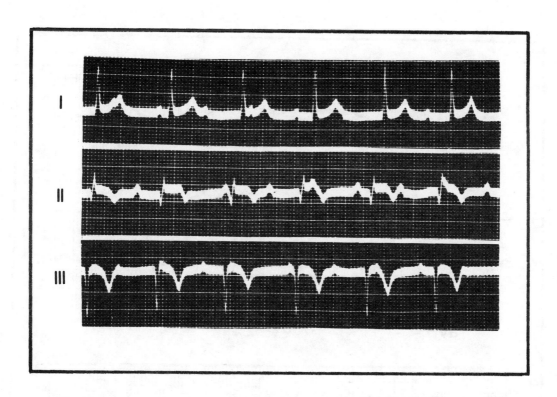

FIGURE 5-30.   *Inferior myocardial infarction. Why are the P-R intervals not constant? See legend for Figure 5-28. (Electrocardiogram reduced in size.)*

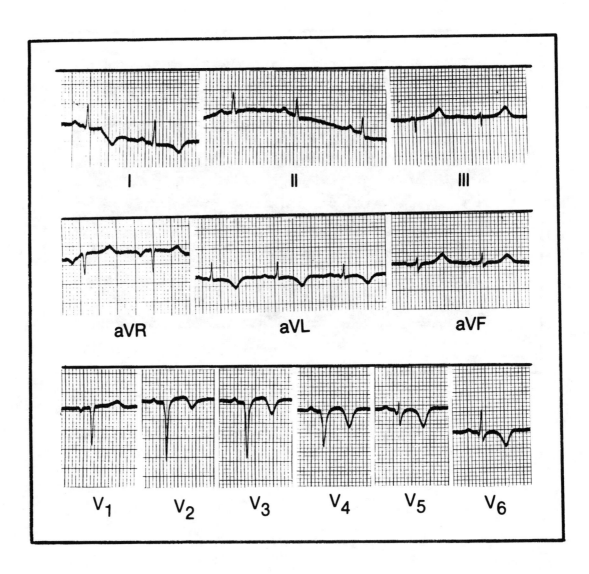

FIGURE 5-31. Anterior myocardial infarction. Could you make this diagnosis without the chest leads?

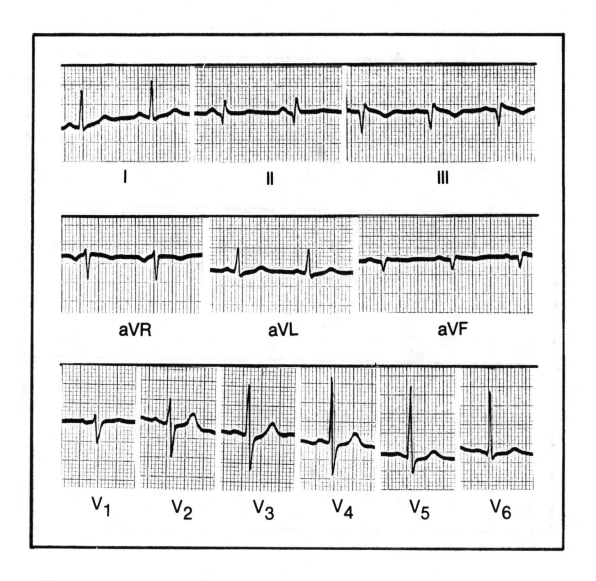

FIGURE 5-32.   Inferior (diaphragmatic) myocardial infarction.

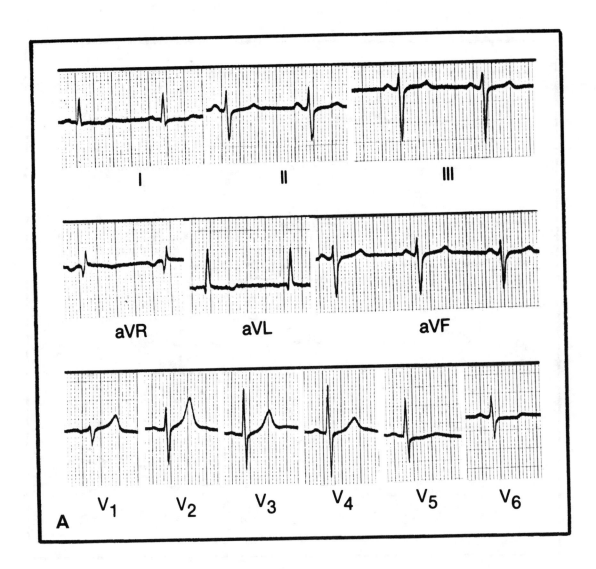

FIGURE 5-33A.   Baseline electrocardiogram prior to myocardial infarction. Describe the abnormalities.

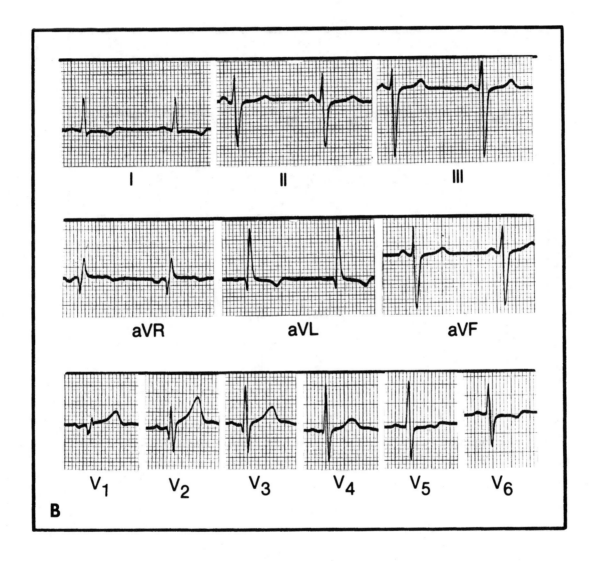

FIGURE 5-33B. Same patient as in Figure 5-33A following anteroseptal myocardial infarction.

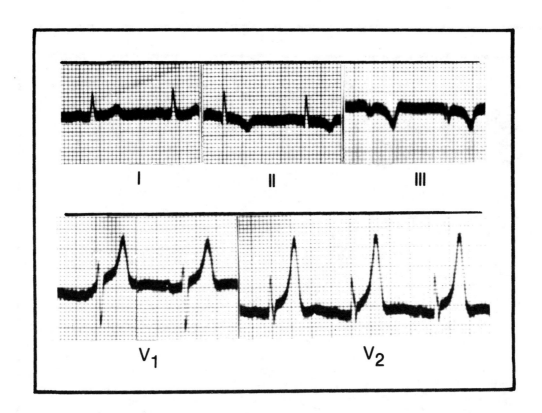

FIGURE 5-34. *Patient with clinical evidence of myocardial infarction. In addition to the deep Q waves in lead III and smaller Q waves in lead II, there is marked peaking of the T waves in leads V$_1$ and V$_2$.[5-12] This patient had sustained an inferior-posterior myocardial infarction.*

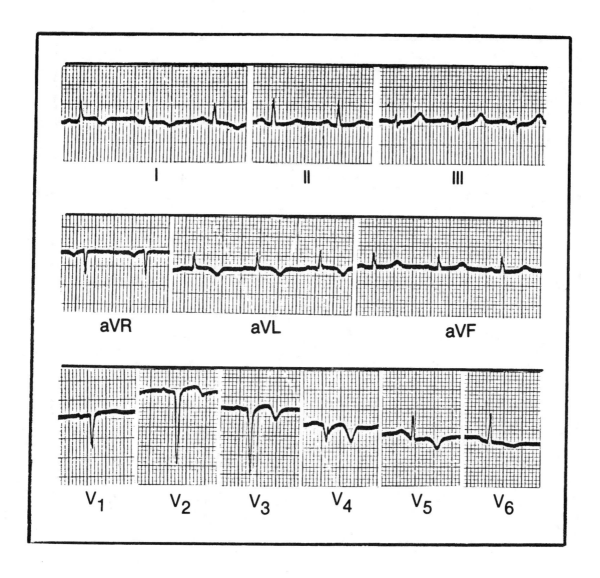

FIGURE 5-35.   *Anterior myocardial infarction. Explain the absence of Q waves in the frontal plane leads.*

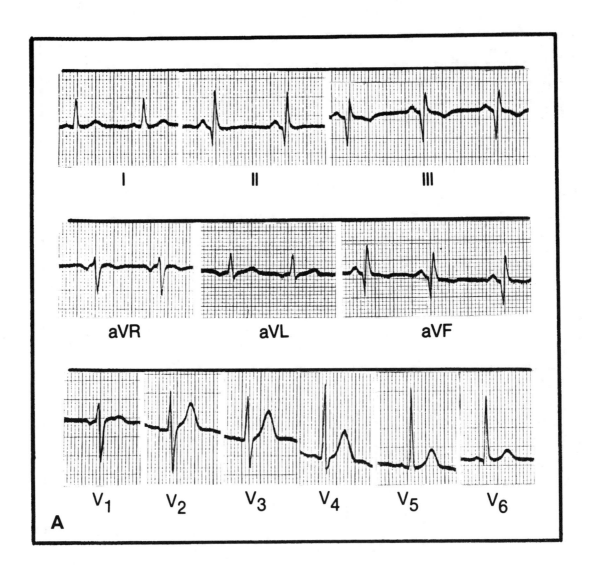

FIGURE 5-36A. Inferior (diaphragmatic) myocardial infarction.

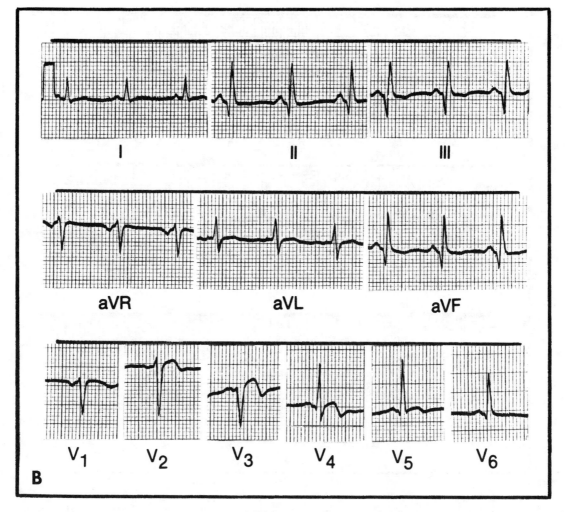

FIGURE 5-36B.   *Same patient as in Figure 5-36A following development of an anteroseptal myocardial infarction. Without the comparison tracings, how would you determine which infarct came before which?*

In addition to the S-T segment and T wave changes of acute myocardial infarction in the precordial leads we see not only "poor R wave progression" (the R wave does not increase in size, as expected, from right to left) but "reversed R wave progression." The R wave in lead V_3 is smaller than in lead V_2. In this case there is no problem with the diagnosis, given the symptoms and the serial electrocardiograms. Zema and associates studied "poor R wave progression" and "reversed R wave progression" and concluded that this pattern, in addition to myocardial infarction, could represent ventricular hypertrophy as well as a normal variant.[5-15]

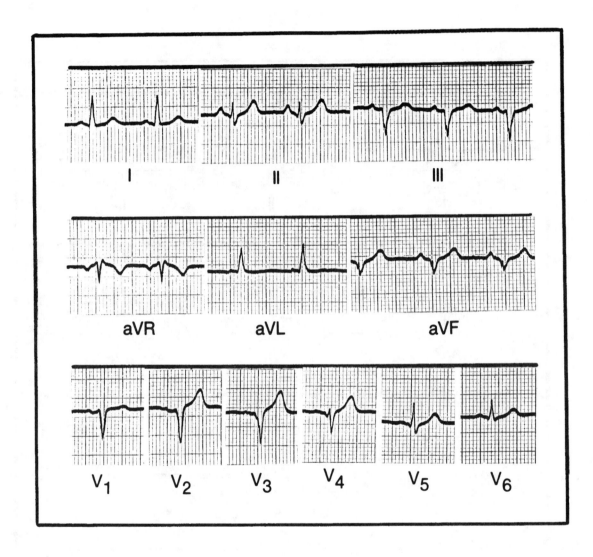

FIGURE 5-37. Infarction of the heart involving the anterior and inferior areas. Were these changes the result of one or more than one myocardial infarction?

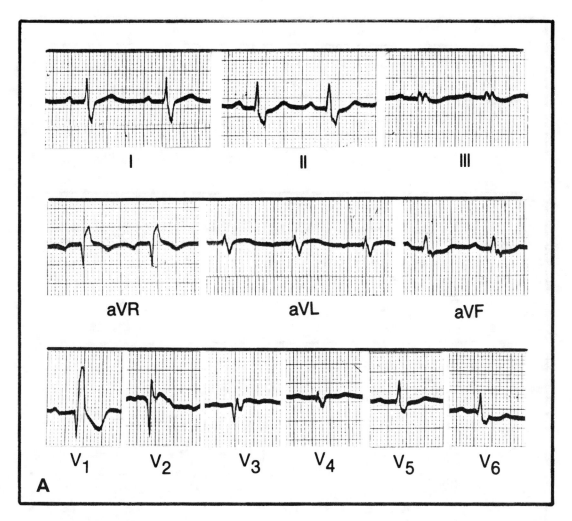

FIGURE 5-38A.   Anteroseptal myocardial infarction in a patient with right bundle branch block. (Bundle branch blocks will be studied in Chapter 6.)

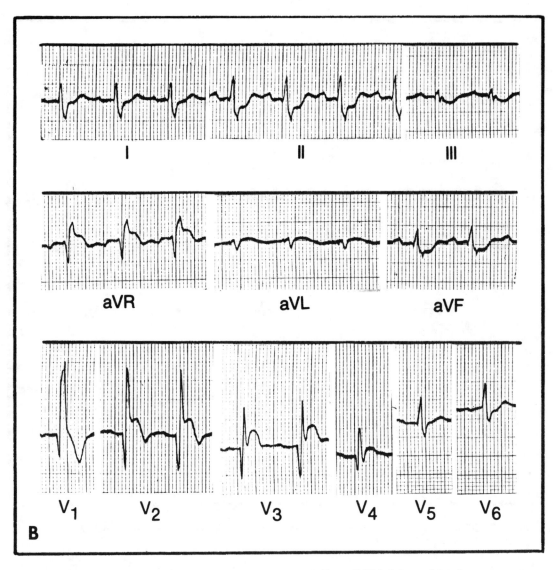

FIGURE 5-38B.   *Acute myocardial infarction in same patient as in Figure 5-38A. Is it possible to have a new myocardial infarction in the area of the old infarction?*

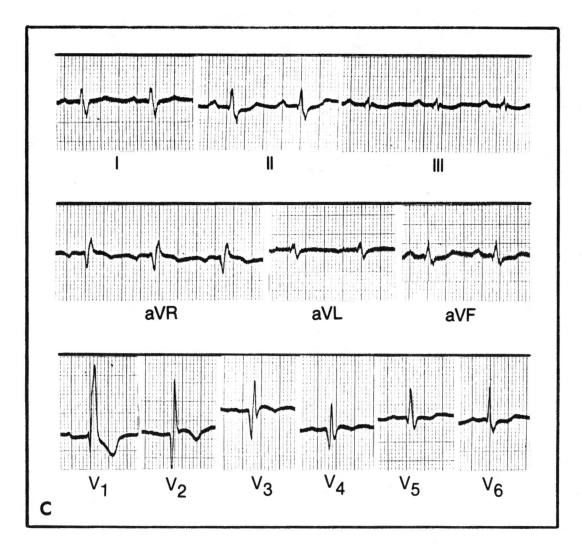

FIGURE 5-38C. Evolutionary changes during recovery from the infarct seen in Figure 5-38B.

> Stop the tape and begin the post-test on the following page.

P O S T · T E S T

DIRECTIONS.   This post-test consists of five electrocardiographic tracings (5-39, 5-40A, 5-41, 5-42, 5-43A) indicative of myocardial infarction. *Proceed without reading the information under the electrocardiograms until you have completed the post-test.* Write your analyses in the spaces indicated.

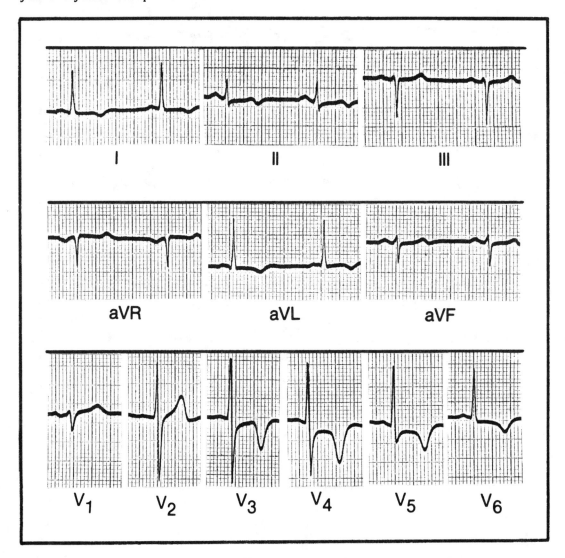

FIGURE 5-39.   Anterior subendocardial infarction. This patient had clinical evidence of myocardial infarction. There are marked repolarization abnormalities, with a very wide QRS-T angle and S-T segment abnormalities. T wave inversion of the magnitude seen in leads V_3 to V_5 are often associated with severe ischemic episodes and anterior myocardial infarction. This is a myocardial infarction without Q waves, often labeled subendocardial infarction. From the post-test directions, you know that this patient had a myocardial infarction. If this electrocardiogram were presented without this information, you could not make a definitive diagnosis of myocardial infarction.

1. Analysis:

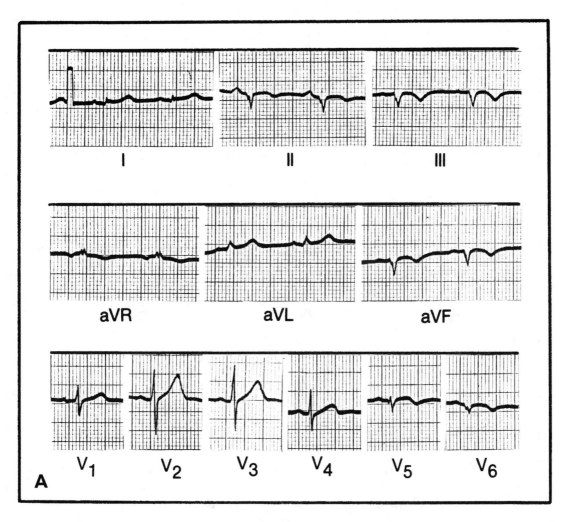

FIGURE 5-40A.   *Evolving changes during recovery from myocardial infarction. Note the Q waves or QS complexes in leads II, III, aVF, V₅, and V₆, representing an inferior-lateral myocardial infarction.*

2.   Analysis:

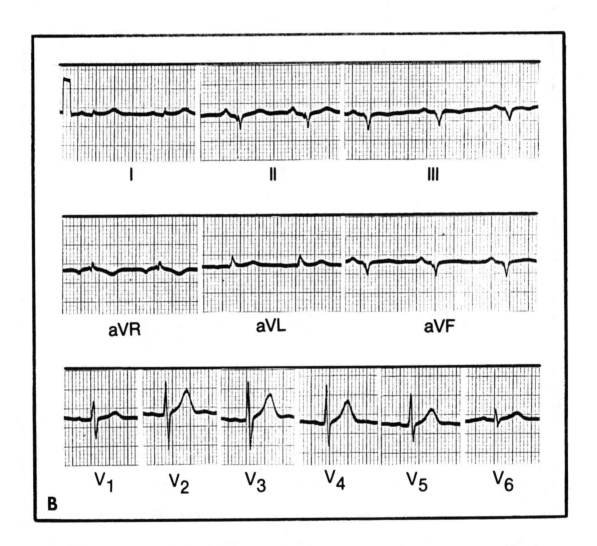

FIGURE 5-40B.   Two months following Figure 5-40A. What happened to the Q waves in leads V_5 and V_6? Did the infarct change location?

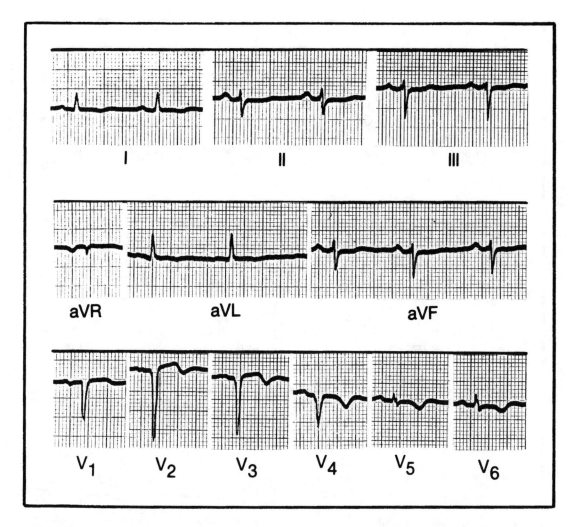

FIGURE 5-41.   Anterior myocardial infarction. This patient had a recent anterior myocardial infarction with QS complexes in leads V₁ to V₄, together with S-T segment and T wave abnormalities. Left axis deviation is also present.

3. Analysis:

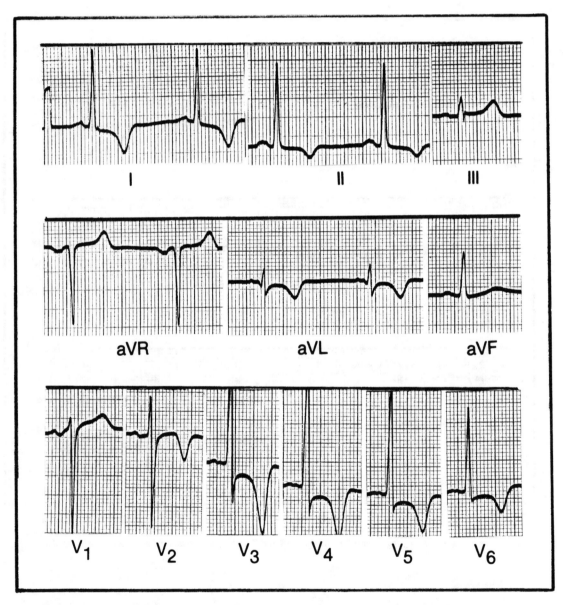

FIGURE 5-42.   *Anterior subendocardial infarction. This electrocardiogram, in a patient with left ventricular hypertrophy and clinical evidence of myocardial infarction, reveals striking repolarization (both S-T segment and T wave) abnormalities. These are additive to the expected repolarization abnormalities of left ventricular hypertrophy. T wave inversion of the magnitude seen in the precordial leads should make you suspect myocardial ischemia or anterior myocardial infarction. As Figure 5-39, this is an example of myocardial infarction without Q waves (subendocardial infarction).*

4. Analysis:

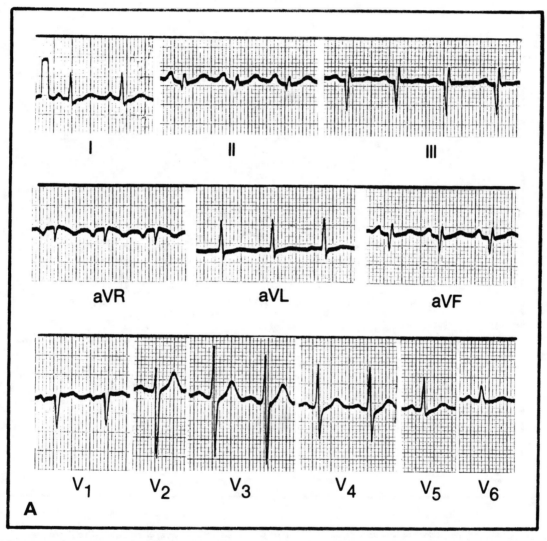

FIGURE 5-43A.   Inferior (diaphragmatic) myocardial infarction. This patient had sustained a myocardial infarction nine years earlier. The significant Q waves in leads II, III, and aVF represent an inferior (diaphragmatic) myocardial infarction.

5. Analysis:

> After completing the post-test, return to each analysis and compare your responses with the analyses under each electrocardiogram and restart the tape.

> On the following pages are additional electrocardiograms for review and practice.

ADDITIONAL REVIEW
ELECTROCARDIOGRAMS

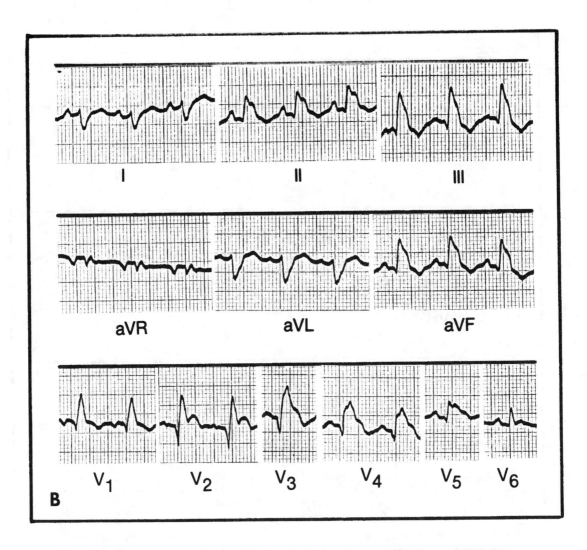

FIGURE 5-43B. *Same patient as in Figure 5-43A, who presented with crushing chest pain with evidence of myocardial infarction. Note the changes which have occurred in both depolarization and repolarization of the ventricles, especially the onset of right bundle branch block and Q waves in leads V₁ to V₅. The right bundle branch block plus the right axis deviation (left posterior hemiblock) is known as bifascicular block and will be studied in the next chapter.*

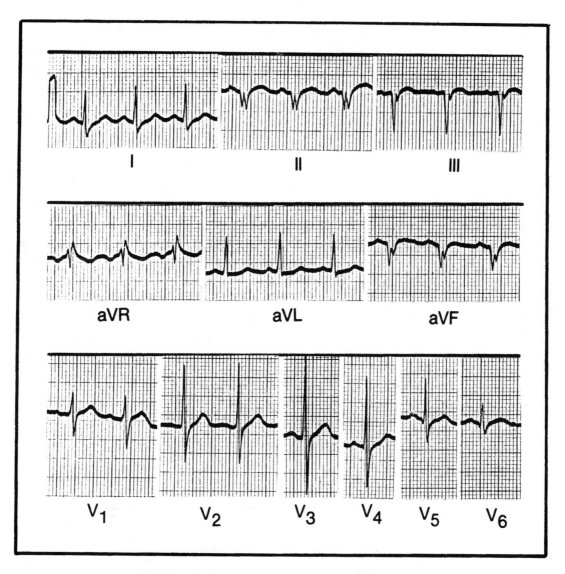

FIGURE 5-44. Inferior-posterior myocardial infarction.

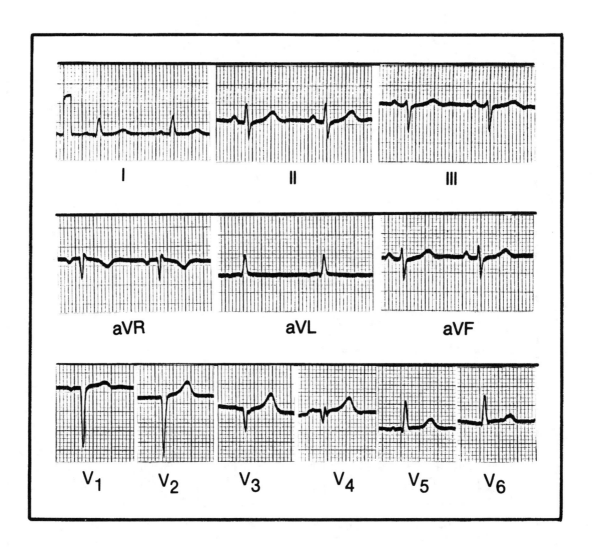

FIGURE 5-45. Anterior myocardial infarction.

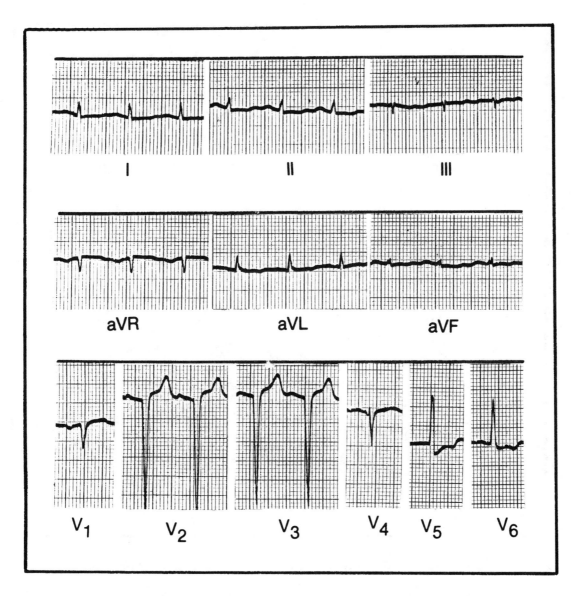

FIGURE 5-46.   Anterior myocardial infarction. Why are the deflections (QRS) in leads I, II, III, aVR, aVL, and aVF so small in a patient with a known large left ventricle? (Review Chapter 3.)

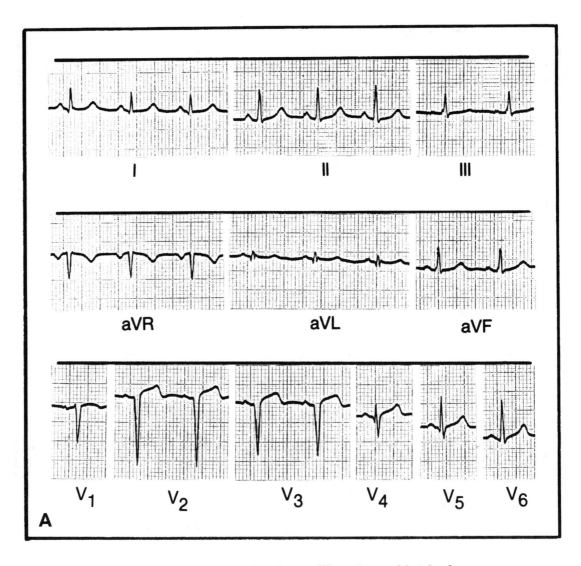

FIGURE 5-47A.   Anterior myocardial infarction. What is the age of the infarct?

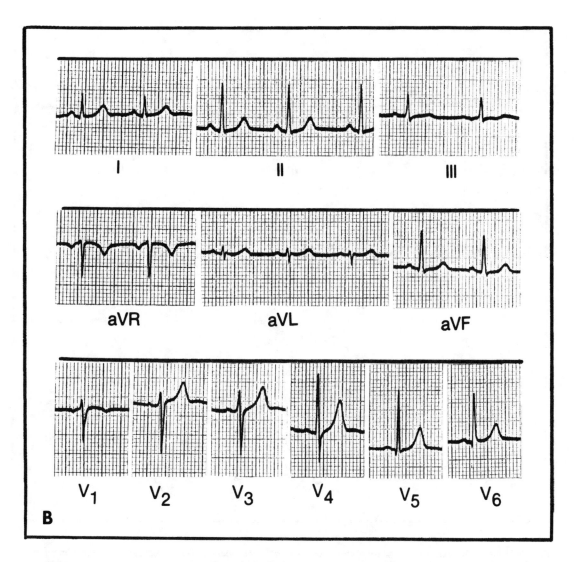

FIGURE 5-47B.   Same patient as in Figure 5-47A. This electrocardiogram was taken 2 weeks before the previous one, just before the onset of clinical symptoms of myocardial infarction.

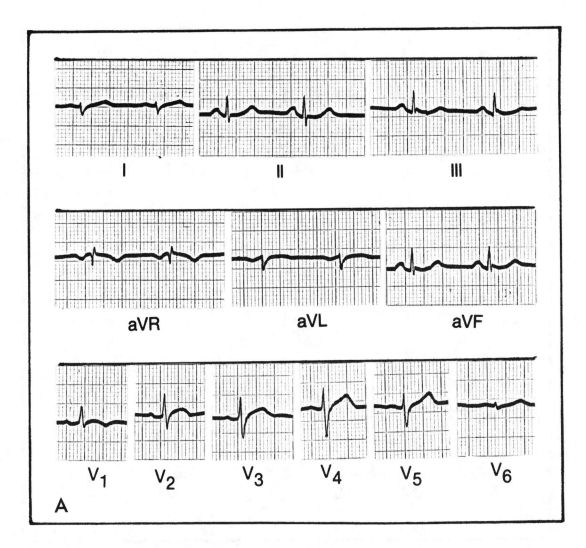

FIGURE 5-48.   *True posterior myocardial infarction. The right axis deviation will be discussed in the section on hemiblocks in Chapter 6. There was no evidence of right ventricular hypertrophy. Electrocardiograms of the same patient will be seen in Figure 6-27A and B.*

NOTES AND REFERENCES

From Page 328:
The Significant Q Wave

The *significant Q wave* is at least *one quarter to one third the height of the QRS complex* and 0.04 sec. in duration (1 small box wide). Lead aVR is the exception, since a large Q wave is normal. See reference to the *pretransitional Q wave* in the precordial leads, pages 349 to 350.

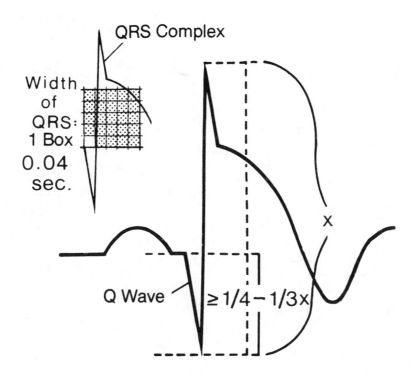

A significant Q wave should be:
    1. ≥ 1/4 − 1/3 height of QRS complex
    2. 0.04 second (one small box wide) in duration

From Page 329:
Right Ventricular Infarction

This electrocardiogram is from an elderly patient with an acute inferior (diaphragmatic) myocardial infarction. As noted on page 329, in the studies of Chou et al.[53] and Erhardt et al.,[54] infarction of the right ventricle should be considered when, in addition to the findings of inferior wall infarction, there is S-T segment elevation in one (lead V_1) or more of the right precordial leads. Leads V_3R and V_4R, with elevated S-T segments (arrows) reveal the involvement of the right ventricle.

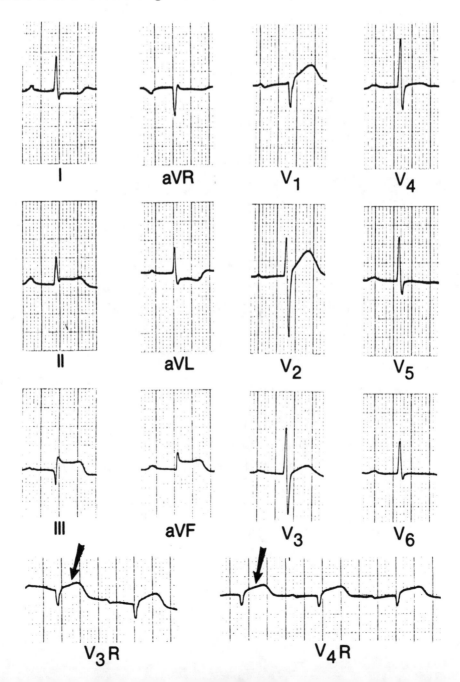

From Page 337:   Reciprocal Changes

Note the Q waves, elevation of the S-T segments, and relatively tall T waves in leads II and III. These are the *indicative* changes in a patient with an early acute inferior (diaphragmatic) myocardial infarction. The depression of the S-T segment and inversion of the T wave in lead I, on the opposite surface of the heart, is an example of *reciprocal* changes. However, following the electrical truth learned in Chapter 1, leads I + III = lead II, the S-T segment and T wave must be negative in lead I, given the more positive S-T segment and T wave in lead III as compared with lead II. A question remains, especially in the precordial leads. Is reciprocity an electrical phenomenon only, or does it represent additional abnormalities? Numerous studies are attempting to answer this question.

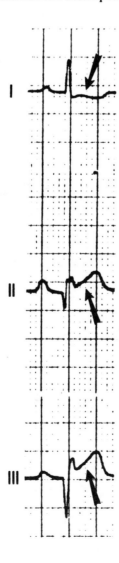

From Page 339:   Evolutionary
Electrocardiographic Changes
Following Blood Flow Obstruction

Note that the S-T segment elevation occurs prior to the formation of the Q wave. During these early hours, interventions are often undertaken to reverse the process. As time passes, the Q wave forms, the S-T segment is less elevated and the T wave inverts. The final outcome varies greatly, depending on the amount of myocardial damage.

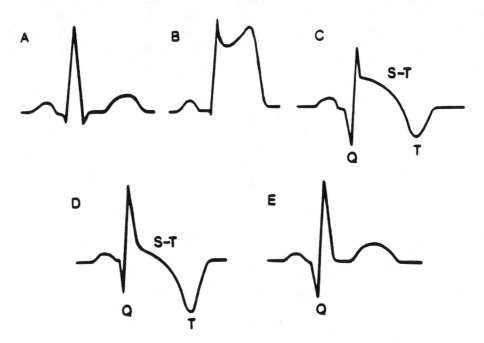

A. Baseline
B. Hyperacute (minutes to hours)
C. Acute (hours to days to weeks)
D. Subacute or recent (weeks to months)
E. Old, stabilized (months to years)

From Page 351: Formation of the Normal Q Wave in Lead III[5-16]
Right Ventricular Infarction

When the QRS vector loop, inscribed clockwise, is nearly parallel with the transition of lead III at +30°, it may, during respiration, shift intermittently into the negative zone of lead III, inscribing a Q wave. Expiration, with the elevation of the diaphragm, tends to shift the QRS vector loop into the negative zone of lead III, inscribing a Q wave (A). Inspiration has the opposite effect, eliminating the Q wave (B).

A. Expiration

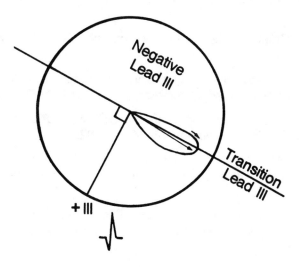

B. Inspiration

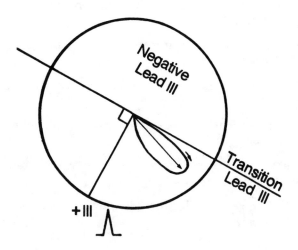

References

5-1. Benchimol, A., et al.: The ventricular premature contraction; its place in the diagnosis of ischemic heart disease. Am. Heart J., *65:*334, 1963.

5-2. Wahl, J.M., et al.: Limitations of premature ventricular complex morphology in the diagnosis of myocardial infarction. J. Electrocardiol., *19:*131, 1986.

5-3. Chou, T.-C., et al.: Electrocardiographic diagnosis of right ventricular infarction. Am. J. Med., *70:*1175, 1981.

5-4. Erhardt, L.R., et al.: Single right-sided precordial lead in the diagnosis of right ventricular involvement in inferior myocardial infarction. Am. Heart J., *91:*571, 1976.

5-5. Beckwith, J.: Grant's Clinical Electrocardiography, 2nd Ed. New York, McGraw-Hill, 1970, p. 160.

5-6. Fulton, M.C., and Marriott, H.J.L.: Acute pancreatitis simulating myocardial infarction in the electrocardiogram. Ann. Intern. Med., *59:*730, 1963.

5-7. Wasserman, A.G., et al.: Prognostic implications of diagnostic Q waves after myocardial infarction. Circulation, *65:*1451, 1982.

5-8. Raunio, H., et al.: Changes in the QRS complex and ST segment in transmural and subendocardial myocardial infarction: a clinicopathologic study. Am. Heart J., *98:*176, 1979.

5-9. Spodick, D.H.: Q-wave infarction versus S-T infarction: nonspecificity of electrocardiographic criteria for differentiating transmural and nontransmural lesions. Am. J. Cardiol., *51:*913, 1983.

5-10. Schamroth, L.: The 12 Lead Electrocardiogram. Oxford, Blackwell Scientific Publications, 1989, p. 184.

5-11. De Zwaan, C., Bär, R.W.H.M., and Wellens, H.J.J.: Characteristic electrocardiographic pattern indicating a critical stenosis high in left anterior descending coronary artery in patients admitted because of impending myocardial infarction. Am. Heart J., *103:*730, 1982.

5-12. Schamroth, L.: The 12 Lead Electrocardiogram. Oxford, Blackwell Scientific Publications, 1989, p. 177.

5-13. Beckwith, J.: Grant's Clinical Electrocardiography, 2nd Ed. New York, McGraw-Hill, 1970, p. 172.

5-14. Marriott, H.J.L.: Practical Electrocardiography, 8th Ed. Baltimore, Williams & Wilkins, 1988, p. 442.

5-15. Zema, M.J., et al.: Electrocardiographic poor R-wave progression: correlation with post mortem findings. Chest, *79:*195, 1981.

5-16. Schamroth, L.: The 12 Lead Electrocardiogram. Oxford, Blackwell Scientific Publications, 1989, p. 158.

6

VENTRICULAR CONDUCTION DISTURBANCES

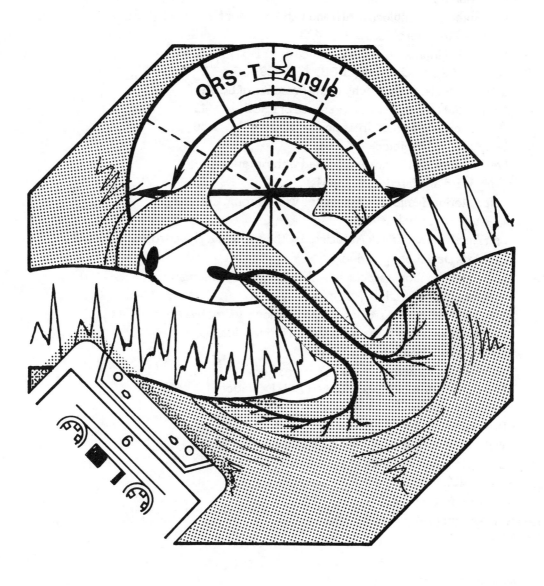

CHAPTER 6
CONTENTS

INTRODUCTION

As noted earlier, the heart possesses its own specialized conduction system. In this chapter the ventricular conduction disturbances will be studied in the following order:

A. Right bundle branch block (RBBB).
B. Left bundle branch block (LBBB).
C. The "hemiblocks" and the "trifascicular" system.
D. $S_I S_{II} S_{III}$ syndrome.
E. Pre-excitation
   Wolff-Parkinson-White (W-P-W) syndrome.
   Lown-Ganong-Levine (L-G-L) syndrome.

OBJECTIVES

Upon completion of this chapter, you should be able to:

1. Recall the electrocardiographic criteria for right bundle branch block.

2. Recognize right bundle branch block in the presence of anterior myocardial infarction.

3. Recall the electrocardiographic criteria for left bundle branch block.

4. State how electrocardiographic manifestations of myocardial infarction may be either simulated or masked by left bundle branch block.

5. State what is meant by "hemiblocks."

6. List the criteria for left anterior and left posterior hemiblock.

7. Recall what is meant by "trifascicular" system.

8. State what is meant by "bifascicular" block.

9. Recognize the $S_I S_{II} S_{III}$ syndrome.

10. Recognize the electrocardiographic manifestations of the Wolff-Parkinson-White syndrome.

DIRECTIONS.   This pretest consists of 10 electrocardiograms. Write a brief analysis of each in the space provided.

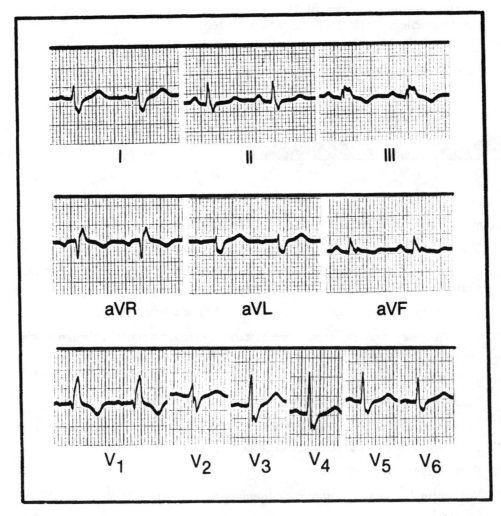

FIGURE 6-3.

1. Analysis:

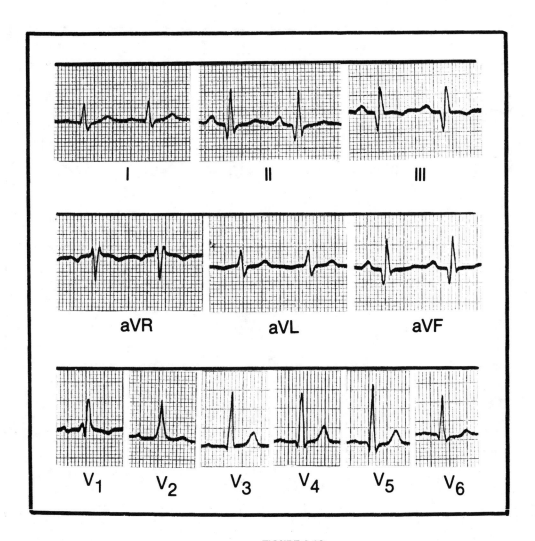

FIGURE 6-10.

2. Analysis:

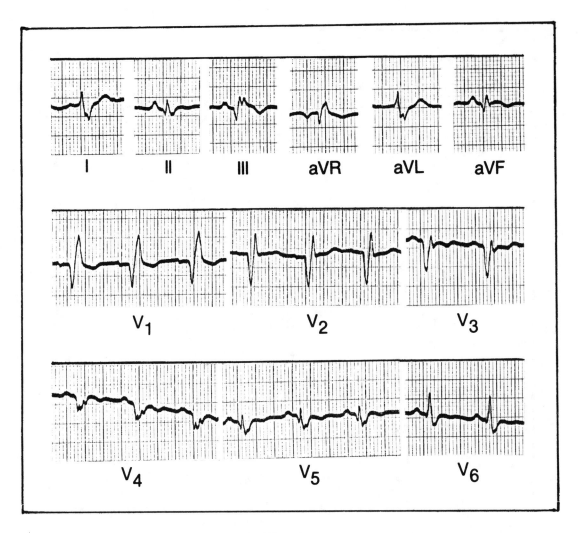

FIGURE 6-12.

2. Analysis:

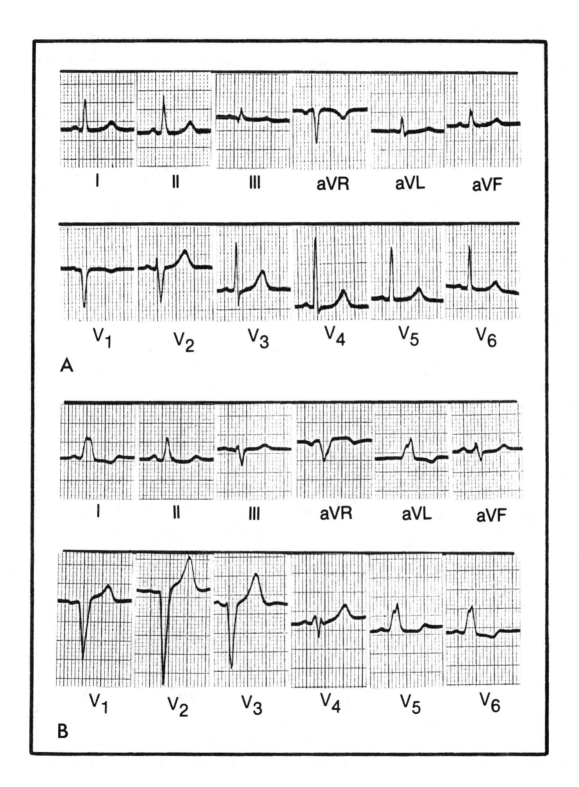

FIGURE 6-14.   *Analyze and describe the changes that have occurred from A to B.*

4. Analysis:

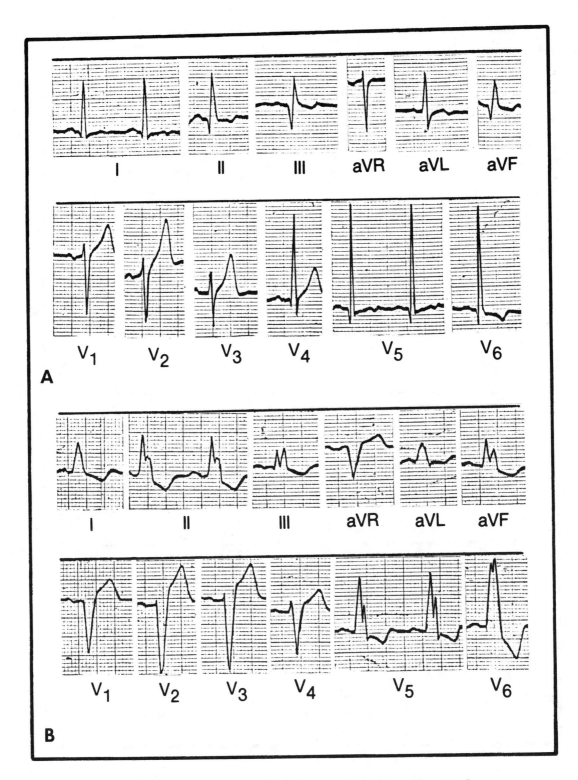

FIGURE 6-19.   Analyze and describe the changes that have occurred from A to B.

5.   Analysis:

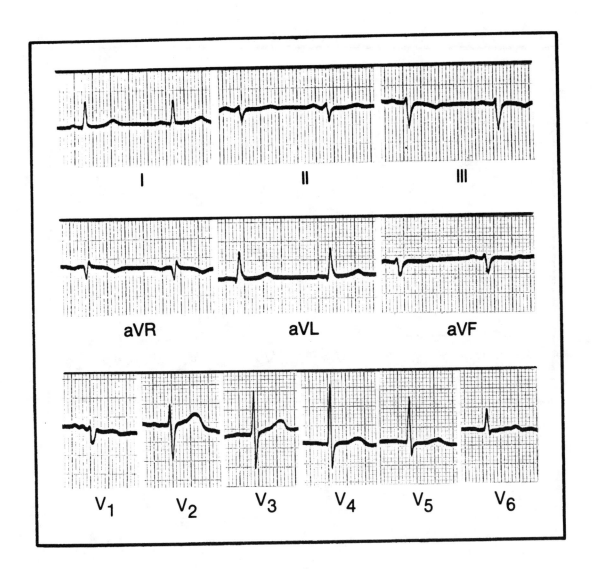

FIGURE 6-22.

6. Analysis:

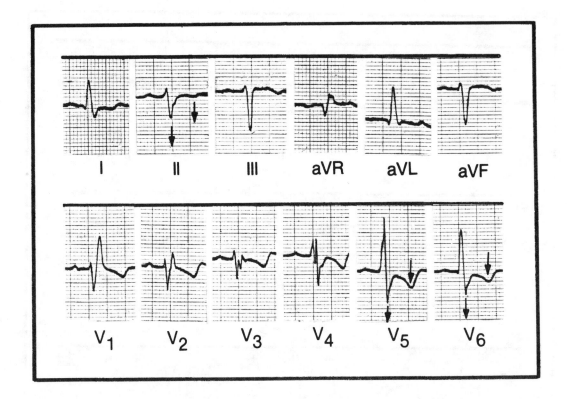

FIGURE 6-30.

2. Analysis:

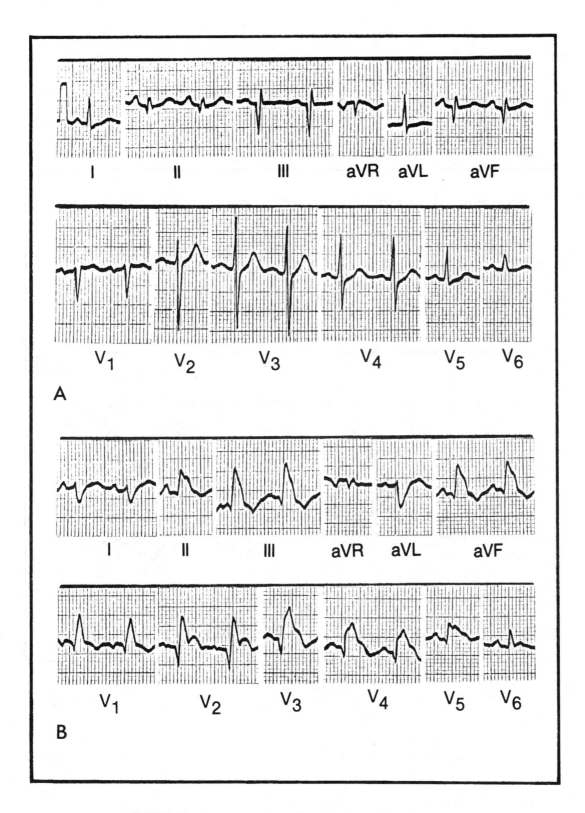

FIGURE 6-32. *Analyze and describe the changes that have occurred from A to B.*

8. Analysis:

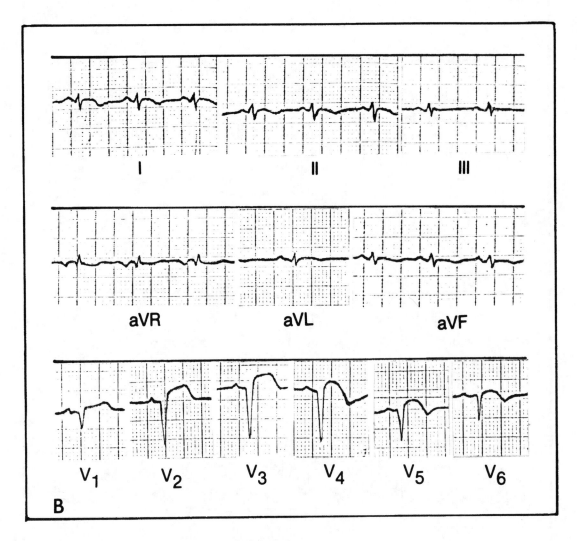

FIGURE 6-39B.

9. Analysis:

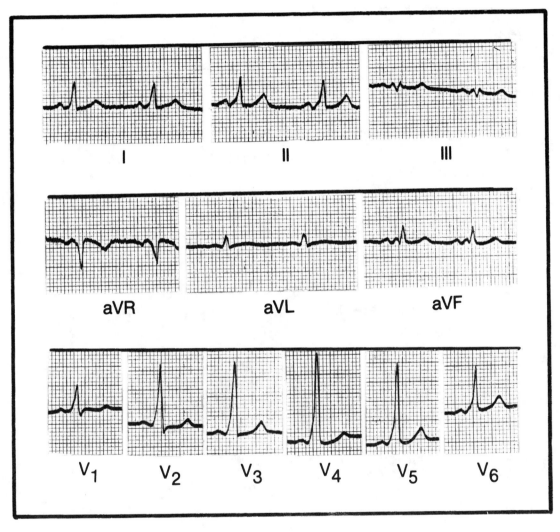

FIGURE 6-42.

10. Analysis:

> Solutions to the pretest will be indicated later in this chapter.

> When you have completed the pretest start Cassette Side 15 and continue on the next page.

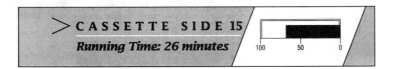

> CASSETTE SIDE 15
> *Running Time: 26 minutes*

100   50   0

VENTRICULAR CONDUCTION
DISTURBANCES

A. *Right Bundle Branch Block (RBBB)*

The atrioventricular (A-V) conduction mechanism of the heart is diagrammed in Figure 6-1. While this diagram is used throughout this chapter, it is only a schematic and should not be construed to reflect strict anatomic accuracy.

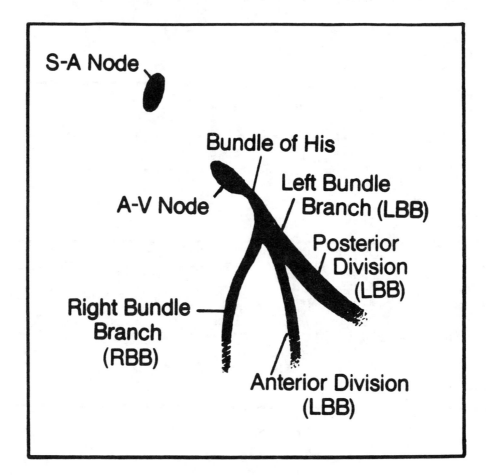

FIGURE 6-1.

Right bundle block refers to a lesion somewhere along the course of the right bundle branch (Figure 6-2).

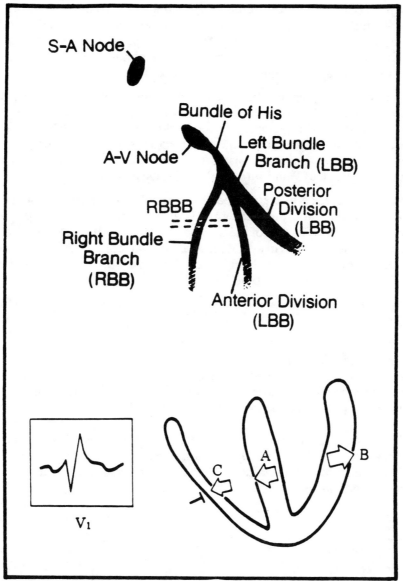

FIGURE 6-2. *Right bundle branch block and sequence of activation of ventricular myocardium.*

Sequence of activation as recorded from lead V_1:

    A. *Septal activation from left to right, inscribing the initial R wave.*
    B. *Activation of the free wall of the left ventricle, inscribing the S wave.*
    C. *Delayed activation of the free wall of the right ventricle, inscribing the terminal R (or R') wave.*

With the interruption of the normal pathway, the impulse must reach the right ventricular myocardium by an intramyocardial spread of activation; hence the prolongation of the QRS complex. Classically, the QRS complex is prolonged to at least 0.12 sec. in "complete" right bundle branch block and up to 0.12 sec. (Marriott suggests 0.09 to 0.10 sec. with right bundle branch block morphology[6-1]) in "incomplete" right bundle branch block. Schamroth points out that in "incomplete" right bundle branch block conduction is still possible, but delayed, through the right bundle branch.[6-2]

Regardless of where the block may be in right bundle branch block, early depolarization will already have occurred from left to right (small Q waves in lead I and left precordial leads). Only the *terminal* QRS vector is affected by right bundle branch block. This is of importance since the electrocardiographic manifestations of initial QRS vector abnormalities, such as Q waves in myocardial infarction, are not obscured. This *terminal delay* is to the *right* (S wave in lead I) and *anterior* (R or R′ wave in lead V_1).

Right bundle branch block is also accompanied by repolarization abnormalities. These are *secondary* to the abnormal depolarization. The T wave orientation is opposite in direction to the *terminal* deflection of the QRS complex. Thus, in lead I, with a terminal S wave, the T wave is upright, and in lead V_1, with a terminal R or R′ wave, the T wave is negative. If this is not found, then primary repolarization abnormalities are evident in addition to the right bundle branch block.

Right bundle branch block may be recognized electrocardiographically by the following principal criteria:

1. Widened QRS complex (0.12 sec. or greater).
2. S wave in leads I, V_5, and V_6.
3. Terminal R or R′ wave in lead V_1 with delayed right ventricular activation time.
4. Repolarization abnormalities (secondary to abnormal depolarization). The T wave is opposite in direction to the terminal deflection of the QRS complex.

Right bundle branch block may be found congenitally without any clinical evidence of heart disease. It may also be found in association with an enlarged right ventricle, myocardial infarction, hypertensive cardiovascular disease, atrial septal defect, and acute pulmonary embolism.

Principal electrocardiographic criteria of right bundle branch block are also summarized and illustrated on page 486.

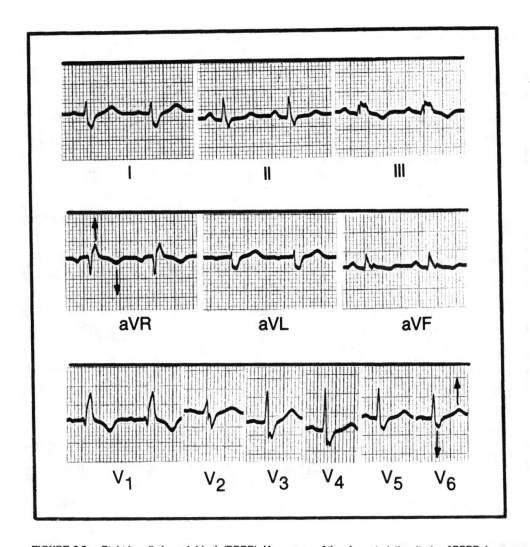

FIGURE 6-3.   Right bundle branch block (RBBB). How many of the characteristic criteria of RBBB do you see here?

1. Widened QRS complex (0.12 sec. or greater).
2. S wave in leads I, V_5, and V_6.
3. Terminal R or R′ wave in lead V_1 with delayed right ventricular activation time.
4. Repolarization abnormalities (secondary to abnormal depolarization). The T wave is opposite in direction to the terminal deflection of the QRS complex (arrows above).

> The analysis of Figure 6-3 in the text and on the tape is the solution to Item 1 on the pretest.

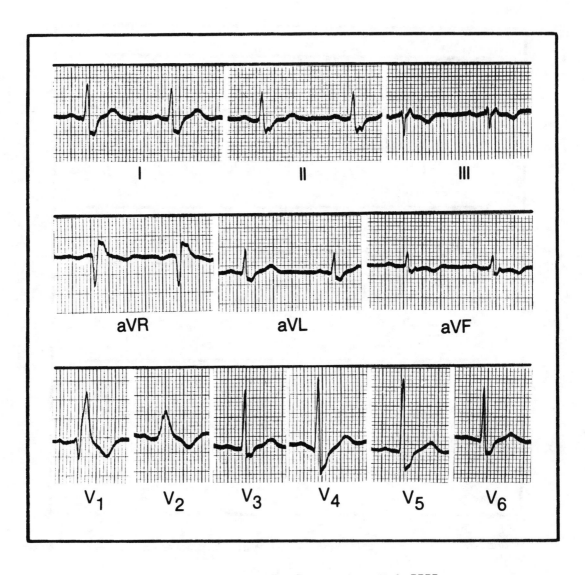

FIGURE 6-4.   Right bundle branch block. Review all the criteria for RBBB.

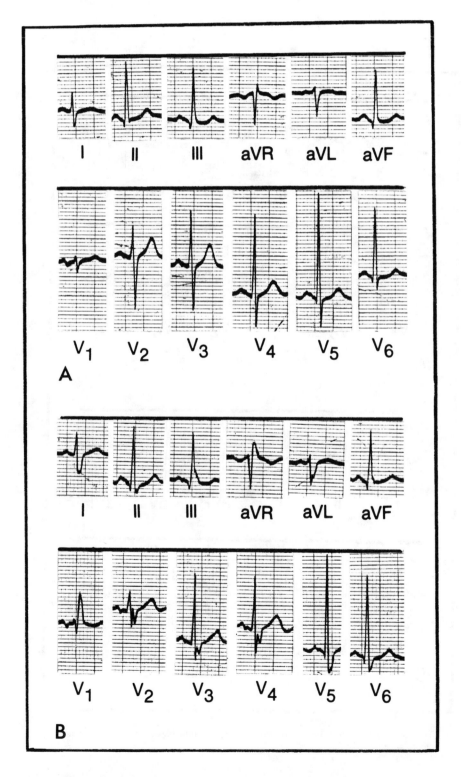

FIGURE 6-5. *Before and after development of right bundle branch block. A, Baseline; B, following onset of RBBB.*

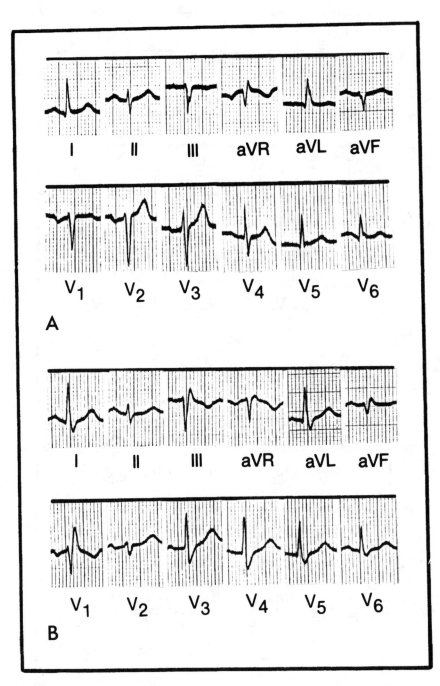

FIGURE 6-6.   *Before and after development of right bundle branch block. A, Baseline; B, following onset of RBBB.*

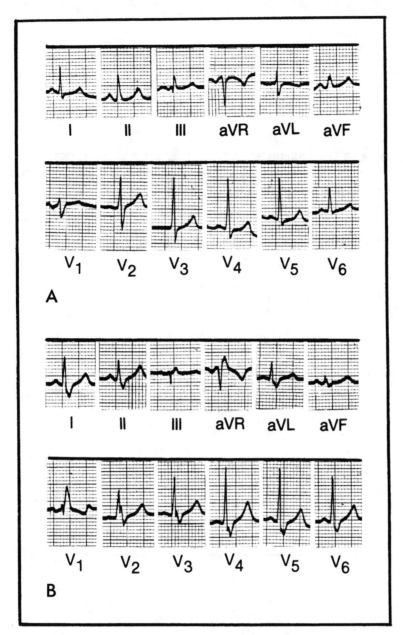

FIGURE 6-7.   Before and after development of right bundle branch block. A, Baseline; B, following onset of RBBB. (Electrocardiogram reduced in size.)

*Left Anterior Hemiblock (LAH) and Left
Posterior Hemiblock (LPH) in the Presence
of RBBB*

LAH and LPH in the presence of RBBB will be studied later in this chapter.

*Myocardial Infarction in the Presence of
RBBB*

Figure 6-8A and B is from a patient with inferior (diaphragmatic) myocardial infarction, before and after development of right bundle branch block. That the initial QRS vectorial forces are *not* affected by the right bundle branch block is of the utmost importance. The Q waves of myocardial infarction are *not* obscured by right bundle branch block.

Figure 6-8A reveals an inferior (diaphragmatic) myocardial infarction prior to the development of right bundle branch block. In Figure 6-8B the findings of inferior myocardial infarction remain in the presence of right bundle branch block.

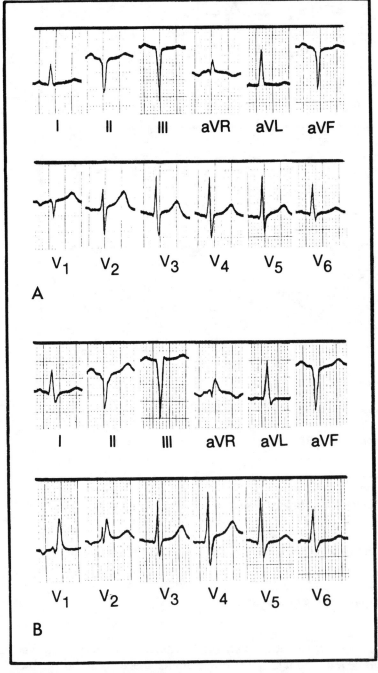

FIGURE 6-8.   Before and after development of right bundle branch block in a patient with inferior myocardial infarction. A, Baseline, with inferior myocardial infarction; B, following onset of RBBB. (Electrocardiogram reduced in size.)

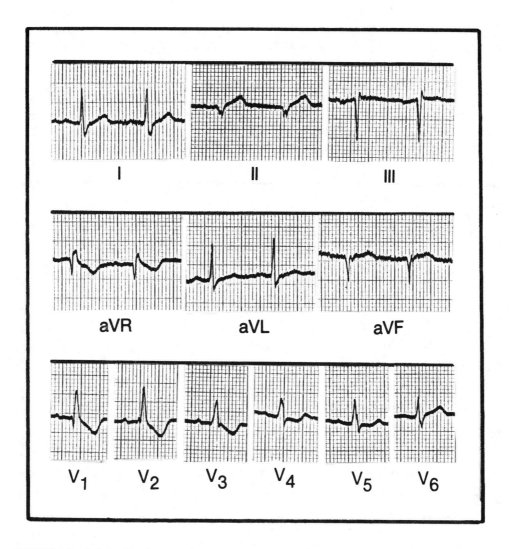

FIGURE 6-9.   *Inferior (diaphragmatic) myocardial infarction in the presence of right bundle branch block.*

In Figure 6-10 are seen the typical findings of inferior (diaphragmatic) myocardial infarction (significant Q waves in leads II, III and aVF). In addition, the principal criteria of RBBB are present.

1. Widened QRS complex (0.12 sec. or greater).
2. S wave in leads I, V_5, and V_6.
3. Terminal R or R' wave in lead V_1 with delayed right ventricular activation time.
4. Repolarization abnormalities (secondary to abnormal depolarization). The T wave is opposite in direction to the terminal deflection of the QRS complex.

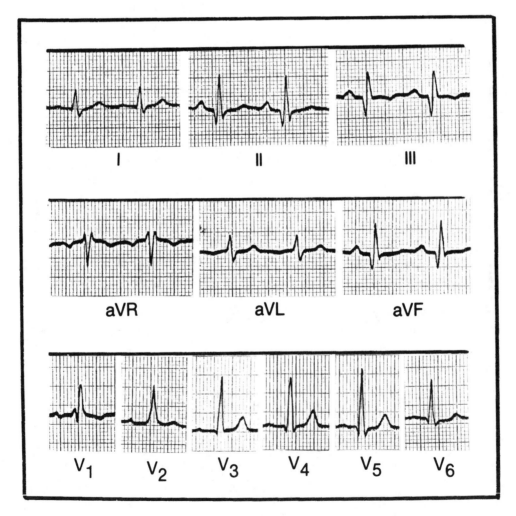

FIGURE 6-10.   *Inferior (diaphragmatic) myocardial infarction in the presence of right bundle branch block.*

> The analysis of Figure 6-10 in the text and on the tape is the solution to Item 2 on the pretest.

The electrocardiographic manifestations of right bundle branch block in the presence of *anterior* myocardial infarction are of special interest. The initial Q wave in lead V_1 is preserved with a resulting QR rather than an RSR' pattern. This should not detract from the diagnosis of right bundle branch block if the other criteria are present; illustrations are presented in Figures 6-11 and 6-12.

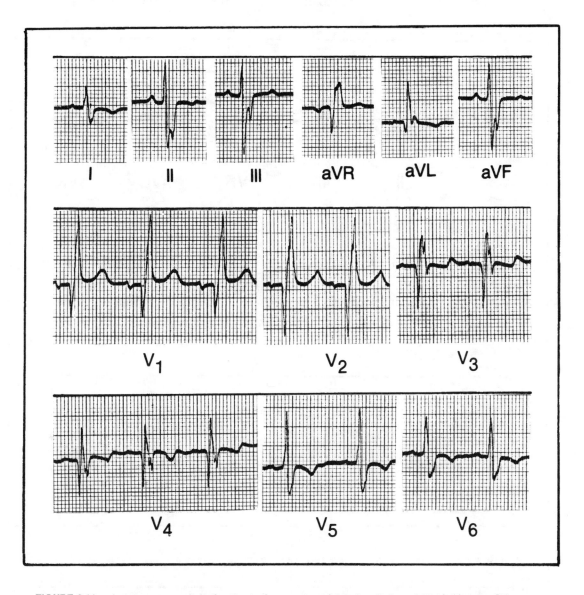

FIGURE 6-11.   *Anterior myocardial infarction in the presence of right bundle branch block. Note the QR pattern in leads V_1, V_2, V_3, and V_4; the QR replaces the RSR' in lead V_1.*

Figure 6-12 presents the findings of anterior myocardial infarction (Q waves or QS complexes in leads V_1 to V_5) and inferior (diaphragmatic) myocardial infarction (Q waves in leads II, III, and aVF). The principal criteria of RBBB include:

1. Widened QRS complex (0.12 sec. or greater).
2. S wave in leads I, V_5, and V_6.
3. Terminal R or R' wave in lead V_1 with delayed right ventricular activation time.
4. Repolarization abnormalities (secondary to abnormal depolarization). The T wave is opposite in direction to the terminal deflection of the QRS complex.

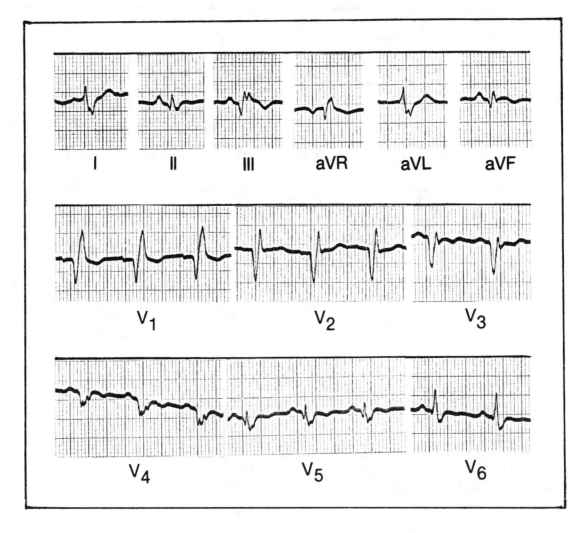

FIGURE 6-12. Anterior and inferior myocardial infarction in the presence of right bundle branch block.

> The analysis of Figure 6-12 in the text and on the tape is the solution to Item 3 on the pretest.

B. Left Bundle Branch Block (LBBB)

In left bundle branch block (Figure 6-13), in contrast to right bundle branch block, the entire sequence of ventricular depolarization is altered. Both the initial and terminal QRS vectorial forces point more leftward and posteriorly in comparison with normal conduction. As with right bundle branch block, Shamroth notes that "complete" left bundle branch block represents a complete interruption of conduction in the left bundle branch while "incomplete" left bundle branch block represents a *delay* of conduction within the left bundle branch.[63] Left bundle branch block is frequently associated with cardiovascular disease although it may be found without other evidence of heart disease. Noble and associates found that hypertension and/or ischemic heart disease was present in 78.5% of their group with left bundle branch block while only one patient was free of any evidence of cardiovascular disease.[64]

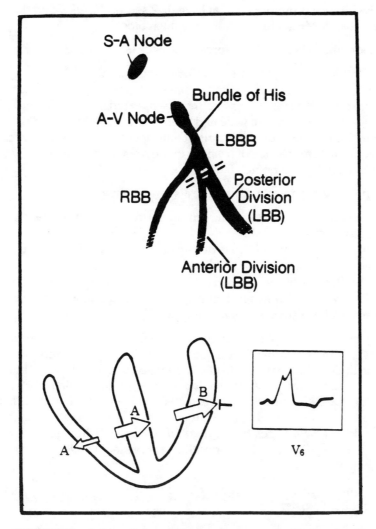

FIGURE 6-13.   Left bundle branch block and sequence of activation of ventricular myocardium.

Sequence of activation as recorded from lead V_6 (see Figure 6-13):

A. Septal activation from right to left and activation of the free wall of the right ventricle inscribing the initial positive deflection. The greater septal forces overshadow the lesser free wall forces. Actually, right septal activation (now unopposed from right to left) is the very first component of left bundle branch block,[63] inscribing a small initial positive deflection before the large positive deflection.

B. Activation of the free wall of the left ventricle, inscribing the terminal positive deflection.

Because of the abnormal sequence of activation the electrocardiographic characteristics of left bundle branch block are as follows:

1. The QRS interval is prolonged to at least 0.12 sec. (if the QRS duration is 0.10 to 0.12 sec. it is "incomplete" left bundle branch block).

2. The major initial QRS vectorial forces are more leftward and posterior.

   a. The initial Q waves disappear in leads I and V_6.
   b. The initial R waves seen in the normal electrocardiogram in leads V_1, V_2, and V_3 are much smaller and have often disappeared in leads V_1 and V_2. The S waves in these leads are wide and deep and, at times, notched.
   Note: Do not make the diagnosis of anterior or anteroseptal myocardial infarction from the lack of R waves in the right precordial leads in the presence of left bundle branch block.

3. The terminal QRS vectorial forces are also more leftward.

   a. The small S waves in lead aVL, during normal conduction, disappear during left bundle branch block.
   b. Lead III has a terminal R wave during normal conduction and a terminal S wave with left bundle branch block.
   c. Lead aVR has a terminal S wave with left bundle branch block.
   d. Leads I, V_5, and V_6 are broad and often notched, positive complexes with delayed left ventricular activation time.

4. Repolarization abnormalities. As in right bundle branch block, abnormalities are *secondary* to the abnormal depolarization. The S-T segment and the T wave are opposite in direction to the main QRS deflection with a wide angle between the QRS complex and the S-T segment and T wave. When the main QRS deflection is positive, the S-T segment is depressed and the T wave is inverted. The opposite is found when the QRS complex is negative. The S-T segment is then elevated and the T wave is positive. If this wide QRS–ST-T divergence is not found, then primary repolarization abnormalities are present in addition to the left bundle branch block.

These criteria are not invariable and may not be found in every case. They do, however, provide important guideposts.

Summary of principal electrocardiographic findings in left bundle branch block.

1. Widened QRS complex (0.12 sec. or greater).
2. QRS complex predominantly negative in leads V_1 and V_2 and predominantly positive in leads V_5 and V_6, often notched with delayed left ventricular activation time.
3. Absence of small normal Q waves in leads I, aVL, V_5, and V_6.
4. Repolarization abnormalities (secondary to abnormal depolarization). The S-T segment and T wave are opposite in direction to the QRS deflection.

Figure 6-14 is from a patient who had intermittent left bundle branch block which was rate dependent. At lower heart rates her conduction was normal. When she reached a *critical rate* (the rate at which her conduction changed), left bundle branch block would occur. This possibility must always be considered, and conduction at different heart rates should be observed. After you have studied the characteristics of the Wolff-Parkinson-White (W-P-W) syndrome, later in this chapter, you will again see the importance of heart rate and its influence on the conduction system of the heart (page 488.)

In answer to pretest Item 4, without the information that the LBBB was rate dependent, the development of LBBB must be noted in Figure 6-14B, outlining the principal criteria as given previously.

> The analysis of Figure 6-14 on this page and on page 432 as well as on the tape is the solution to Item 4 on the pretest.

> Principal electrocardiographic criteria of left bundle branch block are also summarized and illustrated on page 487.

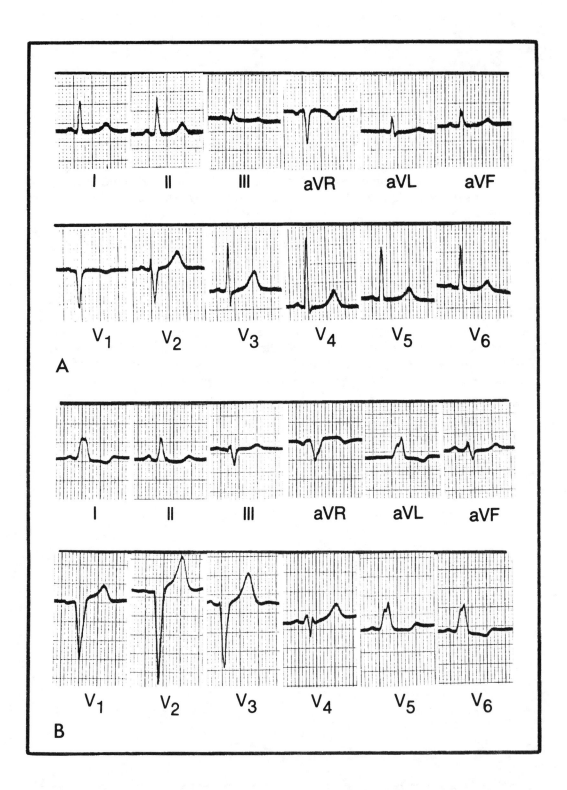

FIGURE 6-14. Before and after development of left bundle branch block. In this patient it was intermittent and rate dependent. How many characteristics of left bundle branch block do you see? A, Baseline; B, following onset of LBBB.

> Another example of rate dependent left bundle branch block is illustrated on page 488.

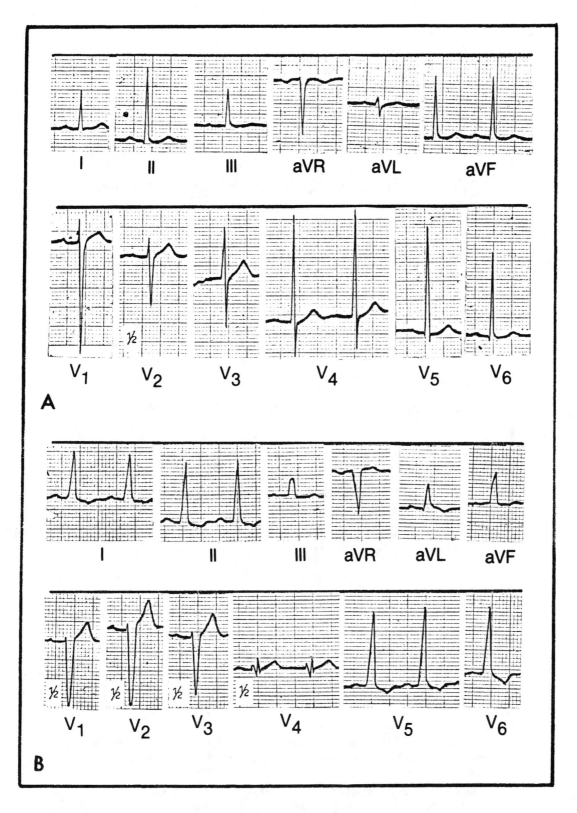

FIGURE 6-15.   Before and after the development of "incomplete" left bundle branch block. The electrocardiogram in B would be listed classically as "incomplete" left bundle branch block, since the above described
changes are present, but the QRS interval is less than 0.12 sec. A, Baseline; B, following onset of "incomplete"
LBBB.

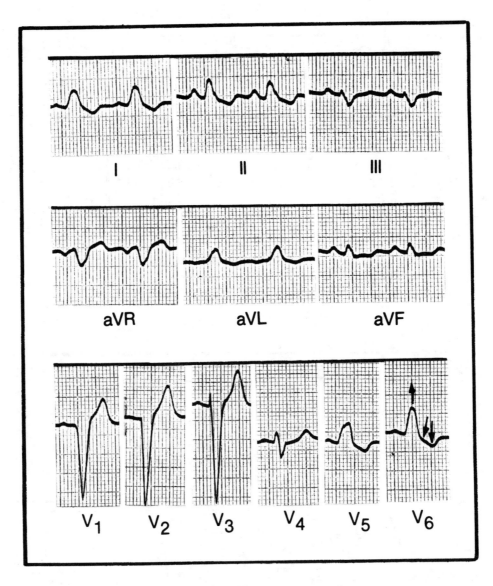

FIGURE 6-16. Left bundle branch block (LBBB). How many of the characteristic criteria of LBBB do you see here?

1. Widened QRS complex (0.12 sec. or greater).
2. QRS complex predominantly negative in leads V_1 and V_2 and predominantly positive in leads V_5 and V_6, often notched with delayed left ventricular activation time.
3. Absence of small normal Q waves in leads I, aVL, V_5, and V_6.
4. Repolarization abnormalities (secondary to abnormal depolarization). The S-T segment and T wave are opposite in direction to the QRS deflection (arrows above).

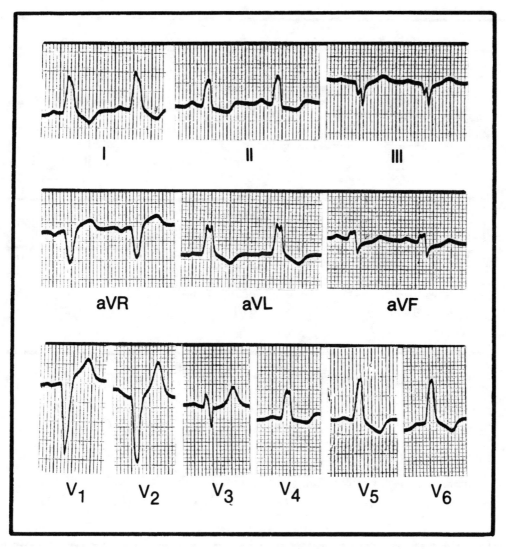

FIGURE 6-17.   Left bundle branch block.

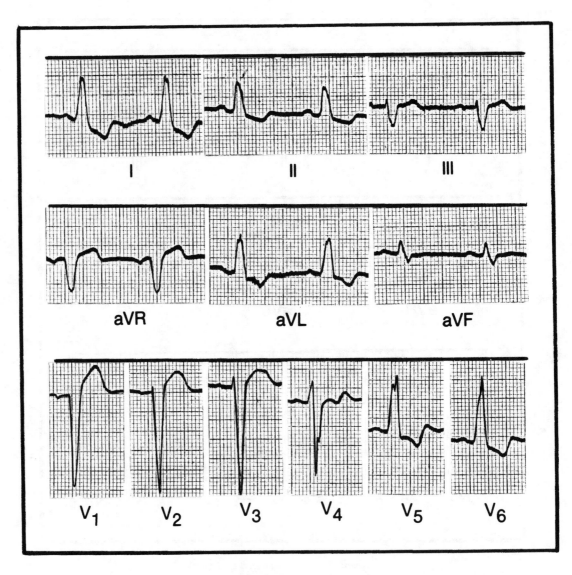

FIGURE 6-18.   Left bundle branch block.

*Left Ventricular Hypertrophy in the Presence
of LBBB*

The electrocardiographic diagnosis of left ventricular hypertrophy in the presence of left bundle branch block remains unsettled. Noble and associates, using echocardiography, found that 89% of their group with left bundle branch block had evidence of left ventricular hypertrophy.[64]

*Myocardial Infarction in the Presence of
LBBB*

Because of the alterations in the initial QRS vectorial forces in left bundle branch block:

1. Myocardial infarction may be simulated (Figure 6-14A and B). In Figure 6-14B, during intermittent left bundle branch block, the small R wave in lead V_1 and the larger R wave in V_2 disappeared entirely. The predominant R wave in V_3 became a predominant S wave. The erroneous diagnosis of anteroseptal myocardial infarction should not be made.
2. Myocardial infarction may be masked (Figure 6-19A and B). Figure 6-19A and B is from a patient with known inferior (diaphragmatic) myocardial infarction (A) who developed left bundle branch block (B). Following development of left bundle branch block, the Q waves in lead II are no longer present, and the Q waves in leads III and aVF have become extremely small.[65]

In answer to pretest Item 5, the development of LBBB in 6-19B must be noted, as well as the masking of electrocardiographic evidence of the inferior myocardial infarction, so clearly seen in Figure 6-19A. The principal criteria of LBBB are outlined on pages 431 and 487.

In spite of the foregoing problems, careful attention may permit the diagnosis of myocardial infarction in the presence of left bundle branch block. In a minority of patients with left bundle branch block, diagnostic Q waves are evident and help in making the diagnosis.[66] Havelda and associates noted that anterior infarction is suggested by a q wave or pathologic Q wave in lead I, a q wave in leads I, V_5, and V_6, or notched S waves in V_3 or V_4.[67]

Repolarization (ST-T) abnormalities will often provide a clue to the presence of myocardial infarction in the presence of left bundle branch block. The acute ST-T changes of myocardial infarction are frequently obvious. It is important to look for ST-T changes beyond the secondary repolarization abnormalities expected with left bundle branch block. This is seen especially well in lead V_6 in Figure 6-19B. The S-T segment depression and T wave inversion are more severe than generally expected.

> The analysis of Figure 6-19 on this page and on page 438 as well as on the tape is the solution to Item 5 on the pretest.

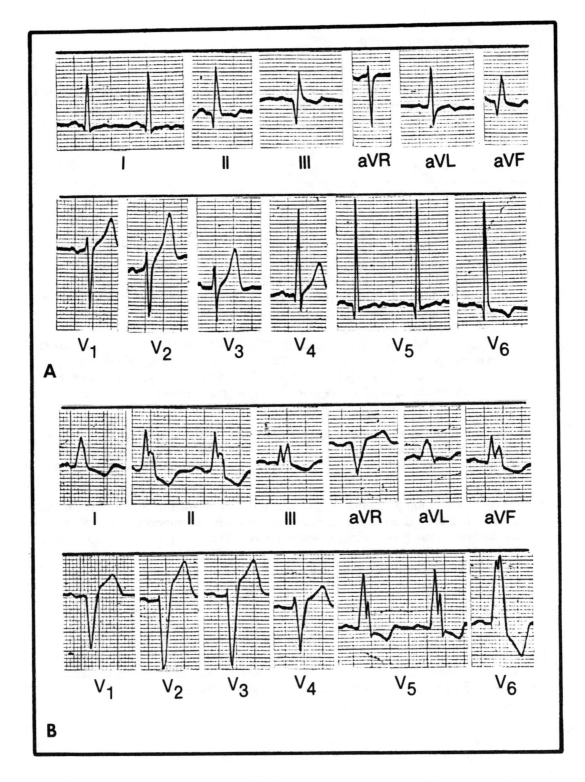

FIGURE 6-19. Development of left bundle branch block in a patient with known inferior (diaphragmatic) myocardial infarction. A, Baseline, with diaphragmatic or inferior myocardial infarction; B, following development of LBBB.

C. The "Hemiblocks" and the "Trifascicular" System

Left axis deviation of the mean QRS vector had, for many years, been considered a major criterion for left ventricular hypertrophy. It has been shown, quite conclusively, that left ventricular hypertrophy, even to a marked degree, is not necessarily accompanied by left axis deviation. Left axis deviation, or perhaps a better term, superiorly oriented QRS vector (in the frontal plane), may be caused by a conduction disturbance in the anterior division of the left bundle branch. Since the left bundle branch comprises two major divisions, the anterior and the posterior division, Rosenbaum,[68] who has helped clarify the subject of intraventricular conduction, recommended the use of the term "hemiblock" to describe a disturbance in either of the divisions. *Left anterior hemiblock* (LAH), therefore, describes a conduction disturbance in the anterior division, and *left posterior hemiblock* (LPH), a disturbance in the posterior division of the left bundle branch. In left anterior hemiblock the mean QRS vector, in the frontal plane, is leftward and superior, or simply superior, and in left posterior hemiblock the mean QRS vector, in the frontal plane, is rightward or frank right axis deviation. Figure 6-20 is a schematic illustration of the hemiblocks.

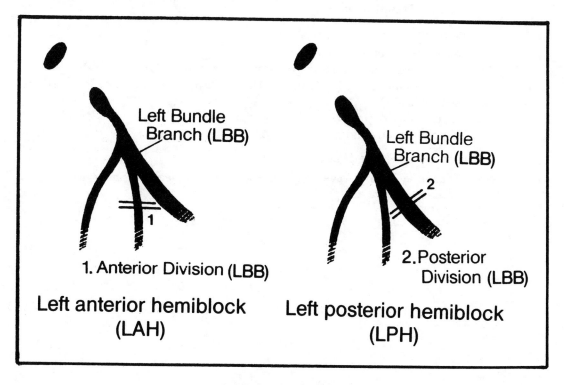

FIGURE 6-20. The "hemiblocks."

TABLE 6-1. Hemiblock Criteria

A. **Left Anterior Hemiblock**

1. *Frontal Plane*
   a. Mean QRS vector usually − 45 to − 75° (often > − 60°)
   b. Small Q wave in leads I and aVL, small R wave in leads II, III, and aVF
   c. QRS interval normal (up to 0.1 sec.) with delayed intrinsicoid deflection (best seen in lead aVL)
   d. Repolarization abnormalities (secondary)

2. *Horizontal Plane* (Criteria not constant)
   a. There may be S waves in leads V_5 and V_6 with absence of Q waves
   b. In right precordial leads there may be a small Q wave or R′

B. **Left Posterior Hemiblock**

1. *Frontal Plane*
   a. Mean QRS vector up to + 120°
   b. Small R wave in leads I and aVL, small Q wave in leads II, III, and aVF
   c. QRS interval normal (up to 0.1 sec.) with delayed intrinsicoid deflection (best seen in lead aVF)
   d. No evidence of right ventricular hypertrophy
   e. Repolarization abnormalities (secondary)

2. *Horizontal Plane* (Criteria not constant)
   a. There may be an R wave or R with small S wave in leads V_5 and V_6 with absence of Q waves

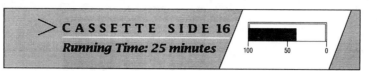

Left Anterior Hemiblock

Left anterior hemiblock is more common than left posterior hemiblock since the anterior division of the left bundle branch is longer, thinner, and has a more tenuous blood supply.

Left Anterior Hemiblock Associated with Anterior Myocardial Infarction. In the study of myocardial infarction it was noted that the *terminal* portion of the QRS complex may *also* be altered by infarction, with no, or almost no, prolongation of the QRS complex itself (Figure 5-22). This is not an infrequent finding in clinical electrocardiography and deserves careful scrutiny. A major cause of *left axis deviation* of the mean QRS vector is an abnormal sequence of depolarization of the left ventricle due to a conduction disturbance in the anterior division of the left bundle branch. Terminal activation must then spread leftward and superiorly from the posterior division, resulting in a leftward and superior orientation of the terminal QRS vector. Before stating that the left anterior hemiblock is due to myocardial infarction, serial electrocardiograms should show that it did not antedate the infarction. Figure 6-21A is from a patient with an acute myocardial infarction. During the recovery phase the mean QRS vector remains oriented abnormally to the left, as seen in Figure 6-21B. Figure 6-21C is the baseline tracing. Eventually, the patient's mean QRS vector returned to the prior state, demonstrating that this disturbance need not be permanent.

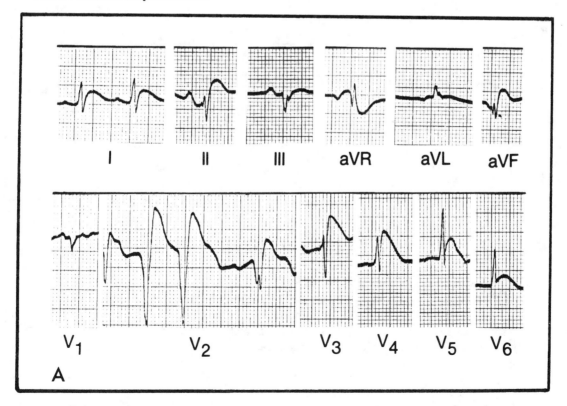

I   II   III   aVR   aVL   aVF

V_1 V_2 V_3 V_4 V_5 V_6

A

FIGURE 6-21A.   Left anterior hemiblock occurring in a patient with an acute myocardial infarction. The mean QRS vector shifted more to the left with the onset of the infarction.

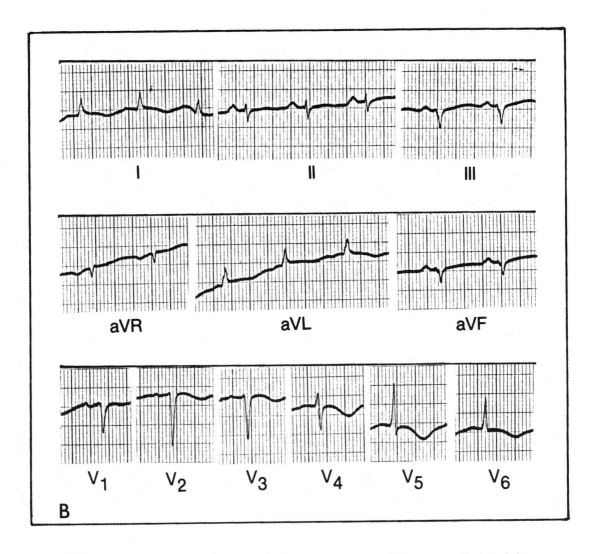

FIGURE 6-21B. Evolutionary changes after myocardial infarction. The mean QRS vector is still oriented abnormally to the left.

Once the major criterion of left axis deviation (-45 to $-75°$) and right axis deviation (up to $+120°$) is evident, researchers will continue to argue whether or not a given electrocardiogram meets the additional criteria of left anterior hemiblock or left posterior hemiblock, respectively. Although additions have been made to Rosenbaum's original criteria, the subject remains a fertile field for continued research.

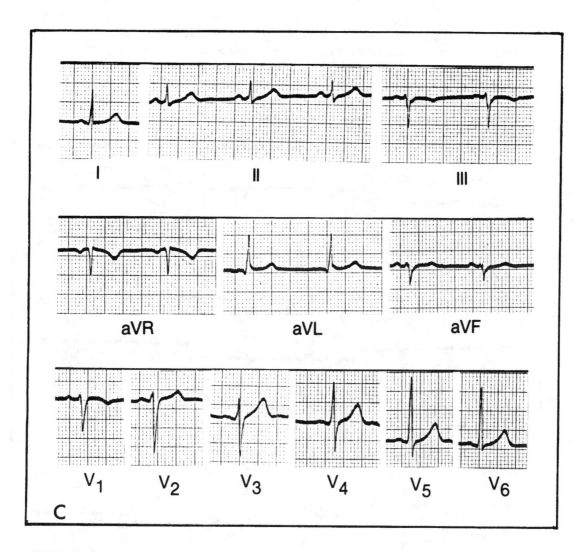

FIGURE 6-21C.   *Baseline electrocardiogram of same patient as in Figures 6-21A and B. Eventually the patient's mean QRS vector returned to the prior state, demonstrating that this disturbance need not be permanent.*

Left Anterior Hemiblock Associated with Chronic Coronary Artery Disease. Frequently, in the absence of myocardial infarction, left anterior hemiblock is present in patients with chronic coronary artery disease. Figure 6-22 is from an elderly patient with angina pectoris and diabetes mellitus. There is no electrocardiographic evidence of myocardial infarction or an enlarged left ventricle. There may, or may not, be repolarization (S-T segment and T wave) abnormalities. It is postulated that the left anterior hemiblock is due to *fibrosis* in the anterior division of the left bundle branch.

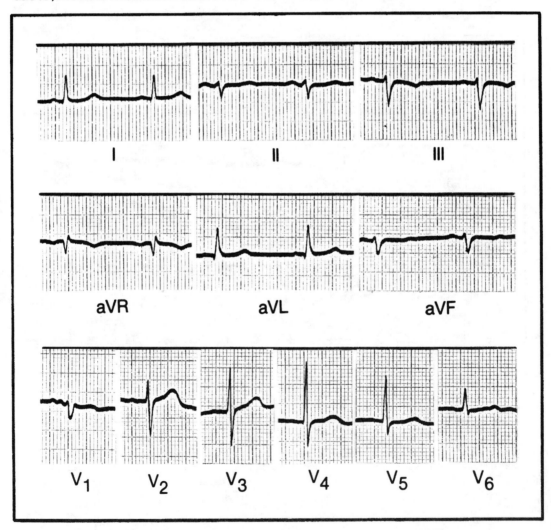

FIGURE 6-22. *Left anterior hemiblock in an elderly patient with chronic coronary artery disease and diabetes mellitus.*

In answering Item 6 on the pretest, since no history was given, the marked left axis deviation (approximately −50°) must be noted.

> The analysis of Figure 6-22 in the text and on the tape is the solution to Item 6 on the pretest.

Left Anterior Hemiblock Associated with Left Ventricular Hypertrophy. Left axis deviation had for many years been considered a major criterion of left ventricular hypertrophy. It is now considered to be a conduction disturbance (left anterior hemiblock) that may or may not accompany left ventricular hypertrophy. In the presence of fibrosis involving the conduction system the two may be found together. Review all the criteria of left ventricular hypertrophy in Figure 6-23.

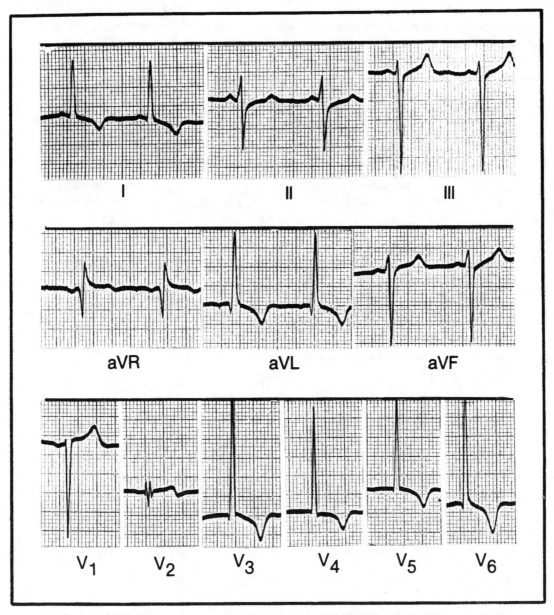

FIGURE 6-23.   Left anterior hemiblock in a patient with left ventricular hypertrophy.

N.B.: Not every abnormal left axis deviation of the mean QRS vector represents left anterior hemiblock.

Left Axis Deviation

Left Axis Deviation Associated with Inferior (Diaphragmatic) Myocardial Infarction. The abnormal leftward axis of the mean QRS vector in Figure 6-24 is due to the Q waves or QS complexes in leads II, III, and aVF, representing the inferior wall myocardial infarction, rather than to large terminal S waves preceded by smaller initial R waves. Review the criteria for left anterior hemiblock. A case, however, could be made for both, inferior myocardial infarction and left anterior hemiblock, with the left axis deviation, terminal R′ wave in lead aVR and absence of a terminal R wave in leads II, III, and aVF.[69] As noted earlier, there is much yet to be learned in the area of intraventricular conduction.

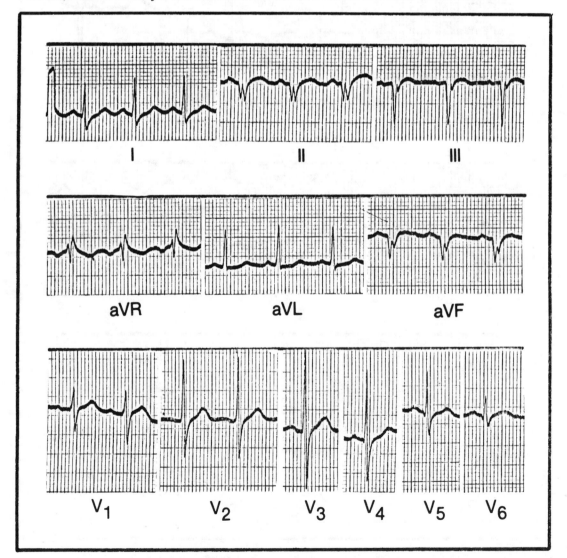

FIGURE 6-24.   Inferior-posterior myocardial infarction.

Left Axis Deviation Associated with Pulmonary Emphysema. Left axis deviation is found in a small percentage of patients with pulmonary emphysema. The mechanism is not clear since, in the majority of patients with emphysema, who have similar deformity of the chest and hyperinflation of the lungs, the mean QRS vector is normal, vertical, or even rightward. Figure 6-25 is from a patient with severe, chronic obstructive lung disease. Recognized authorities have argued that the left axis deviation associated with pulmonary emphysema is really left anterior hemiblock and may be the only indication of disease of the left ventricle. Research in this area is in progress. Low QRS complex amplitude is common in patients with emphysema.

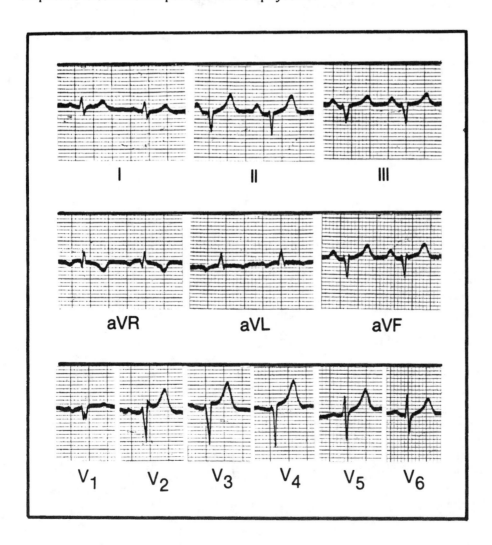

FIGURE 6-25.   *Left axis deviation in a patient with pulmonary emphysema.*

Left Axis Deviation in the "Otherwise Normal" Patient. Left axis deviation is sometimes found in a young "otherwise normal" patient. Figure 6-26 is from a 30-year-old "healthy" man. Laboratory studies and chest x-ray were within normal limits. Although the left axis deviation is abnormal, the criteria for left anterior hemiblock are not clearly met. Still, the possibility of a congenital block in the anterior division of the left bundle branch must be considered. Thorough follow-up of these patients for many years is needed for evaluation of this entity.

Although discussion of these is beyond the scope of our present study, left axis deviation has also been associated with various congenital heart lesions.

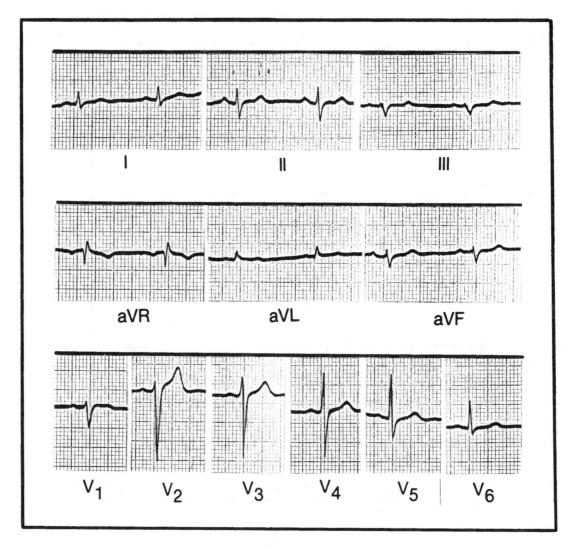

FIGURE 6-26. Left axis deviation in an "otherwise normal" patient.

Left Posterior Hemiblock

Left posterior hemiblock is less common than left anterior hemiblock because of the more secure blood supply to the posterior division of the left bundle branch. Figure 6-27A is from a patient with true posterior myocardial infarction who developed left posterior hemiblock. Review the criteria for left posterior hemiblock at this point. The criteria for left posterior hemiblock, especially in the precordial leads, are not strictly met on this electrocardiogram; however, a major change in the orientation of the mean

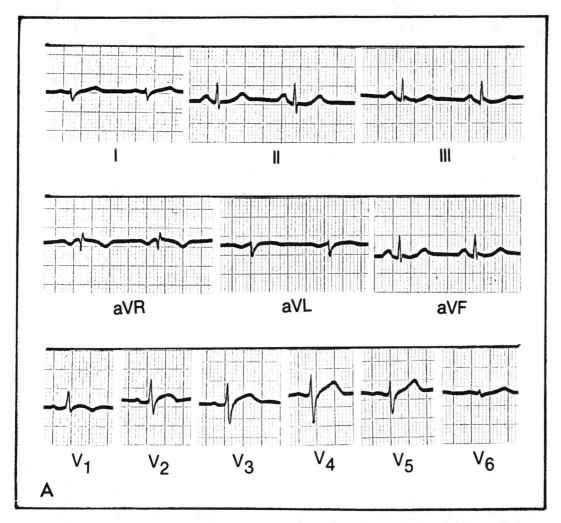

FIGURE 6-27A.   *Right axis deviation in a patient with true posterior myocardial infarction, presumed left posterior hemiblock. Although the criteria for left posterior hemiblock are not strictly met, there was neither right ventricular hypertrophy nor increased pressure in the right atrium, right ventricle, or pulmonary artery.*

QRS vector took place which cannot be explained on the basis of the myocardial infarction alone. There was no right ventricular hypertrophy or increased pressure in the right atrium, right ventricle, or pulmonary artery. The left posterior hemiblock is presumed here. As clearly stated by Rosenbaum, LPH cannot be a pure electrocardiographic diagnosis; it must necessarily be a clinical-electrocardiographic diagnosis.

At the time of the myocardial infarction the patient also had an atrioventricular conduction disturbance known as Mobitz I block. This is illustrated in Figure 6-27B and will be seen again in Chapter 7 (Figure 7-42).

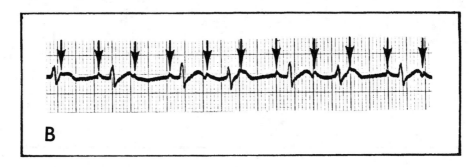

FIGURE 6-27B.   Same patient as in Figure 6-27A. Atrioventricular conduction disturbance at time of true posterior myocardial infarction. The arrows point to the P waves.

Trifascicular System

Both divisions of the left bundle branch (1 and 2 in Figure 6-28) plus the right bundle branch (3) have been termed the "trifascicular" system of intraventricular conduction. Each of the three component parts is called a fascicle. For example, right bundle branch block plus left anterior hemiblock or right bundle branch block plus left posterior hemiblock could be called *bifascicular* block. Examples and diagrams will be seen in the figures to follow. Block in all three fascicles would result in complete atrioventricular (A-V) block.

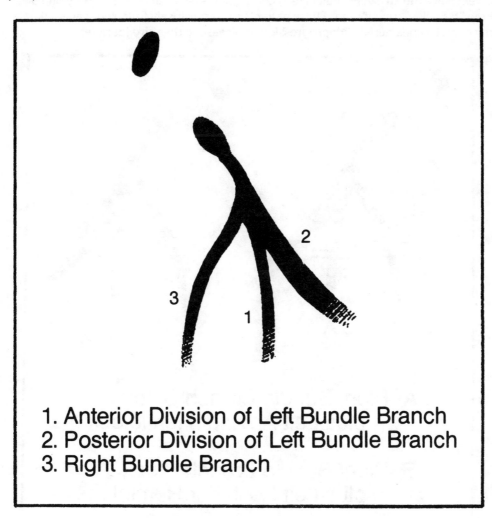

1. Anterior Division of Left Bundle Branch
2. Posterior Division of Left Bundle Branch
3. Right Bundle Branch

FIGURE 6-28. The "trifascicular" system.

Left anterior hemiblock is much more common than left posterior hemiblock, as already noted, since the anterior division of the left bundle branch is longer, thinner, and has a more tenuous blood supply.

The combination of right bundle branch block (RBBB) plus left anterior hemiblock (LAH) is seen in Figures 6-29A, 6-30, and 6-31. Right bundle branch block plus left posterior hemiblock (LPH) is seen in Figures 6-29B and 6-32B. This combination may augur ill for the patient since the atrioventricular (A-V) conduction system depends on only one of the three "fascicles" functioning. These patients must be closely followed; pacemaker therapy must be considered with progression of disease to the third fascicle.

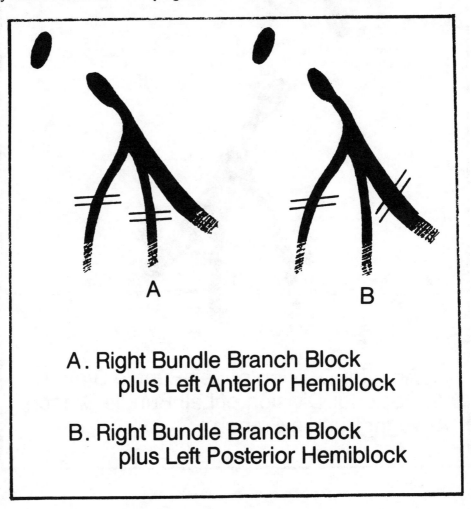

A. Right Bundle Branch Block plus Left Anterior Hemiblock

B. Right Bundle Branch Block plus Left Posterior Hemiblock

FIGURE 6-29. Types of "bifascicular" block.

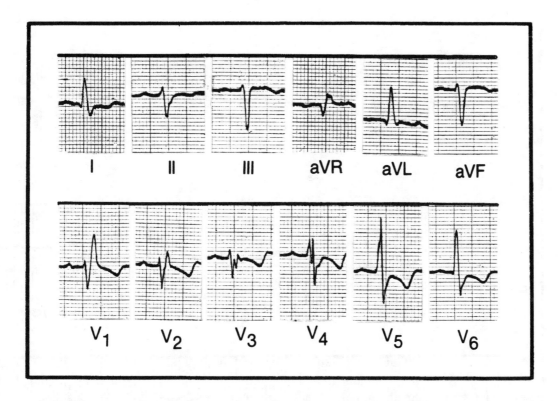

FIGURE 6-30.   *Bifascicular block. Right bundle branch block plus left anterior hemiblock is not an infrequent association. What may follow this state? Note also that the repolarization abnormalities are primary (arrows).*

In answer to Item 7 on the pretest it should be noted that:

1. Bifascicular block is present (RBBB + (LAH).

2. Primary repolarization abnormalities are evident. As noted on page 418, *secondary* repolarization abnormalities are expected with RBBB. The T wave is *opposite* in direction to the terminal deflection of the QRS complex. In Figure 6-30 it is noted, however, that the T waves are in the *same* direction as the terminal QRS deflections, especially well seen in leads V_5 and V_6; these represent primary repolarization abnormalities.

> The analysis of Figure 6-30 in the text and on the tape is the solution to Item 7 on the pretest.

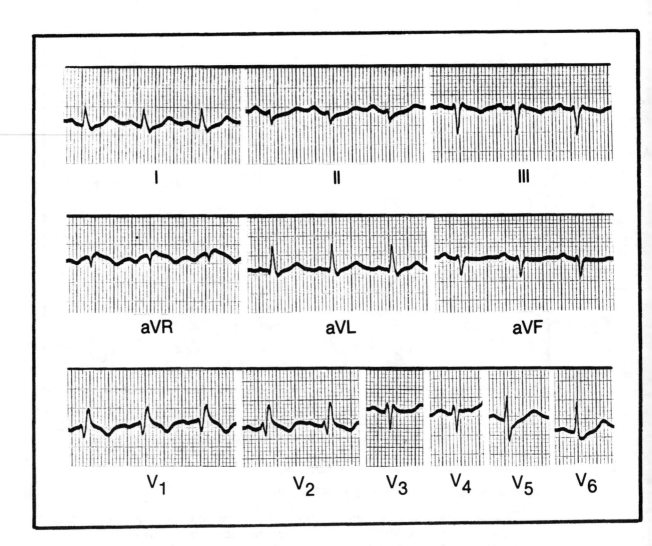

FIGURE 6-31.   Right bundle branch block plus left anterior hemiblock. In this combination of conduction distur-bances the S wave in lead I is often quite small and the QRS complex might resemble that of a left bundle branch block. The RSR' in lead V₁, however, remains the key to the correct diagnosis.

In answering Item 8 on the pretest (Figure 6-32) the following should be noted:

A. Inferior myocardial infarction (Q waves in leads II, III, and aVF).

B. 1. Acute anterior myocardial infarction (Q waves and repolarization abnormalities in leads V_1 to V_5).

    2. RBBB (see principal criteria on pages 418 and 486).

    3. Right axis deviation (left posterior hemiblock); RBBB + LPH represents a bifasci-cular block.

The analysis of Figure 6-32 on this page and next as well as on the tape is the solution to Item 8 on the pretest.

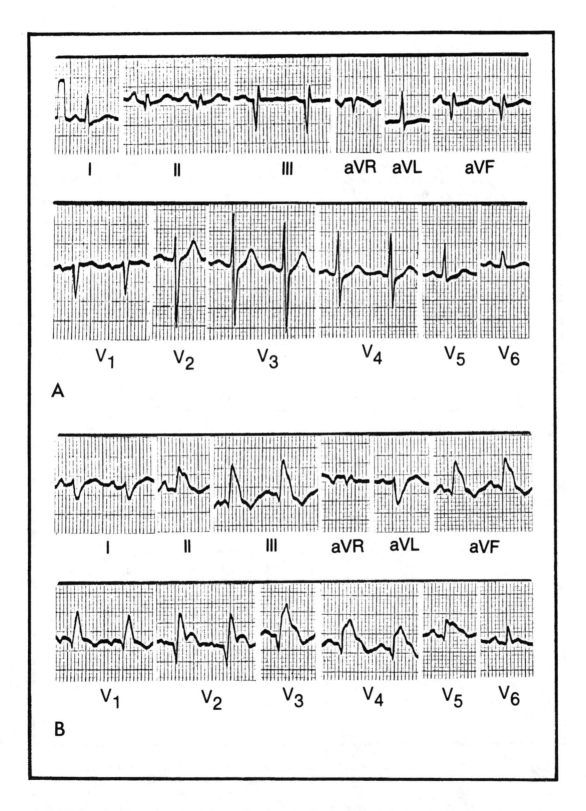

FIGURE 6-32.   *Development of* right bundle branch block *plus* left posterior hemiblock *with acute anterior myocardial infarction in a patient with a history of old inferior (diaphragmatic) myocardial infarction. Note the marked shift of the mean QRS axis to the right in B. A, Baseline, with inferior myocardial infarction; B, following acute onset of anterior myocardial infarction, RBBB with right axis deviation.*

Figure 6-33 (A to E) is from a patient who in the course of an anterior myocardial infarction (B) developed right bundle branch block plus left anterior hemiblock (C). Cardiac pacing was required with the development of complete atrioventricular block (D). When the patient's sinus rhythm returned spontaneously he no longer had left anterior hemiblock but left posterior hemiblock plus right bundle branch block (E). This series comprises a review of the subject of fascicular blocks.

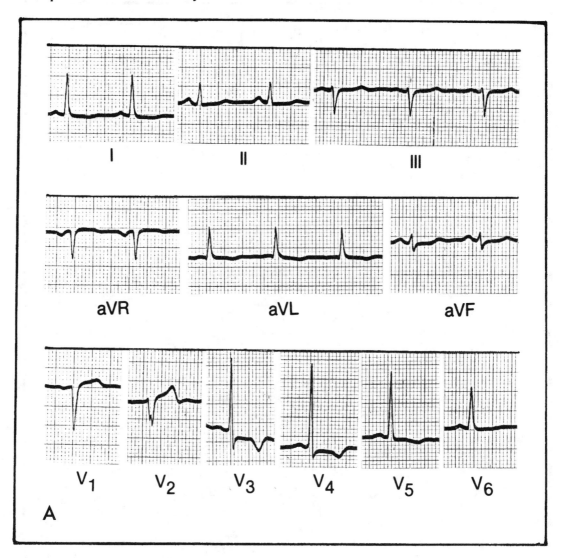

FIGURE 6-33A.   Baseline. Figures 6-33B to E are from the same patient during an anterior wall myocardial infarction. The mean QRS vector is at 0° in the frontal plane, with the transition at lead aVF.

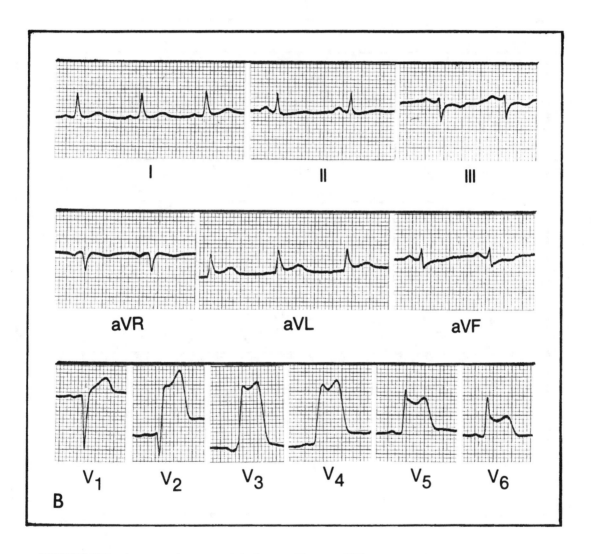

B

FIGURE 6-33B.   Acute anterior myocardial infarction. The mean QRS vector remains essentially unchanged.
Note the hyperacute ST-T changes with the infarction. See page 400 for the evolutionary changes of myocardial
infarction.

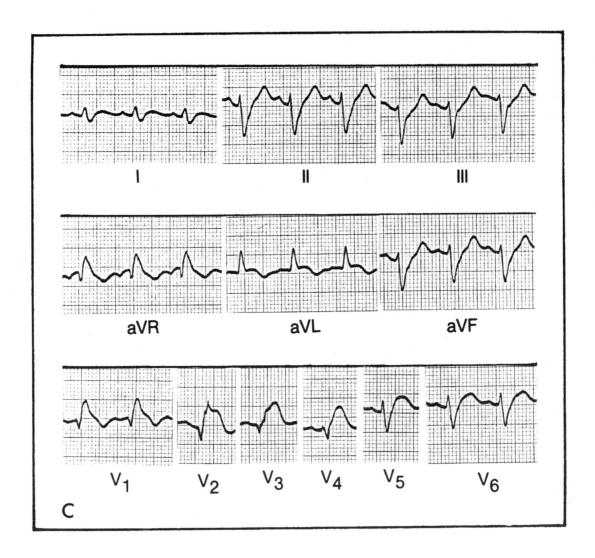

FIGURE 6-33C. *Bifascicular block (right bundle branch block plus left anterior hemiblock) one day after Figure 6-33B.*

REVIEW—Describe the electrocardiographic findings in

1. Anterior myocardial infarction with evolutionary changes
2. RBBB ⎱ bifascicular block
3. LAH ⎰

The mean QRS vector in the frontal plane shifted markedly to the *left* with the onset of *left anterior hemiblock (LAH)*. Note the wide QRS complex, the broad S wave in lead I and the terminal R wave in lead V_1, signifying *right bundle branch block (RBBB)*. The patient developed *bifascicular block* (RBBB + LAH). The evolutionary changes of myocardial infarction are also evident.

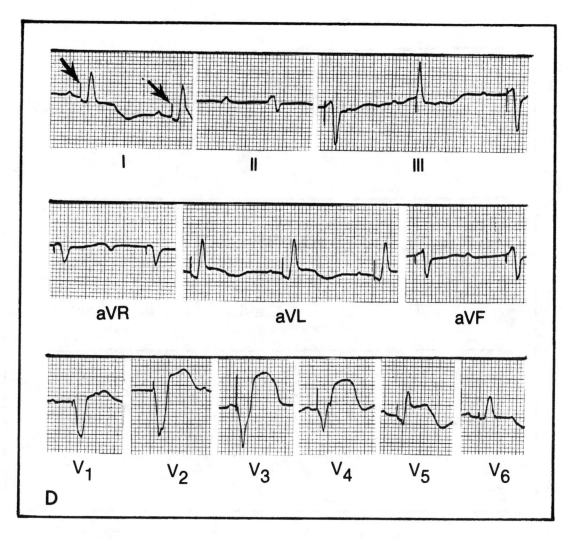

FIGURE 6-33D.   Cardiac pacing due to complete A-V block. The arrows in lead I point to the pacemaker impulses. The middle beat in lead III is conducted, with a prolonged P-R interval. Same evening as Figure 6-33C. When the patient developed block in the third fascicle, the left posterior fascicle, resulting in trifascicular block, electrical pacing was necessary.

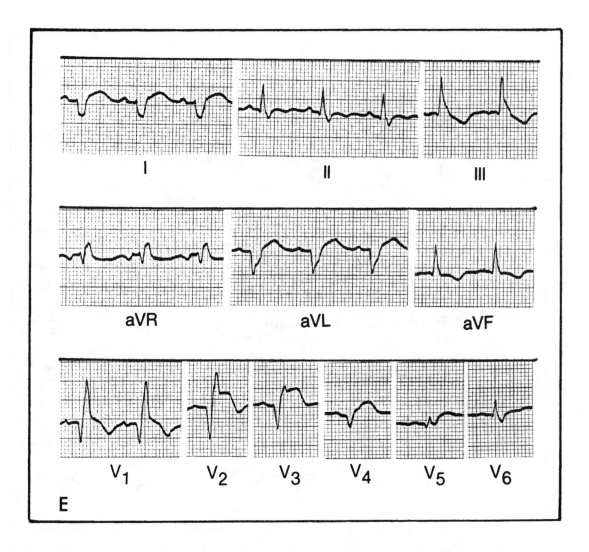

FIGURE 6-33E.   Bifascicular block (right bundle branch block plus left posterior hemiblock) 1 week after Figure 6-33D.

REVIEW—Describe the electrocardiographic findings in LPH + RBBB (bifascicular block)

Following several days of pacing, the *left anterior fascicle* recovered and the patient had 1:1 atrioventricular conduction. The mean QRS vector in the frontal plane shifted markedly to the *right* with the onset of left posterior hemiblock.

Left Bundle Branch Block Plus
Left Axis Deviation

In studying the onset of left bundle branch block, in contrast to left anterior or left posterior hemiblock, we noted some shifting of the mean QRS vector in the frontal plane without the development of either frank left axis deviation or frank right axis deviation. Our series revealed some movement either to the left or to the right as seen in Figures 6-14 (A and B), 6-15 (A and B), and 6-19 (A and B). Where we did find a combination of left bundle branch block plus left axis deviation, the left axis deviation antedated the left bundle branch block. The significance of this combination has been the subject of various studies.[6-10,6-11] Dhingra and associates found that among patients with left bundle branch block, those with left axis deviation had a greater incidence of myocardial dysfunction, more advanced conduction disease, and greater cardiovascular mortality than those with a normal axis.[6-12] This combination is seen in Figures 6-34 through 6-36.

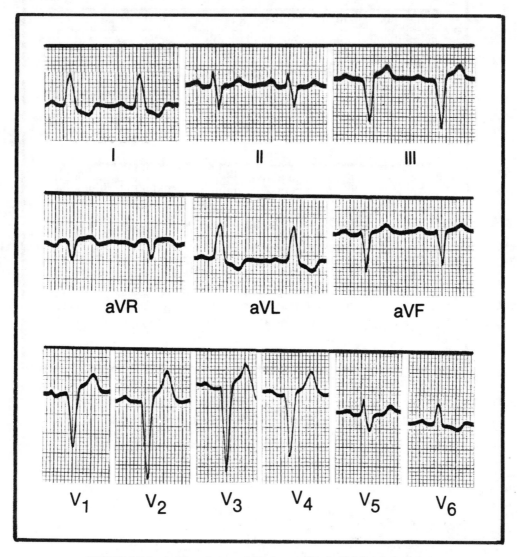

FIGURE 6-34.   Left bundle branch block associated with left axis deviation.

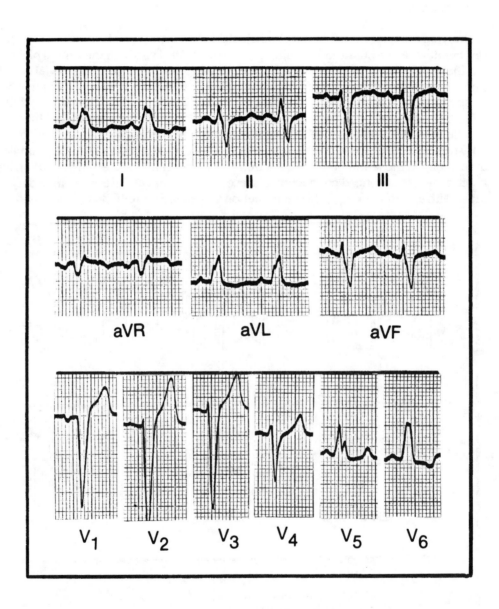

FIGURE 6-35. *Left bundle branch block associated with left axis deviation.*

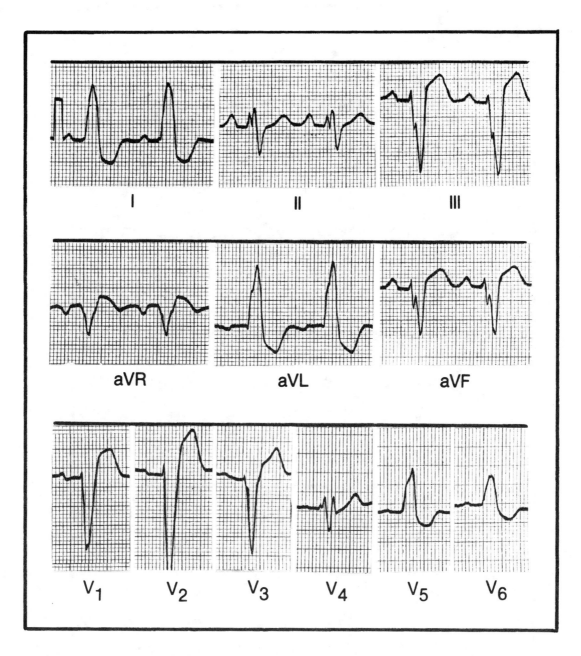

FIGURE 6-36.   *Left bundle branch block associated with left axis deviation.*

D. $S_I S_{II} S_{III}$ SYNDROME

The $S_I S_{II} S_{III}$ syndrome,[6-13] in which there are prominent S waves in the three standard leads with no prolongation of the QRS interval and, at times, with an R′ in lead V_1 (terminal QRS vector which is to the right, superior, and sometimes anterior) has been found:

1. In normal patients.

2. In patients with right ventricular hypertrophy, both congenital and acquired (such as cor pulmonale).

3. In patients with acute myocardial infarction without complicating cor pulmonale.

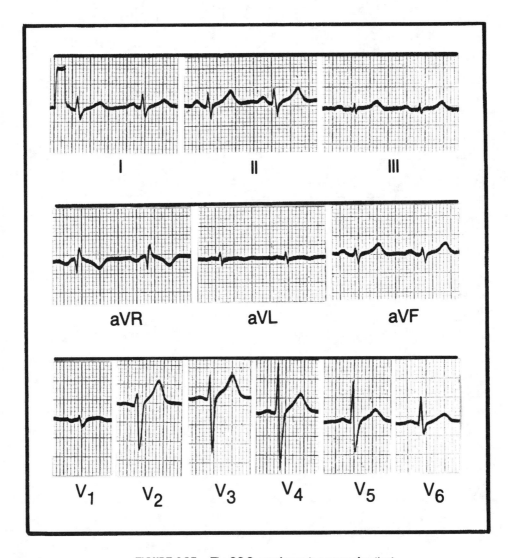

FIGURE 6-37.   The $S_I S_{II} S_{III}$ syndrome in a normal patient.

Figure 6-37 is from a "normal" patient with the $S_I S_{II} S_{III}$ syndrome. The patient was normotensive with no evidence of heart disease by history, on physical examination, chest x-ray, and laboratory studies.

Figure 6-38 is from a patient with severe chronic obstructive lung disease and cor pulmonale, and Figure 6-39A and B is from a patient who developed the $S_IS_{II}S_{III}$ syndrome with acute anterior myocardial infarction.

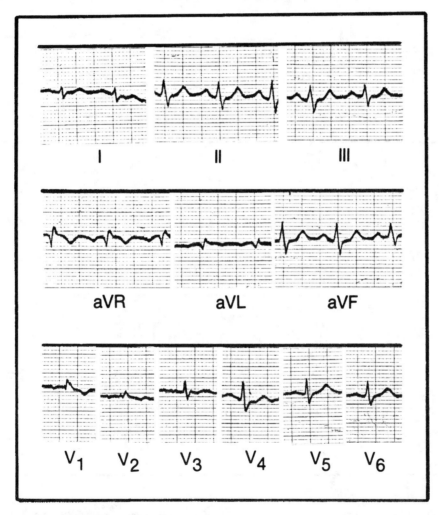

FIGURE 6-38.   The $S_IS_{II}S_{III}$ syndrome in a patient with severe chronic obstructive lung disease and cor pulmonale. Note the small QRS deflections in all the leads, not uncommon in patients with severe hyperinflation of the lungs (pulmonary emphysema).

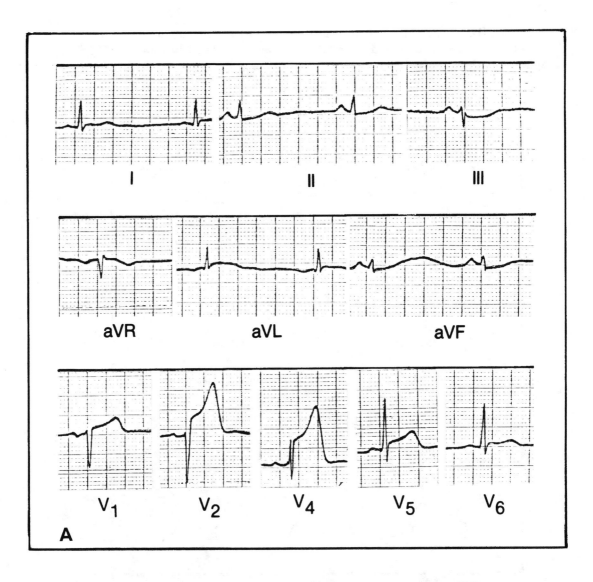

FIGURE 6-39A.   Patient with acute anterior myocardial infarction. Note the mean QRS vector.

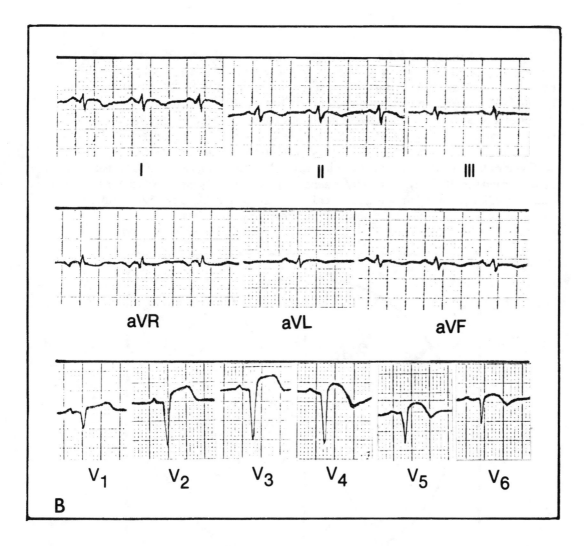

FIGURE 6-39B.　Same patient as in Figure 6-39A, with onset of $S_IS_{II}S_{III}$ syndrome during the acute myocardial infarction.

Item 9 on the pretest, since Figure 6-39A was not available, requires that the following be noted:

1. The presence of the $S_IS_{II}S_{III}$ syndrome.

2. Anterior myocardial infarction. The infarction appears to be recent with repolarization (S-T segment and T wave) abnormalities in addition to the QS complexes across the precordium. However, since no history was given, it could represent a ventricular aneurysm following an old myocardial infarction. An example was seen in the study of myocardial infarction (Figure 5-18).

> The analysis of Figure 6-39B in the text and on the tape is the solution to Item 9 on the pretest.

In Figures 6-37, 6-38, and 6-39B it is not possible to plot a mean QRS vector in the frontal plane using the entire QRS complex, since in every lead of the frontal plane the QRS complex is biphasic. To plot the QRS vectorial forces properly, the QRS complexes must be divided into initial and terminal vectors. In Figure 6-40 it is seen that the initial QRS vectorial forces are approximately along the axis of positive lead II and the terminal QRS vectorial forces are along the axis of negative lead II, in the opposite direction. In summary, in the $S_I S_{II} S_{III}$ syndrome the initial QRS is to the left and inferior, and the terminal QRS vector is to the right and superior in the frontal plane. Bayés de Luna and associates have studied the $S_I S_{II} S_{III}$ syndrome by means of spatial-velocity electrocardiograms and thallium-201 myocardial imaging to elucidate the electrophysiology.[6-14] A complete explanation has not been given, however, and research continues.

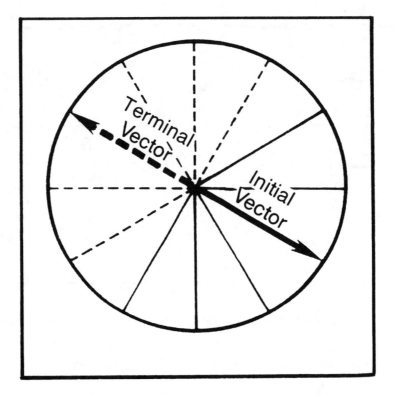

FIGURE 6-40. *Initial and terminal vectorial forces of the QRS in the $S_I S_{II} S_{III}$ syndrome.*

E. Pre-excitation

Wolff-Parkinson-White (W-P-W) Syndrome

In 1930 Louis Wolff, John Parkinson, and Paul Dudley White published their classic study of eleven cases entitled: "Bundle branch block with short P-R interval in healthy young people prone to paroxysmal tachycardia."[6-15] This is known universally as the Wolff-Parkinson-White or W-P-W syndrome. It does not represent bundle branch block as was once thought. Wolff, in a later paper, enumerated the various names given to this syndrome as the Wolff-Parkinson-White (W-P-W) syndrome, anomalous atrioventricular excitation, the syndrome of the short P-R interval with abnormal QRS complexes and paroxysmal tachycardia, pre-excitation, and the bundle of Kent syndrome.[6-16] The electrocardiographic pattern is characterized by a:

1. Short P-R interval (0.12 sec. or less).
2. Prolonged QRS interval (greater than 0.1 sec.).
3. Slurring of the upstroke by a *delta* wave.

The mechanism responsible for this syndrome is illustrated in Figure 6-41.[6-17] There is an accessory atrioventricular pathway, the bundle of Kent, in addition to the A-V node. Conduction from the atria to the ventricles through the accessory pathway occurs before the normal conduction through the A-V node resulting in pre-excitation of the ventricles. Pre-excitation refers to the earlier activation of the ventricles than would normally be expected. Conduction through the accessory pathway bypasses the A-V node and its normal delay. Since this pre-excitation results in asynchronous activation of the ventricles, a wide and abnormal appearing QRS deflection is inscribed. Usually, before completion of this deflection, the remainder of ventricular activation is through the normal conduction system. The resulting QRS complex, therefore, begins with a slurred upstroke known as the *delta* wave (conduction through the bundle of Kent).

The early classification of W-P-W pattern in type A and type B is still used today:

Type A: The R wave is the main ventricular deflection in, at least, leads V_1 and V_2.

Type B: The S wave or the QS complex is the main ventricular deflection in, at least, lead V_1.

Grant suggested a classification on the basis of the axis of the delta wave,[6-18] while Sherf and Neufeld recommended a classification based on the combination of the frontal and horizontal planes.[6-19]

The important features of the Wolff-Parkinson-White syndrome include the following:

1. The association of the W-P-W syndrome with supraventricular tachycardias—namely reentrant (reciprocating) supraventricular tachycardia, atrial fibrillation and atrial flutter. An example of an arrhythmia associated with an accessory pathway is seen in Figure 6-44A. These arrhythmias will receive further attention in the next chapter, and reentry is explained and illustrated in Chapter 7 (pages 597 to 599).

2. The alternation of normal conduction with the W-P-W syndrome is frequent and can make the search for the etiology of a supraventricular tachycardia a difficult one.

3. The electrocardiogram must be carefully scrutinized since:

    a. A negative delta wave may cause Q waves or QS complexes simulating myocardial infarction (Figure 6-43: QS complexes are seen in leads III and V_1).

    b. The delta wave may obscure the electrocardiographic evidence of myocardial infarction.

    c. The tall R waves in lead V_1 in the W-P-W syndrome, type A (Figure 6-42), may cause the diagnosis of true posterior myocardial infarction or right ventricular hypertrophy to be made.

    d. Secondary S-T segment and T wave abnormalities occur and may obscure primary abnormalities.

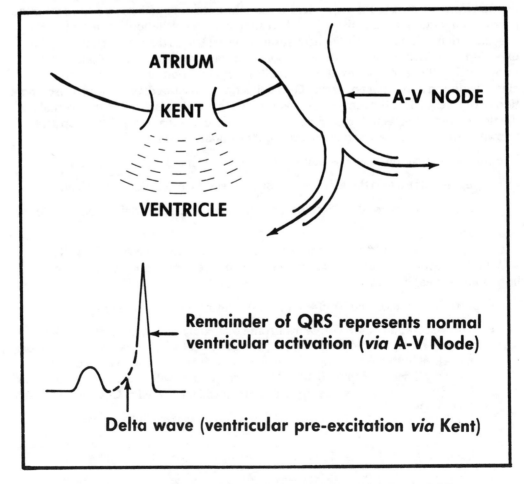

FIGURE 6-41.   Pre-excitation—the Wolff-Parkinson-White or W-P-W syndrome.[6-17]

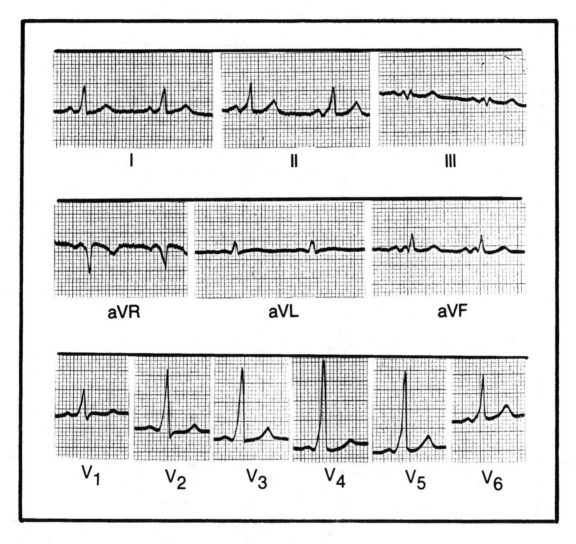

FIGURE 6-42. *Wolff-Parkinson-White syndrome, type A. Note that all the precordial complexes are upright. Describe the typical findings in this syndrome.*

The electrocardiographic criteria of the W-P-W syndrome, type A is characterized by a (an):

1. Short P-R interval (0.12 sec. or less).
2. Prolonged QRS interval (greater than 0.1 sec.).
3. Slurring of the upstroke by a *delta* wave.
4. R wave that is the main ventricular deflection in, at least, leads V_1 and V_2.

> The analysis of Figure 6-42 in the text and on the tape is the solution to Item 10 on the pretest.

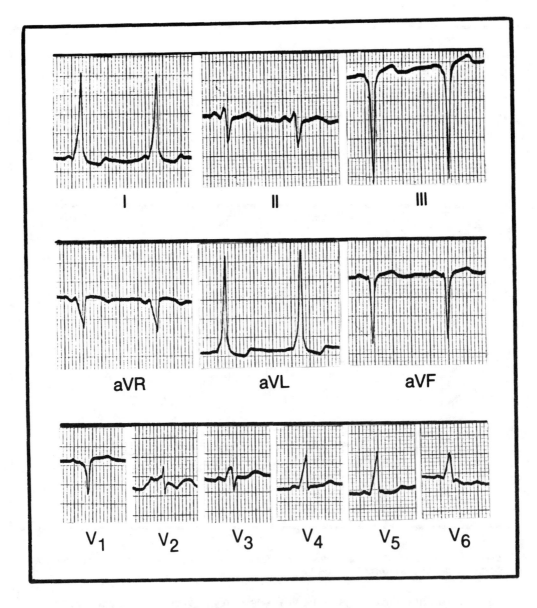

FIGURE 6-43.   Wolff-Parkinson-White syndrome, type B. Note that the QRS complex in lead V₁ is negative, in contrast to Figure 6-42. A negative delta wave may cause Q waves or QS complexes simulating myocardial infarction. QS complexes are present in leads III and V₁.

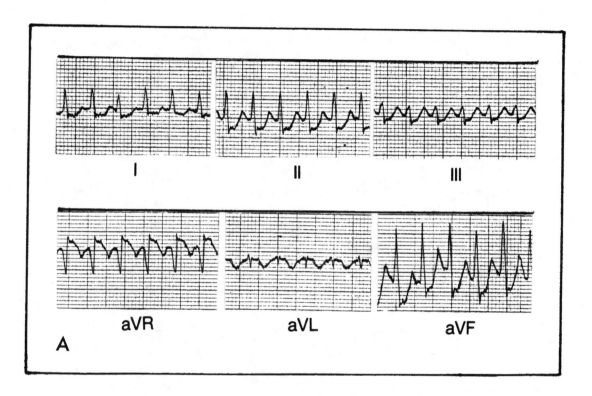

FIGURE 6-44A.   *Electrocardiogram of an 18-year-old patient who came to the emergency room because of rapid heart action. Diagnosis?*

The patient presented with a heart rate of more than 200 beats per minute. Even an 18-year-old patient may be quite symptomatic at this heart rate. Following cardioversion, the W-P-W syndrome became apparent. Figure 6-44B shows both the normal conduction and conduction through an accessory pathway. The negative delta waves in leads I and aVL may be mistaken for an anterolateral or lateral myocardial infarction. The prominent R waves in lead V_1 may simulate right ventricular hypertrophy or true posterior myocardial infarction. On the following day (Figure 6-44C) we see conduction only through the accessory pathway.

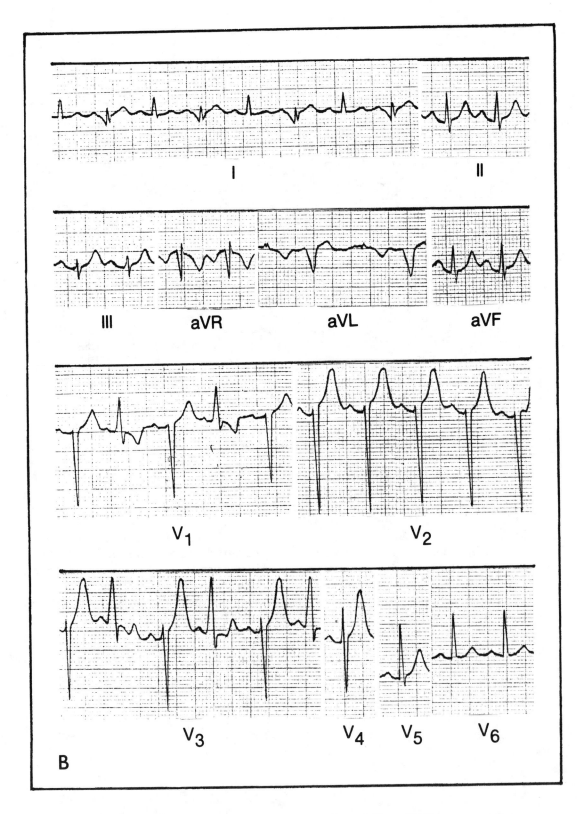

B

FIGURE 6-44B.   After cardioversion: same patient as in Figure 6-44A.

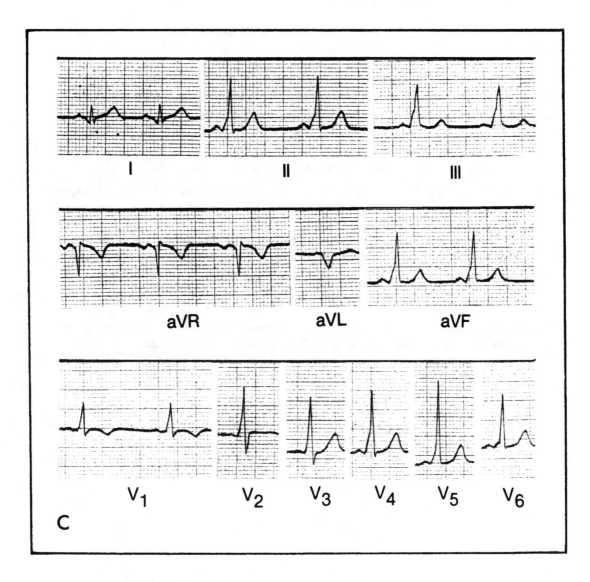

FIGURE 6-44C.   Same patient as in Figure 6-44A and B (W-P-W, Type A).

Review: In Chapter 2 you learned that the differential diagnosis of an R wave which is the main ventricular deflection in lead V_1 includes:

1. Right ventricular hypertrophy.
2. True posterior myocardial infarction.
3. Right bundle branch block.
4. Wolff-Parkinson-White syndrome, type A.

> A QRS complex with a "delta-like" wave is illustrated on page 488. It may be mistaken for the W-P-W syndrome at a certain *critical rate.*

Lown-Ganong-Levine (L-G-L) Syndrome

Lown, Ganong, and Levine described the syndrome of the short P-R interval (less than 0.12 sec.), *normal* QRS complex, and paroxysmal rapid heart action.[620] An example of the L-G-L syndrome is seen in the next chapter (Figure 7-11B). Caracta and associates studied 18 patients with a short P-R interval (<0.12 sec.) and normal QRS complex.[621] Eight had a history of supraventricular tachycardia. Among the possible explanations for the short P-R interval were the following:

1. Total or partial bypass of the A-V node.
2. An anatomically small A-V node.
3. Short or rapidly conducting intranodal pathway.

Benditt and associates demonstrated that A-V nodal refractory periods were shorter, and enhanced A-V conduction more frequent in L-G-L patients compared with normal controls.[622] Josephson and Kastor studied the mechanism of the abbreviated A-V nodal conduction time and paroxysmal supraventricular tachycardia in six patients with the L-G-L syndrome.[623] Their findings included dual A-V nodal pathways and suggested that preferential rapidly conducting A-V nodal fibers and intranodal reentry are the responsible mechanisms in these patients with the L-G-L syndrome and reciprocating tachycardia.

Of historical interest, Katz and Pick called this rhythm the *coronary nodal rhythm* stating that "it is diagnosed when, with the P-R interval between 0.02 and 0.10 second, the P waves in leads I and II are upright. Usually the P-R interval is nearer 0.10 second."[624]

> Stop the tape and begin the post-test on the next page.

P O S T · T E S T

DIRECTIONS.   Supply the information requested in each of the following.

1. Explain why the electrocardiographic manifestations of myocardial infarction may be both (a) simulated and (b) masked in the presence of left bundle branch block (LBBB) and in the Wolff-Parkinson-White (W-P-W) syndrome.

2. Why is left anterior hemiblock more common than left posterior hemiblock?

3. State the electrocardiographic criteria for left anterior hemiblock and left posterior hemiblock in both the frontal and horizontal planes.

4. What is the "trifascicular" system of intraventricular conduction?

5. What is the $S_I S_{II} S_{III}$ syndrome? Where is it found and why is it not possible to plot a mean QRS vector in the frontal plane?

6. Explain what is mean by the "hemiblocks."

7. (a) Are the initial QRS vectorial forces affected by RBBB? Why is this important?

   (b) Why are the electrocardiographic manifestations of right bundle branch block in the presence of anterior myocardial infarction of special interest?

8. List three electrocardiographic findings in the Wolff-Parkinson-White (W-P-W) syndrome.

9. List three QRS alterations that occur with the onset of right bundle branch block.

10. Explain the common QRS changes that occur with the onset of left bundle branch block (QRS interval, initial and terminal QRS vectorial alterations).

> Check your responses on the following pages.

ANSWERS TO
POST-TEST

1. Left Bundle Branch Block

   Because of the alterations in the initial QRS vectorial forces in left bundle branch block, myocardial infarction may be simulated or masked.

   a. In Figure 6-14B, during intermittent left bundle branch block, the small R wave in lead V_1 and the larger R wave in V_2 disappeared entirely. The predominant R wave in V_3 became a predominant S wave. The erroneous diagnosis of anteroseptal myocardial infarction should not be made.

   b. Figure 6-19A and B is from a patient with known diaphragmatic myocardial infarction (A) who developed left bundle branch block (B). Following development of left bundle branch block the Q waves in lead II are no longer present and the Q waves in leads III and aVF have become extremely small.

   Wolff-Parkinson-White Syndrome

   a. The delta waves may cause Q waves and QS complexes resembling myocardial infarction (Figure 6-43: QS complexes are seen in leads III and V_1).

   b. The delta waves may obscure the electrocardiographic evidence of myocardial infarction.

   c. The tall R waves in lead V_1 in the W-P-W syndrome, type A (Figure 6-42), may cause the diagnosis of posterior myocardial infarction or right ventricular hypertrophy to be made.

2. Left anterior hemiblock is much more common than left posterior hemiblock since the anterior division of the left bundle branch is longer, thinner, and has a more tenuous blood supply.

3. **TABLE 6-1.   HEMIBLOCK CRITERIA**

   A. Left Anterior Hemiblock
   1. *Frontal Plane*
      a. Mean QRS vector usually -45 to $-75°$ (often $> -60°$)
      b. Small Q wave in leads I and aVL, small R wave in leads II, III, and aVF
      c. QRS interval normal (up to 0.1 sec.) with delayed intrinsicoid deflection (best seen in lead aVL)
      d. Repolarization abnormalities (secondary)
   2. *Horizontal Plane* (Criteria not constant)
      a. There may be S waves in leads V_5 and V_6 with absence of Q waves
      b. In right precordial leads there may be a small Q wave or R'

   B. Left Posterior Hemiblock
   1. *Frontal Plane*
      a. Mean QRS vector up to $+120°$
      b. Small R wave in leads I and aVL, small Q wave in leads II, III, and aVF
      c. QRS interval normal (up to 0.1 sec.) with delayed intrinsicoid deflection (best seen in lead aVF)
      d. No evidence of right ventricular hypertrophy
      e. Repolarization abnormalities (secondary)
   2. *Horizontal Plane* (Criteria not constant)
      There may be an R wave or R with small S wave in leads V_5 and V_6 with absence of Q waves

4. The "Trifascicular" System

   Both divisions of the left bundle branch (1 and 2 in Figure 6-28) plus the right bundle branch (3) have been termed the "trifascicular" system of intraventricular conduction. Each of the three component parts is called a fascicle.

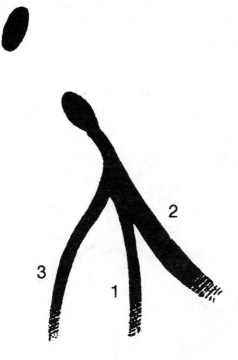

   # 1. Anterior Division of Left Bundle Branch
   # 2. Posterior Division of Left Bundle Branch
   # 3. Right Bundle Branch

   FIGURE 6-28.   The "trifascicular" system.

5. The $S_I S_{II} S_{III}$ syndrome, in which there are prominent S waves in the three standard leads with no prolongation of the QRS interval and, at times, with an R' in lead V_1 (terminal QRS vector which is to the right, superior and sometimes anterior) has been found in:

   a. Normal patients.

   b. Patients with right ventricular hypertrophy, both congenital and acquired (such as cor polmonale).

   c. Patients with acute myocardial infarction without complicating cor pulmonale.

It is not possible to plot a mean QRS vector in the frontal plane using the entire QRS complex, since in every lead of the frontal plane the QRS complex is biphasic. To plot the QRS vectorial forces properly, the QRS complexes must be divided into initial and terminal vectors. As seen in Figure 6-40 the initial QRS vectorial forces are approximately along the axis of + lead II and the terminal QRS vectorial forces are along the axis of − lead II, in the opposite direction. In summary, in the $S_IS_{II}S_{III}$ syndrome the initial QRS vector is to the left and inferior, and the terminal QRS vector is to the right and superior in the frontal plane.

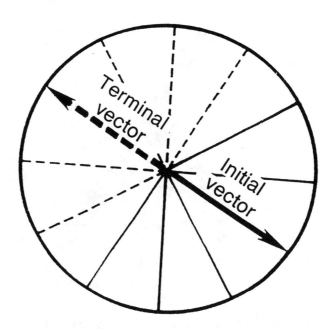

FIGURE 6-40.   Initial and terminal vectorial forces of the QRS in the $S_IS_{II}S_{III}$ syndrome.

6. Left axis deviation of the mean QRS vector had, for many years, been considered a major criterion for left ventricular hypertrophy. It has been shown, quite conclusively, that left ventricular hypertrophy, even to a marked degree, is not necessarily accompanied by left axis deviation. Left axis deviation, or perhaps a better term, superiorly oriented QRS vector (in the frontal plane), may be caused by a conduction disturbance in the anterior division of the left bundle branch. Since the left bundle branch comprises two major divisions, the anterior and the posterior division, Rosenbaum, who has helped clarify the subject of intraventricular conduction, recommended the use of the term "hemiblock" to describe a disturbance in either of the divisions. *Left anterior hemiblock* (LAH), therefore, describes a conduction disturbance in the anterior division, and *left posterior hemiblock* (LPH), a disturbance in the posterior division of the left bundle branch. In left anterior hemiblock the mean QRS vector, in the

frontal plane, is leftward and superior, or simply superior, and in left posterior hemiblock the mean QRS vector, in the frontal plane, is rightward or frank right axis deviation.

Figure 6-20 is a schematic illustration of the hemiblocks.

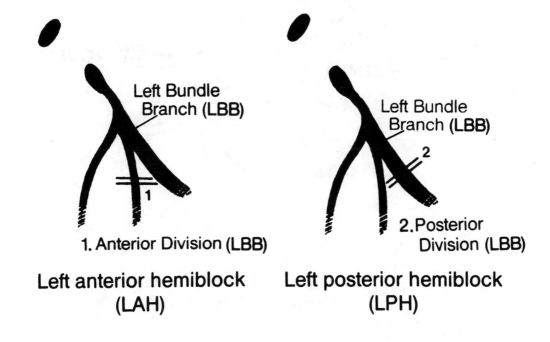

FIGURE 6-20.   The "hemiblocks."

7. a. The initial QRS vectorial forces are *not* affected by right bundle branch block; this is of the utmost importance. The Q waves of myocardial infarction are *not* obscured by right bundle branch block. Figure 6-8A reveals a diaphragmatic myocardial infarction prior to the development of right bundle branch block. In Figure 6-8B the findings of diaphragmatic myocardial infarction remain in the presence of right bundle branch block.

    b. The electrocardiographic manifestations of right bundle branch block in the presence of *anterior* myocardial infarction are of special interest. The initial Q wave in lead V_1 is preserved with a resulting QR rather than an RSR' pattern. This should not detract from the diagnosis of right bundle branch block if the other criteria are present; an illustration is presented in Figure 6-11. In Figure 6-12 right bundle branch block is seen in the presence of both anterior and inferior myocardial infarction.

8. a. Short P-R interval (0.12 sec. or less).
   b. Prolonged QRS interval (greater than 0.1 sec.).
   c. Slurring of the upstroke of the QRS complex by a delta wave.

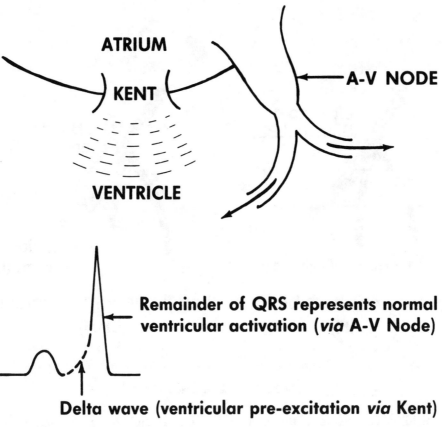

FIGURE 6-41. Pre-excitation—the Wolff-Parkinson-White or W-P-W syndrome.[6-17]

9. a. Widened QRS complex (beyond 0.10 sec.).
   b. S wave in lead I.
   c. R' wave in lead V_1.

10. In left bundle branch block (Figure 6-13), in contrast to right bundle branch block, the entire sequence of ventricular depolarization is altered. Both the initial and the terminal QRS vectorial forces point more leftward and posteriorly in comparison with normal conduction.

The characteristics of left bundle branch block follow.

   a. The QRS interval is prolonged to 0.12 sec. or more (if the QRS duration is 0.10 to 0.12 sec. it is labeled "incomplete").

   b. The initial QRS vector is changed in orientation to have a more leftward and posterior orientation, so that:

      1. The initial Q waves disappear in leads I and V_6.
      2. The initial R waves seen in the normal electrocardiogram in leads V_1, V_2, and V_3 are much smaller and have often disappeared in leads V_1 and V_2.

      Note: Do not make the diagnosis of myocardial infarction from the lack of R waves in the right precordial leads in the presence of left bundle branch block.

   c. The terminal vector has changed in orientation pointing more leftward, so that:

      1. The small S waves in lead aVL, during normal conduction, disappear during left bundle branch block.

      2. Lead III has a terminal R wave during normal conduction and a terminal S wave with left bundle branch block.

      3. Lead aVR has a terminal S wave with left bundle branch block.

NOTES AND
REFERENCES

FROM PAGE 418:
Right Bundle Branch Block, Principal
Criteria Review

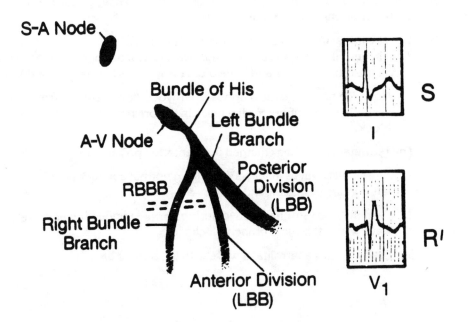

1. QRS Interval 0.12 sec. or Greater
2. S Wave in Leads I, V5 and V6
3. Terminal R or R' Wave in Lead V1
4. Repolarization Abnormalities

FROM PAGE 431:
Left Bundle Branch Block, Principal
Criteria Review

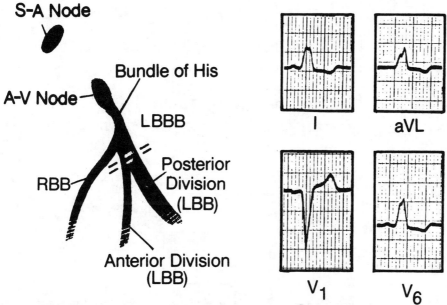

1. QRS Interval 0.12 sec. or Greater.
2. QRS Complex
    a. Predominantly Negative in Leads V1, V2
    b. Predominantly Positive in Leads V5, V6
        and Often Notched
3. Absence of Small Normal Q Waves
        in Leads I, aVL, V5 and V6
4. Repolarization Abnormalities

FROM PAGES 431-432 AND 475:
Rate Dependent Left Bundle
Branch Block

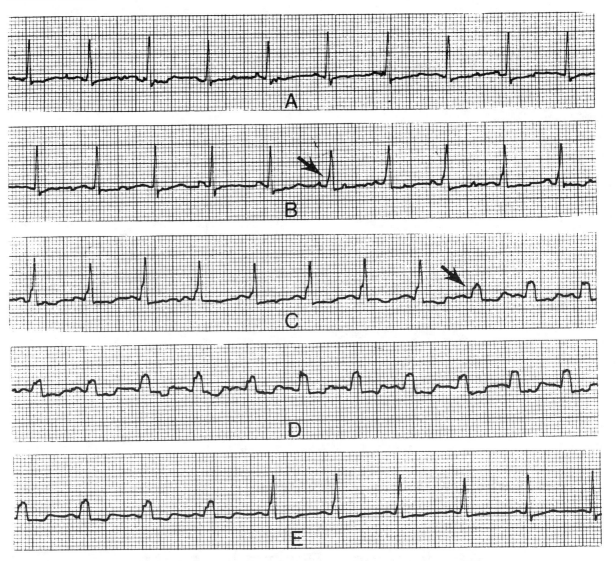

In panel A, at a heart rate of 90 to 93 beats per minute, the QRS complex is normally narrow. As the heart rate increases to a *critical rate* of 95, the QRS complex begins to widen with the appearance of a "delta-like" wave which persists up to a rate of 100 (arrow in panel B). An electrocardiogram taken at a rate of 96 could lead to the erroneous diagnosis of the Wolff-Parkinson-White (W-P-W) syndrome. At a rate of approximately 100, the pattern of left bundle branch block is obvious (arrow in panel C). As the rate begins to slow, the left bundle branch block persists to a rate of 87, followed by the "delta-like" wave for several beats, then by the normally narrow QRS complex. Note that the *critical rate* is different as the heart rate slows (panel E). The "delta-like" wave does not represent the W-P-W syndrome but is a step along the way toward the development of left bundle branch block at the *critical rate*. Within a few beats at *critical rates* three different conclusions may be reached:

1. Conduction with a normally narrow QRS complex.
2. Erroneous diagnosis of the W-P-W syndrome.
3. Left bundle branch block.

Earlier, you saw illustrated (Figure 6-14 A and B) an example of rate-dependent left bundle branch block. Once again, heart rate must be given due emphasis and conduction at different heart rates should be observed.

References

6-1. Marriott, H.J.L.: Practical Electrocardiography, 8th Ed. Baltimore, Williams & Wilkins, 1988, p. 78.

6-2. Schamroth, L.: The 12 Lead Electrocardiogram. Oxford, Blackwell Scientific Publications, 1989, p. 51.

6-3. Schamroth, L.: The 12 Lead Electrocardiogram. Oxford, Blackwell Scientific Publications, 1989, p. 56.

6-4. Noble, L.M., et al.: Left ventricular hypertrophy in left bundle branch block. J. Electrocardiol., *17*:157, 1987.

6-5. Gilchrist, I.C., et al.: Left bundle branch block eliminates Q waves of inferior infarction: confirmation by ventriculography. Am. J. Noninvas. Cardiol., *1*:206, 1987.

6-6. Horan, L., et al.: The significance of diagnostic Q waves in the presence of bundle branch block. Chest, *58*:214, 1970.

6-7. Havelda, C.J., et al.: The pathologic correlates of the electrocardiogram: complete left bundle branch block. Circulation, *65*:445, 1982.

6-8. Rosenbaum, M.B.: The hemiblocks: diagnostic criteria and clinical significance. Mod. Concepts Cardiovasc Dis., *39*:141, 1970.

6-9. Marriott, H.J.L.: Practical Electrocardiography, 8th Ed. Baltimore, Williams & Wilkins, 1988, p. 99.

6-10. Blondeau, M.: Complete left bundle branch block with marked left axis deviation of QRS: clinical and anatomic study. Adv. Cardiol., *14*:25, 1975.

6-11. Schneider, J.F., et al: Clinical-electrocardiographic correlates of newly acquired left bundle branch block: the Framingham Study. Am. J. Cardiol., *55*:1332, 1985.

6-12. Dhingra, R.C., et al.: Significance of left axis deviation in patients with chronic left bundle branch block. Am. J. Cardiol., *42*:551, 1978.

6-13. Schamroth, L.: The 12 Lead Electrocardiogram. Oxford, Blackwell Scientific Publications, 1989, p. 78.

6-14. Bayés de Luna, A., et al.: Electrophysiological mechanisms of the $S_IS_{II}S_{III}$ electrocardiographic morphology. J. Electrocardiol., *20*:38, 1987.

6-15. Wolff, L., Parkinson, J., and White, P.D.: Bundle branch block with short P-R interval in healthy young people prone to paroxysmal tachycardia. Am. Heart J., *5*:685, 1930.

6-16. Wolff, L.: Syndrome of short P-R interval with abnormal QRS complexes and paroxysmal tachycardia (Wolff-Parkinson-White syndrome). Circulation, *10*:282, 1954.

6-17. Fox, W., and Stein, E.: Cardiac Rhythm Disturbances: A Step-by-Step Approach. Philadelphia, Lea & Febiger, 1983, p. 162.

6-18. Grant, R.P., et al.: Ventricular activation in the pre-excitation syndrome (Wolff-Parkinson-White). Circulation, *18*:355, 1958.

6-19. Sherf, L., and Neufeld, H.N.: The Pre-excitation Syndrome: Facts and Theories. New York, Yorke Medical Books, 1978, p. 48.

6-20. Lown, B., Ganong, W.F., and Levine, S.A.: The syndrome of short P-R interval, normal QRS complex and paroxysmal rapid heart action. Circulation, *5*:693, 1952.

6-21. Caracta, A.R., et al.: Electrophysiologic studies in the syndrome of short P-R interval, normal QRS complex. Am. J. Cardiol., *31*:245, 1973.

6-22. Benditt, D.G., et al.: Characteristics of atrioventricular conduction and the spectrum of arrhythmias in Lown-Ganong-Levine syndrome. Circulation, *57*:454, 1978.

6-23. Josephson, M.E., and Kastor, J.A.: Supraventricular tachycardia in Lown-Ganong-Levine syndrome: atrionodal versus intranodal reentry. Am. J. Cardiol., *40*:521, 1977.

6-24. Katz, L.N., and Pick, A.: Clinical Electrocardiography: The Arrhythmias. Philadelphia, Lea & Febiger, 1956, p. 102.

7

ARRHYTHMIAS

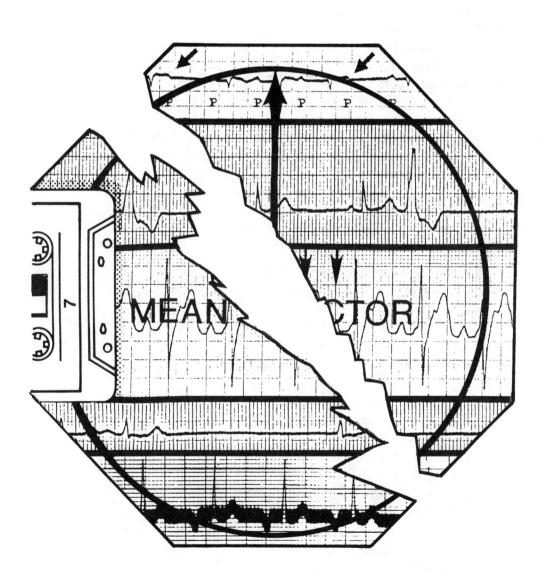

CHAPTER 7
CONTENTS

INTRODUCTION

All the heartbeat disorders have been under intensive investigation. Proliferation of coronary care units has given great impetus to this study; many arrhythmias arising in the patient with a myocardial infarction may be stopped or prevented entirely. New methods have been developed that help in the interpretation of arrhythmias and facilitate understanding of the underlying electrophysiologic principles. Among these has been the technique of His bundle recording for clinical use, which was developed in our laboratory and which represents one of the great advances in cardiology.[7.1] Some of the illustrations are from our other books on arrhythmias.[7.2,7.3] I am very grateful to Drs. William Fox and David B. Propert for their contributions.

Once the basics in this chapter are learned, the other concepts may be easily acquired from works devoted specifically to arrhythmias and by keeping abreast of the current literature. The arrhythmias will be described in the classic manner. Be ready, however, to revise these concepts as knowledge, which may nullify time-honored ideas, accumulates.

In the previous chapters we have been studying the 12-lead electrocardiogram using leads I, II, III, aVR, aVL, aVF, and V_1 to V_6. In the monitoring of arrhythmias, single leads are used often, in addition to the 12-lead electrocardiogram. The single leads commonly used are leads II (modified), MCL_1 and MCL_6. Lead II is a modified lead II since the positive and negative electrodes are not placed on the respective extremities, but on the chest. In lead MCL_1 the positive electrode is placed on the chest in the position of lead V_1. In lead MCL_6 the positive electrode is placed on the chest in the position of lead V_6. These leads are illustrated on pages 595 and 596. We will analyze arrhythmias following the steps enumerated in this list:

Rhythm Analysis

1. P Wave:

2. P-R Interval:

3. QRS Complex:

4. Rhythm:

5. Rate:

Impression and Comment:

O B J E C T I V E S

Upon completion of this chapter, you should be able to:

1. List the criteria of "normal sinus rhythm."

2. Recognize the characteristics of sinus arrhythmia, sinus tachycardia, and sinus bradycardia.

3. Recognize the difference between S-A block and sinus arrest.

4. Recall the association of the short P-R interval and the Wolff-Parkinson-White (W-P-W) syndrome with arrhythmias.

5. Recognize the electrocardiographic manifestations of coronary sinus rhythm (ectopic atrial rhythm).

6. State what is meant by bigeminy.

7. Recognize premature beats of the atria, atrial tachycardia, atrial flutter, and atrial fibrillation.

8. Identify the group of patients among which multifocal (chaotic) atrial tachycardia is most often found.

9. Recognize the contribution of His bundle studies to the understanding of arrhythmias.

10. Recognize premature beats of the ventricle, ventricular tachycardia, ventricular flutter, and ventricular fibrillation.

11. State what is meant by first, second, and third degree A-V block.

12. State the differences between A-V dissociation and A-V block.

P R E T E S T

DIRECTIONS. This pretest consists of 10 electrocardiograms from patients with a history of arrhythmias. Write a brief analysis of each in the space provided.

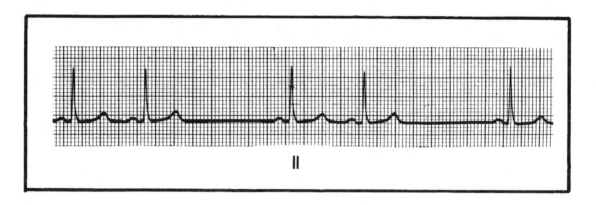

II

FIGURE 7-8.

1. Analysis:

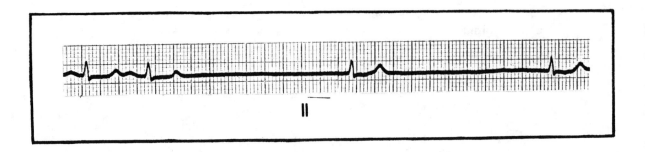

FIGURE 7-9.

2. Analysis:

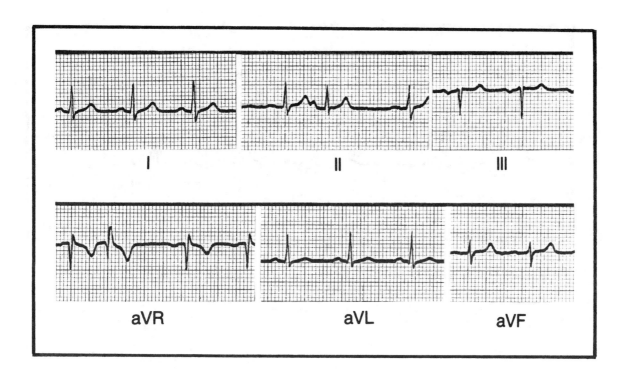

FIGURE 7-15.

3. Analysis:

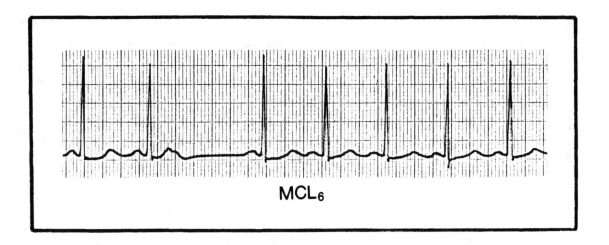

FIGURE 7-16.

4. Analysis:

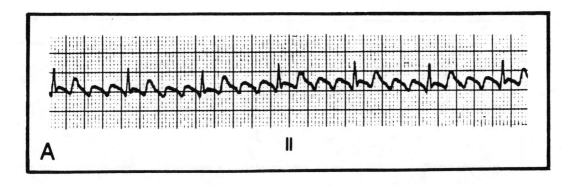

FIGURE 7-20A.

5. Analysis:

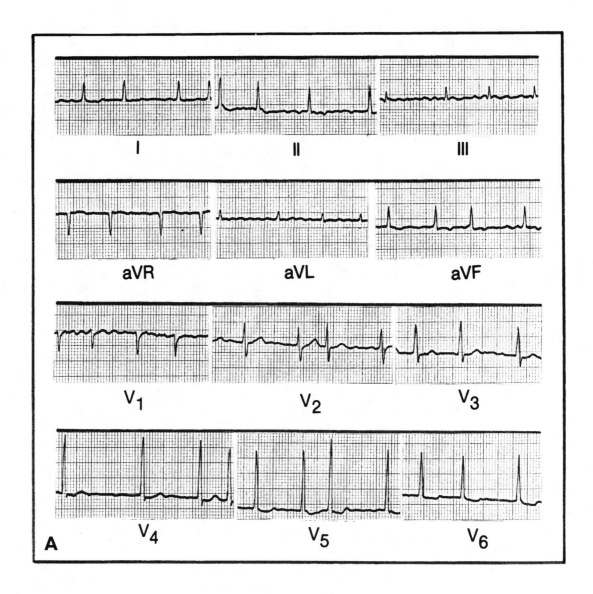

FIGURE 7-22A.

6. Analysis:

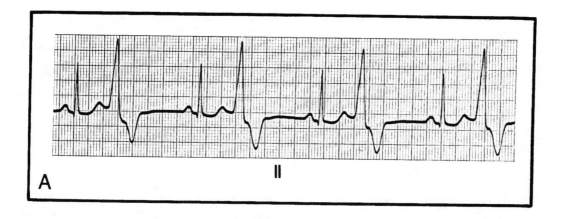

FIGURE 7-35A.

7. Analysis:

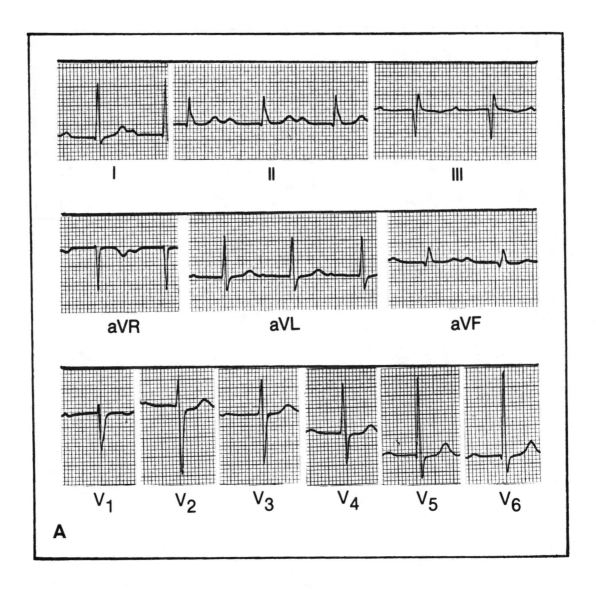

FIGURE 7-40A.

8. Analysis:

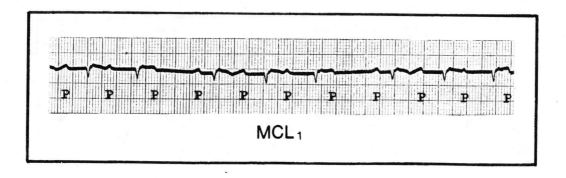

FIGURE 7-41.

9. Analysis:

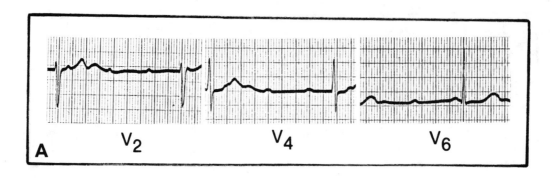

FIGURE 7-44A.

10. Analysis:

> Solutions to the pretest will be indicated later in this chapter.

> When you have completed your analyses start Cassette Side 17 and continue on the next page.

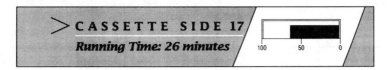

> CASSETTE SIDE 17
Running Time: 26 minutes
100   50   0

NORMAL AND ABNORMAL RHYTHMS OF THE HEART

The *sinoatrial (S-A) node* is normally the site of origin of the electrical impulse, leading to depolarization of the atria. The impulse then spreads through the *atrioventricular (A-V) node* and *bundle of His* to the *left (LBB)* and *right (RBB) bundle branches* and then to the ventricles through the *Purkinje fiber network,* leading to ventricular depolarization. If the S-A node fails, a lower pacemaker may become dominant. If that one fails, a still lower pacemaker may become dominant. Although the dominant pacemaker of the heart is the S-A node, under various circumstances and stimuli any part of the specialized conduction system may become the dominant pacemaker. There may be 2 or more pacemakers propagating impulses at the same time. The S-A node emits from 60 to 100 impulses per minute, the A-V junction from 40 to 60 impulses per minute, and still lower pacemakers, such as idioventricular pacemaker, fewer than 40 per minute.

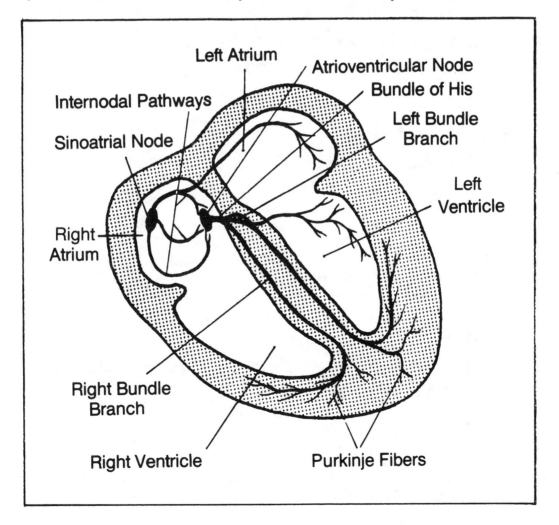

FIGURE 7-1. Electrical conduction system of the heart.

Normal Sinus Rhythm

1. P Wave:

The P waves are positive (upright) and uniform in leads I and II. Every P wave is followed by a QRS complex.

2. P-R Interval:

The normal P-R interval (from the beginning of the P wave to the beginning of the QRS complex) is constant between 0.12 and 0.2 sec.

3. QRS Complex:

The QRS complex duration is 0.1 sec. or less. Every QRS complex is preceded by a P wave.

4. Rhythm:

The rhythm is regular.

5. Rate:

The rate is between 60 and 100 per minute. It is quite constant at a given rate, varying less than 10%.

A. Sinoatrial (S-A) Node and Atria: Normal Sinus Rhythm

The sinoatrial (S-A) node is normally the site of origin of the electrical impulse (as noted on page 505), leading to depolarization of the atria. The P waves are constant and upright in at least leads I and aVF or I and II. Each P wave is followed by a QRS complex and each QRS complex is preceded by a P wave. The P-R interval is from 0.12 to 0.2 second (3 to 5 small boxes), and constant from beat to beat. The heart rate is regular, between 60 and 100 beats per minute. When the word "nodal" is used, it refers to the A-V node and *not* to the S-A node; "nodal" is never an abbreviation for the S-A node. Any beat or rhythm originating outside the S-A node is an *ectopic beat* or *rhythm, ectopic* in that it does not originate in the normal site.

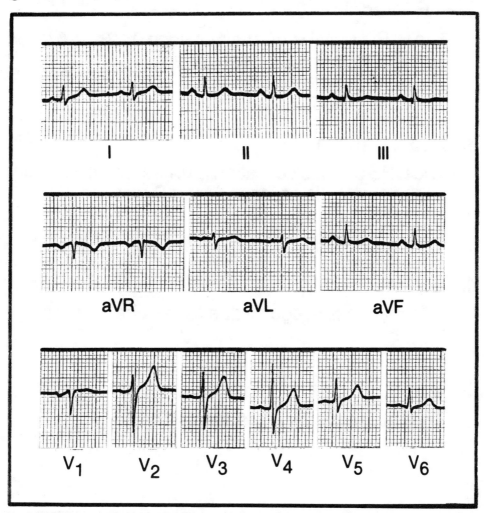

FIGURE 7-2. Normal sinus rhythm.

> The *ladder diagram* or *laddergram* of normal sinus rhythm was introduced in Chapter 1, page 129. Please study it since other laddergrams will be seen in this chapter.

Sinus Arrhythmia

1. P Wave:

The P waves are positive and uniform in leads I and II. Every P wave is followed by a QRS complex.

2. P-R Interval:

The P-R interval is normal between 0.12 and 0.2 sec. and is constant from beat to beat.

3. QRS Complex:

The QRS complex duration is 0.1 sec. or less. Every QRS complex is preceded by a P wave.

4. Rhythm:

The rhythm is irregular due to the changing rate.

5. Rate:

The rate varies by more than 10%.

1. Sinus Arrhythmia

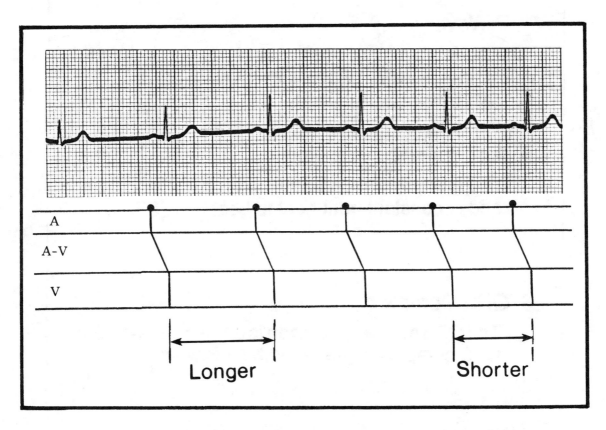

FIGURE 7-3.   *Sinus arrhythmia. The same characteristics as described under normal sinus rhythm apply, except that there may be marked variation in rate that is often, but not always, associated with the respiratory cycles. It is commonly seen in the young. The P-R intervals are constant, but the R-R intervals are continually changing.*

Sinus Tachycardia

1. P Wave:

The P waves are positive and uniform in leads I and II. Every P wave is followed by a QRS complex.

2. P-R Interval:

The P-R interval is normal between 0.12 and 0.2 sec. and is constant from beat to beat.

3. QRS Complex:

The QRS complex duration is 0.1 sec. or less. Every QRS complex is preceded by a P wave.

4. Rhythm:

The rhythm is regular.

5. Rate:

The rate is constant above 100 (100-160) per minute.

2. *Sinus Tachycardia*

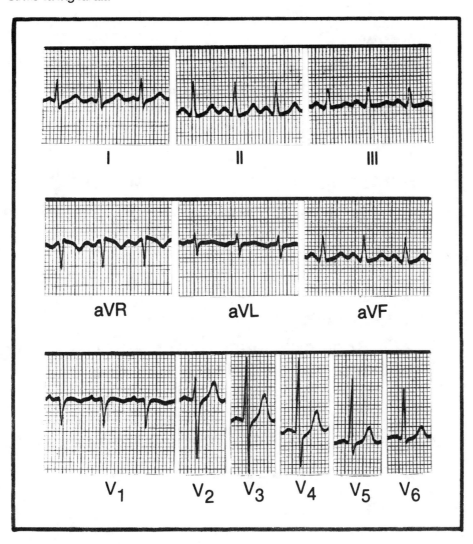

FIGURE 7-4. Sinus tachycardia. As in normal sinus rhythm, except that the rate is greater than 100 beats per minute, usually 100 to 160 beats per minute.

Sinus Bradycardia

1. P Wave:

The P waves are positive and uniform in leads I and II. Every P wave is followed by a QRS complex.

2. P-R Interval:

The P-R interval is normal between 0.12 and 0.2 sec. and is constant from beat to beat.

3. QRS Complex:

The QRS complex duration is 0.1 sec. or less. Every QRS complex is preceded by a P wave.

4. Rhythm:

The rhythm is regular.

5. Rate:

The rate is constant below 60 per minute.

3. *Sinus Bradycardia*

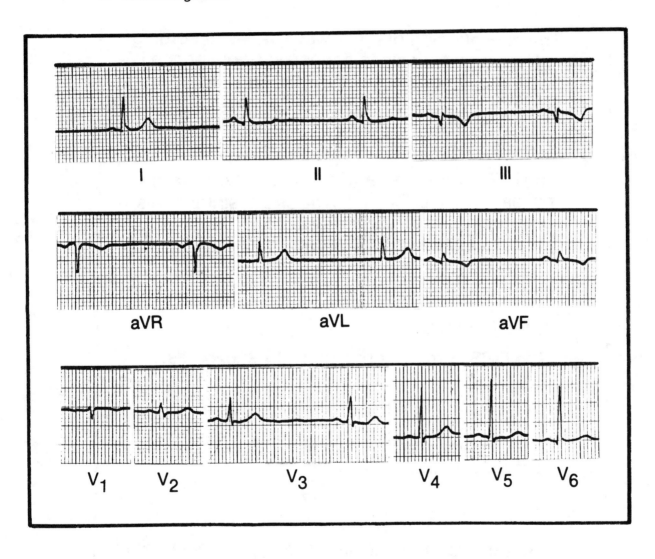

FIGURE 7-5. Sinus bradycardia. As in normal sinus rhythm, except for a rate under 60 beats per minute.

Wandering Pacemaker

1. P Wave:

The configuration of the P wave varies according to the pacemaker, since pacemaker dominance is shared by more than one pacemaker.

2. P-R Interval:

The P-R interval depends on the dominant pacemaker. The P-R interval of the sinus beats is between 0.12 and 0.2 sec., and the P-R interval of the junctional beats* is 0.12 sec. or less.

3. QRS Complex:

The QRS complex duration is 0.1 sec. or less.

4. Rhythm:

The rhythm may be slightly irregular with the shifting pacemaker sites.

5. Rate:

The rate may vary with the shifting pacemaker sites.

*Figure 7-7.

4. Wandering Pacemaker

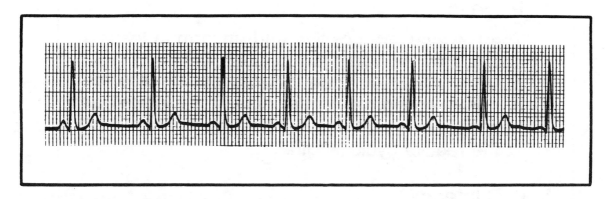

FIGURE 7-6.   Wandering atrial pacemaker. The P wave contours vary with the different sites of impulse formation. Note also the variation in rate.

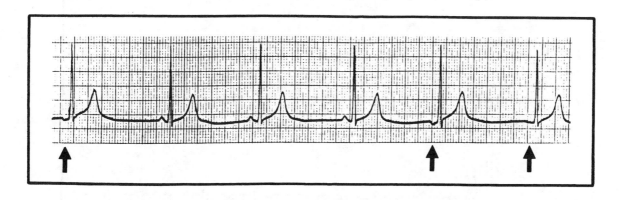

FIGURE 7-7.   Wandering pacemaker. The P wave polarity varies as the site of impulse formation shifts back and forth from a lower to a higher pacemaker. (Electrocardiogram reduced in size.)

Sinoatrial (S-A) Block

1. P Wave:

The P waves are positive and uniform in leads I and II. However, an entire cycle (P, QRS and T) is missing. The S-A node initiates an impulse, but it is not propagated to the atria; it is blocked and hence there is no P wave. The pause is a multiple of the regular cycle length.

2. P-R Interval:

The P-R interval is normal between 0.12 and 0.2 sec. and is constant from beat to beat except during the pause, when an entire cycle is missing.

3. QRS Complex:

The QRS complex duration is 0.1 sec. or less except during the pause, when an entire cycle is missing.

4. Rhythm:

The rhythm may be regular or irregular, according to the number and position of the missing cycles.

5. Rate:

The rate may be constant or varying, according to the number and position of the missing cycles.

5. Sinoatrial (S-A) Block

In sinoatrial block the S-A node initiates an impulse but the propagation is blocked, so that the atria are not depolarized and, therefore, there is no P wave. The pause is a multiple of the regular P-P interval. Figure 7-8 reveals a 2:1 S-A block. The block, represented by the letter B, is seen where the P wave should normally be. "Block" refers to a delay or interruption of conduction of an impulse.

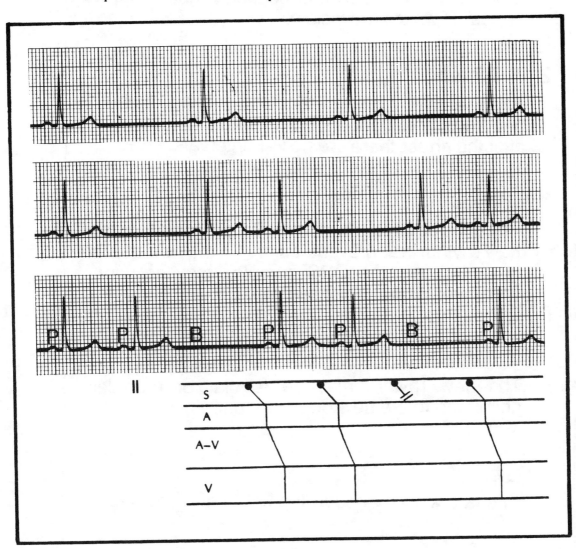

FIGURE 7-8.   Sinoatrial (S-A) block. The "S" on the ladder diagram refers to the S-A node.

> The analysis of Figure 7-8 in the text and on the tape is the solution to Item 1 on the pretest.

Sinus Arrest

1. P Wave:

Since the S-A node has ceased functioning, no "sinus" P waves are visible.

2. P-R Interval:

The P-R interval depends on the pacemaker that becomes dominant. In the example given, after the arrest, there are no P-R intervals.

3. QRS Complex:

The QRS complex duration is 0.1 sec. or less if the new rhythm is supraventricular. If the new rhythm is ventricular, the QRS complex may be very wide, greater than 0.12 sec. and bizarre.

4. Rhythm:

The new rhythm may be regular or irregular according to the new dominant pacemaker.

5. Rate:

The rate will vary according to the new rhythm.

6. Sinus Arrest, Escape Beats, and Escape Rhythms

Sinus arrest is a failure of the S-A node to initiate an expected impulse; it is a failure of impulse *formation* rather than a failure of impulse *propagation*. If no other pacemaker becomes dominant at this point, death follows quickly. The "escape" beat is usually from a lower pacemaker. When the S-A node fails to initiate an impulse, a lower pacemaker may become dominant. The beat that follows the "arrest" is then called an "escape" beat. If the pacemaker originating the escape beat remains the dominant one, the rhythm may then be called an escape rhythm. The QRS complex of the escape beat is similar to the QRS complexes of sinus origin but is not preceded by a P wave (Figure 7-9). The escape beat and rhythm are of junctional origin. Junctional rhythm will be studied later in this chapter. Escape rhythms, either of junctional or of ventricular origin, for example, are safety rhythms although they are ectopic. They must not be suppressed since the patient may not have another effective pacemaker.

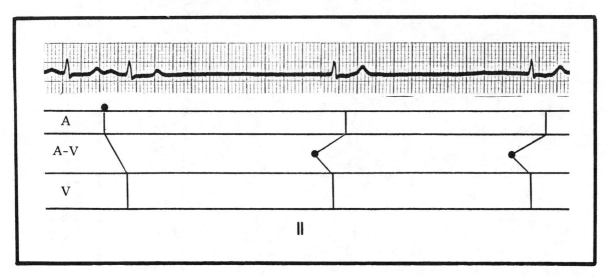

FIGURE 7-9.   *Sinus arrest with "escape" of lower pacemaker.*

> The analysis of Figure 7-9 in the text and on the tape is the solution to Item 2 on the pretest.

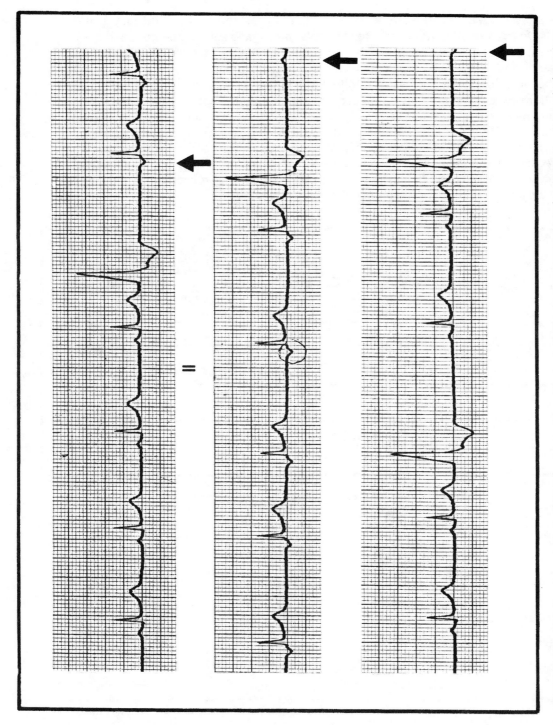

FIGURE 7-10. Note the change in rhythm following interruption of the basic rhythm by premature ventricular contractions, sinus rhythm to junctional rhythm, again sinus rhythm followed by junctional rhythm. Junctional rhythm and premature ventricular contractions will be discussed later in this chapter.

7. Pre-excitation

Wolff-Parkinson-White (W-P-W) Syndrome. In the W-P-W syndrome there is an accessory atrioventricular pathway, the bundle of Kent, in addition to the A-V node. Conduction from the atria to the ventricles through the accessory pathway occurs before the normal conduction through the A-V node, resulting in pre-excitation and asynchronous activation of the ventricles, inscribing a wide and abnormal QRS complex. The QRS complex begins with a slurred upstroke known as the *delta* wave (conduction through the bundle of Kent). Refer to Chapter 6, pages 469 to 475 for discussion of pre-excitation. The W-P-W syndrome has been associated with supraventricular tachycardias, namely, reentrant (reciprocating) supraventricular tachycardia, atrial fibrillation, and atrial flutter. It is important, at this time, to become familiar with the concept of *reentry* since it is the mechanism of most supraventricular tachycardias and many ventricular tachycardias. Refer to pages 597 to 599 for the explanation and illustration of reentry and reentrant circuits using the A-V node and bundle of Kent.

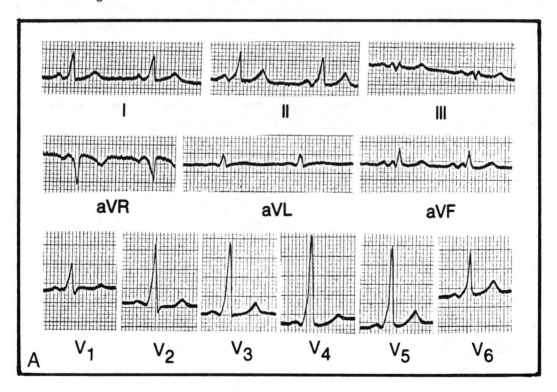

FIGURE 7-11A.   Wolff-Parkinson-White (W-P-W) syndrome.

> Reentry is explained and illustrated on pages 597 to 599.

Short P-R Interval Syndrome or the Lown-Ganong-Levine (L-G-L) Syndrome. The syndrome of the short P-R interval with the normal QRS complex has characteristics of normal sinus rhythm except for the short P-R interval (usually 0.1 sec. or less). The P wave is usually upright in leads I, II, and aVF. There is no delta wave, as in the W-P-W syndrome. This syndrome, also known as coronary nodal rhythm in years past (see page 476), is included in the study of arrhythmias since it has been associated with reentrant (reciprocating) tachycardias.

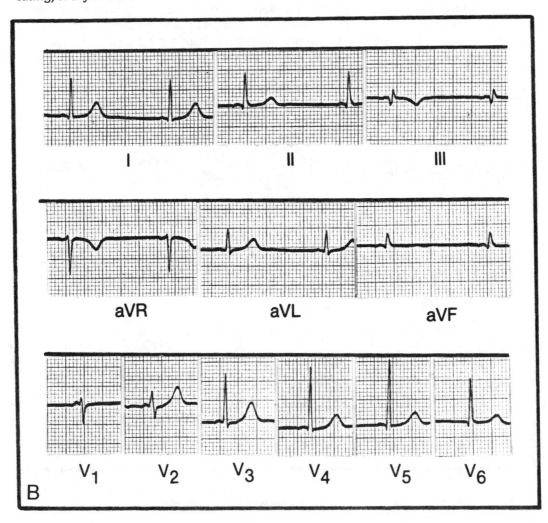

FIGURE 7-11B.   The short P-R interval or Lown-Ganong-Levine (L-G-L) syndrome.

8. Coronary Sinus Rhythm (Ectopic Atrial Rhythm)

This rhythm, with *retrograde* activation of the atria and a *normal* P-R interval, is now better known as an *ectopic atrial rhythm.* Of historical interest, Borman and Meek concluded, in 1931, that the "nodal tissue of the coronary sinus apparently acts as a reserve mechanism, as a pacemaker under conditions of experimental destruction of the sino-auricular node . . . "[7-4] Scherf and Gurbuzer stated, in 1958, that this rhythm originates in the extension of the A-V node toward the area of the orifice of the coronary sinus vein, an area which has a high degree of automatism."[7-5]

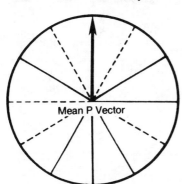

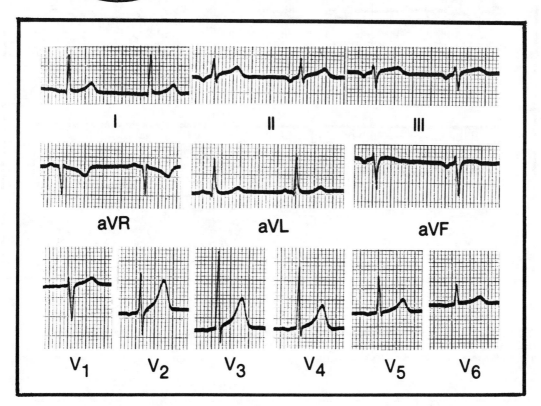

FIGURE 7-12.   *Coronary sinus rhythm. Note the* retrograde *activation of the atria with negative P waves in leads II, III, and aVF. The P-R interval is of normal duration, at least 0.12 sec.*

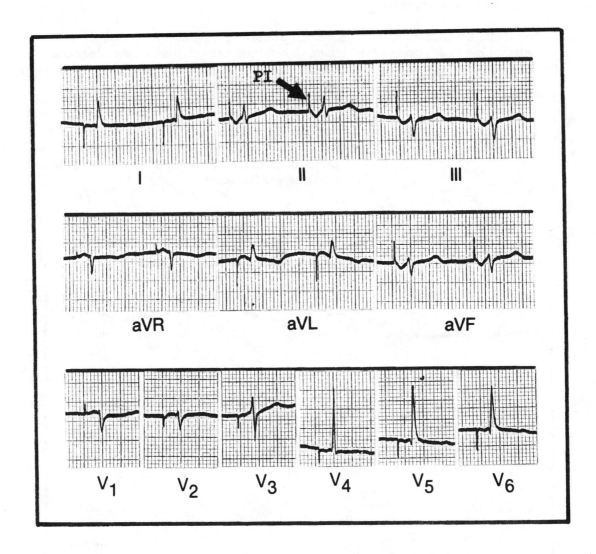

FIGURE 7-13.   This electrocardiogram is from a patient who was treated with electrical pacing of the coronary sinus. Note the characteristic mean P vector of coronary sinus rhythm. The narrow deflection preceding each P wave is the pacemaker impulse (labeled PI in lead II).

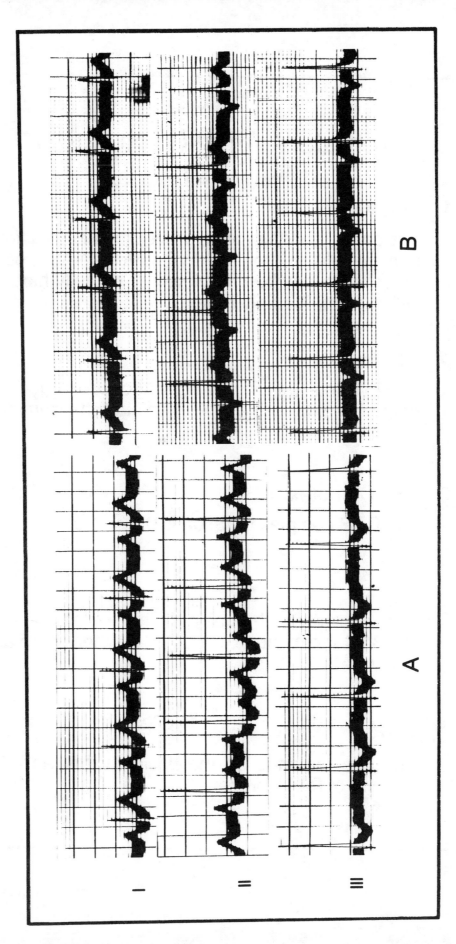

FIGURE 7-14.   Onset of coronary sinus rhythm (B) in a patient taking digitalis; there is no significant change in heart rate. (Electrocardiogram enlarged.)

Premature Atrial Contraction (PAC)

1. P Wave:

The configuration of the P wave of the PAC differs from that of the dominant rhythm. If the PAC is early, the P wave may be completely or partially hidden within the preceding T wave.

2. P-R Interval:

The P-R interval may be normal or prolonged and often differs from the P-R interval of the dominant rhythm.

3. QRS Complex:

The QRS complex duration is 0.1 sec. or less.

4. Rhythm:

The regularity of the basic rhythm is disturbed by the PAC. It may be quite irregular when there are many PACs.

5. Rate:

The rate depends on the basic rhythm and the number of PACs present.

9. Premature Atrial Contraction (PAC)

Premature beats of the atria are seen when an atrial impulse is propagated before the next normal beat is due. The premature beat may be conducted to the ventricles as seen below in lead II (arrow). The P waves of the premature beat differ from the sinus P waves

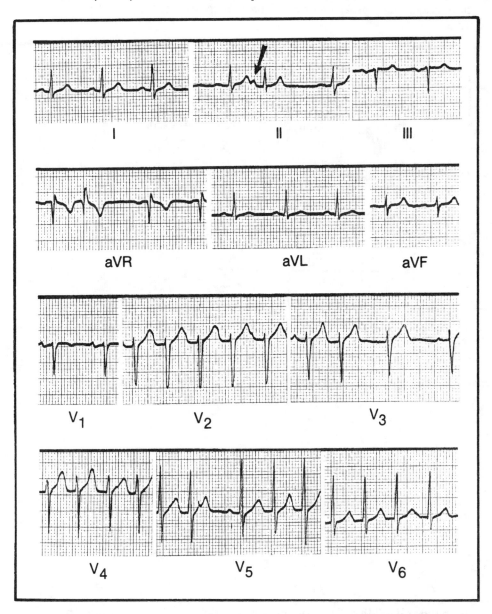

FIGURE 7-15.   Premature atrial contractions. (Electrocardiogram reduced in size.)

> The analysis of Figure 7-15 in the text and on the tape is the solution to Item 3 on the pretest.

in contour. In general, following atrial premature beats, the P-R interval may be normal or prolonged, and the QRS complexes may be of normal contour and duration or of changed configuration and prolonged, depending upon the state of refractoriness of the conduction tissue. The premature beats of the atria may herald "runs" of atrial tachycardia.

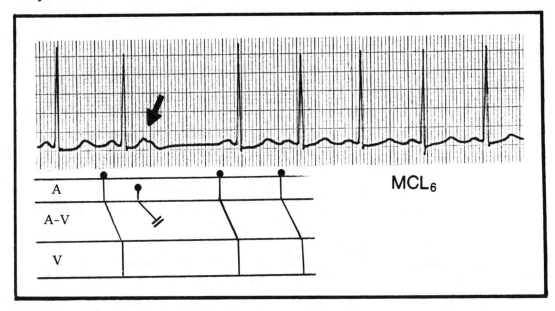

FIGURE 7-16. *Blocked atrial premature beat. If the premature beat of the atria does not conduct to the ventricles, it is said to be blocked and is not followed by a QRS complex. The arrow above points to the blocked atrial premature beat. Absolute and relative refractory periods are explained and illustrated on page 600.*

Absolute and relative refractory periods are explained and illustrated on page 600.

The analysis of Figure 7-16 in the text and on the tape is the solution to Item 4 on the pretest.

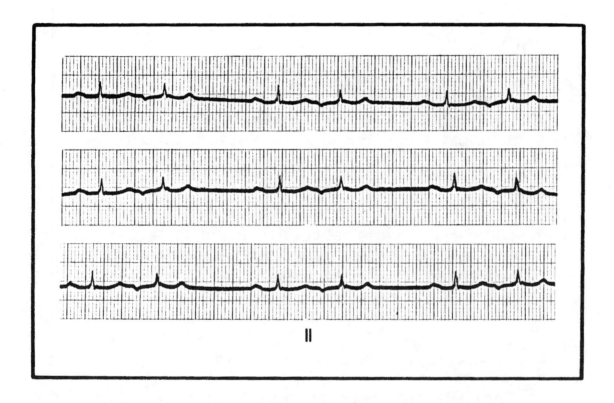

FIGURE 7-17.   Bigeminy. Bigeminy refers to heart beats that occur in groups of two. In this case the second beat in each pair is an ectopic atrial beat. You must describe what you see since the word "bigeminy" does not give you any clue as to the component parts of a pair.

Atrial Tachycardia

1. P Wave:

The P wave differs in configuration from the sinus P wave. It may, however, be hidden in the preceding T wave and not be seen as a separate entity due to the rapid rate.

2. P-R Interval:

The P-R interval is between 0.12 and 0.2 sec. and is constant from beat to beat. The P-R interval may not be measurable if the P wave is partially or completely hidden in the preceding T wave.

3. QRS Complex:

The QRS complex duration is 0.1 sec. or less. Every QRS complex is preceded by a P wave.

4. Rhythm:

The rhythm is regular.

5. Rate:

The rate is constant between 160 and 250 per minute.

10. Atrial Tachycardia

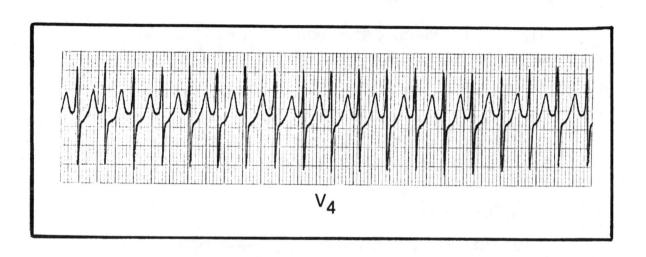

FIGURE 7-18.   *Atrial tachycardia. The pacemaker responsible for the premature beats of the atria is capable of becoming the dominant pacemaker, superseding the S-A node. It is usually characterized by a rapid (160 to 250 beats per minute) rate and regular rhythm. The P waves, when seen, differ from the sinus P waves in contour but are usually upright in leads I and II. The P waves often are not seen without an esophageal lead or intra-atrial recording.*

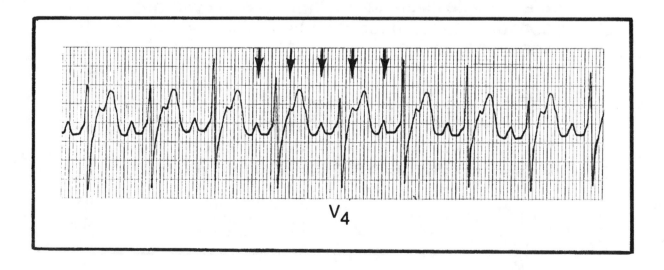

FIGURE 7-19.   *Atrial tachycardia with 2:1 A-V block is seen with alternate blocked P waves. Arrows point to the P waves.*

Atrial Flutter

1. P Wave (F Wave):

The atrial deflections, which often have a "saw-tooth" appearance, are known as F or flutter waves.

2. P-R Interval:

Because of the characteristic appearance of the flutter waves, it is often difficult to determine the P-R interval. It is therefore not measured.

3. QRS Complex:

The QRS complex duration is 0.1 sec. or less.

4. Rhythm:

The rhythm may be regular or irregular, depending on the relationship of atrial to ventricular beats. In the example given the rhythm is regular with a 4:1 conduction ratio (four atrial beats for every ventricular beat).

5. Rate:

The atrial rate is constant between 250 and 350 per minute. The ventricular rate depends on the conduction ratio between the atria and ventricles.

11. Atrial Flutter

The fluttering atria are represented by the undulating atrial waves, at times with a saw-tooth appearance, and uniform morphology. In Figure 7-20A there are 4 atrial deflections (F or flutter waves) for each QRS complex, hence atrial flutter with a 4:1 conduction ratio. In each case, determine in the usual manner, the atrial rate and the ventricular rate, to set up the ratio. In this electrocardiogram the atrial rate is 300 per minute and the ventricular rate is 75 per minute. The atrial rate in atrial flutter is usually 250 to 350 per minute.

On page 532 it is stated that the P-R interval, or more correctly, the F-R interval, is not measured. Since there are numerous atrial impulses, it is not always certain which impulses reach the ventricles. Besoain-Santander, Pick, and Langendorf, studying A-V conduction in atrial flutter, found long A-V conduction times (F-R intervals), 0.26 to 0.46 sec. in atrial flutter with a constant 2:1 conduction ratio.[7,8] This was ascribed to concealed conduction of the nonconducted atrial impulses. In patients with a constant 4:1 conduction ratio, the conduction time was 0.33 to 0.43 sec.

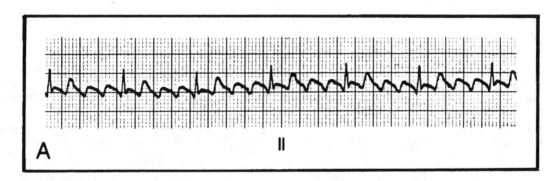

FIGURE 7-20A.   *Atrial flutter. The A-V conduction ratio is 4:1 with an atrial rate of 300 and a ventricular rate of 75. Note the saw-tooth appearance of the atrial waves (F or flutter waves).*

> The analysis of Figure 7-20A in the text and on the tape is the solution to Item 5 on the pretest.

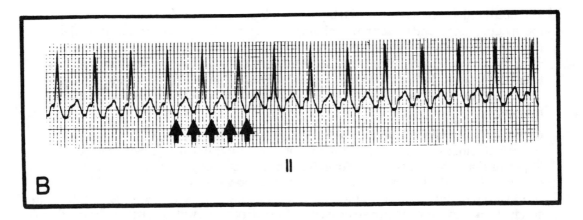

FIGURE 7-20B. *Atrial flutter. The series of arrows point to the flutter waves. The A-V conduction ratio is 2:1, with the resulting ventricular rate of 150 beats per minute.*

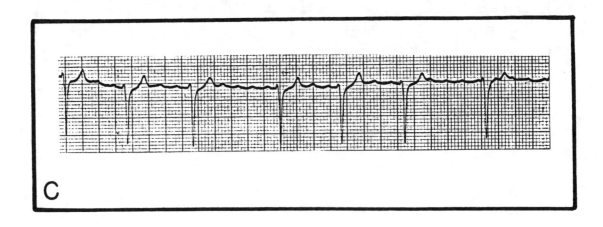

FIGURE 7-20C. *Atrial flutter with varying A-V block. (Electrocardiogram reduced in size.)*

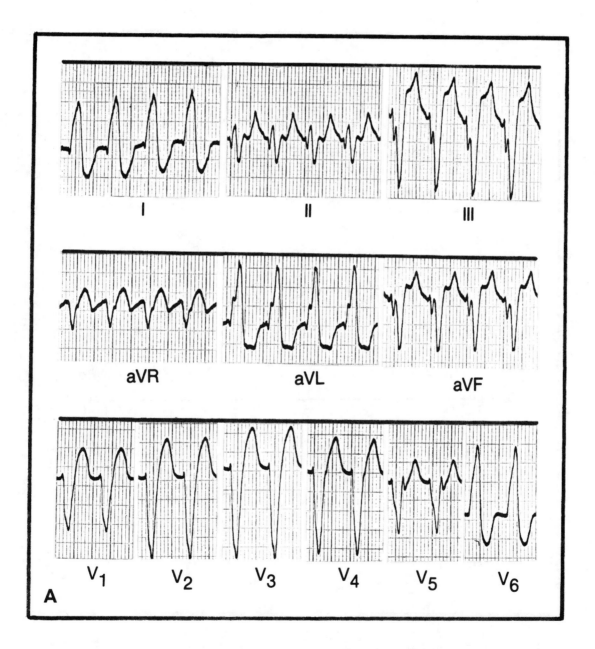

FIGURE 7-21A.   The elaboration on the following patient will serve as an example of how difficult an arrhythmia problem may be. A 67-year-old man with hypertensive, atherosclerotic heart disease presented with a heart rate of 145 beats per minute and the electrocardiogram above. The ventricular rate was rapid and the QRS complexes wide. What was the underlying rhythm? Was this a ventricular tachycardia or supraventricular tachycardia with a conduction disturbance? Try to answer these questions before proceeding.

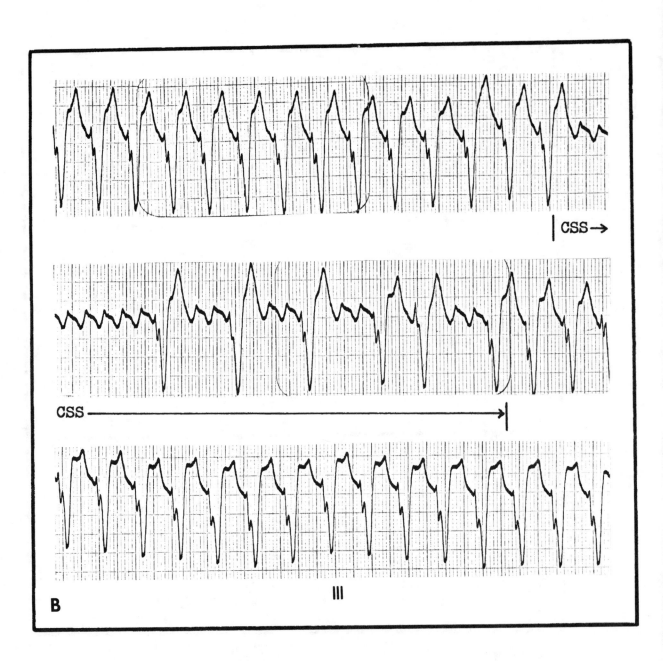

FIGURE 7-21B.   *Carotid sinus stimulation (CSS above) was used, with caution, and the atrial flutter became evident. The flutter waves have the often described "saw-tooth" appearance.*

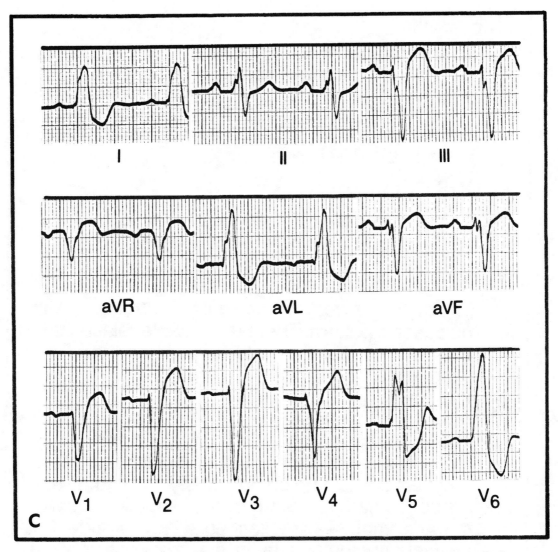

FIGURE 7-21C. *After resumption of his previous rhythm, it became clear that left bundle branch block was responsible for the wide QRS complexes. Did you answer the questions in Figure 7-21A correctly?*

Atrial Fibrillation

1. P Wave:

There are no identifiable P waves, only fibrillatory waves, irregular movements of the baseline.

2. P-R Interval:

Since there are no identifiable P waves, there is no measurable P-R interval.

3. QRS Complex:

The QRS complex duration is 0.1 sec. or less.

4. Rhythm:

The rhythm is irregularly irregular, i.e. irregular with no specific pattern. There is no stable relationship between the fibrillatory atrial waves and the QRS complexes.

5. Rate:

The atrial rate is above 350 (350-600) per minute with a chaotic rhythm. The ventricular response is irregular, depending on how many of the impulses are conducted, irregularly, to the ventricles. Most of the atrial impulses are blocked at the A-V node. The optimal ventricular rate, in the presence of atrial fibrillation, is between 60 and 100 per minute. If it is below 60 it is considered a slow ventricular response; if it is over 100 it is considered a rapid ventricular response.

12. Atrial Fibrillation

Disorganized, ineffective contractions of the atria (350 to 600 per minute) characterize atrial fibrillation. No P waves are seen, and the ventricular response is irregular, depending on how many of the 350 to 600 impulses are conducted to the ventricles. If the atrial rate is 500 per minute and the ventricular rate is 125 per minute, it means that 1 in every 4 atrial impulses is conducted, irregularly, to the ventricles.

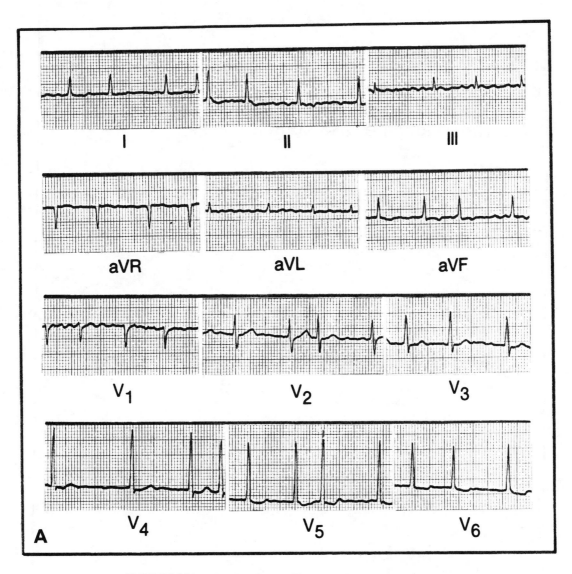

FIGURE 7-22A.   Atrial fibrillation. (Electrocardiogram reduced in size.)

> The analysis of Figure 7-22A in the text and on the tape is the solution to Item 6 on the pretest.

Multifocal Atrial Tachycardia

1. P Wave:

The P waves vary in configuration, with multiple atrial foci initiating impulses.

2. P-R Interval:

The P-R intervals vary from normal to prolonged. There is no stable relationship between the P waves and the QRS complexes.

3. QRS Complex:

The QRS complex duration is 0.1 sec. or less.

4. Rhythm:

The rhythm is irregularly irregular and resembles atrial fibrillation except that P waves are clearly visible.

5. Rate:

The rate is not constant from beat to beat because of multiple atrial foci, often above 170 per minute.

The discussion from sinus tachycardia (up to 160/minute) to atrial tachycardia (160 to 250/minute) to atrial flutter (250 to 350/minute), to atrial fibrillation (350 to 600/minute) has included rate as a criterion. These classic figures should be considered as guideposts rather than as rigid absolutes, for there is much overlap.

13. Multifocal Atrial Tachycardia

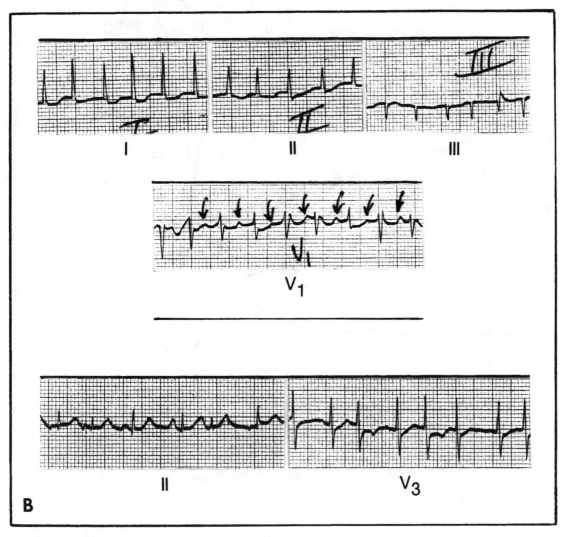

B

FIGURE 7-22B. *Two patients with multifocal (chaotic) atrial tachycardia. Leads I, II, and III in the first patient and lead V₃ in the second patient, at a quick glance, might appear to be examples of atrial fibrillation. Leads V₁ and II, respectively, show that the rhythm is not atrial fibrillation. This rhythm is frequently found in patients with chronic obstructive pulmonary disease with hypoxia.*

B. Atrioventricular (A-V) Node (Historical Interest)

We do not refer to these rhythms today as "nodal rhythms" but as "junctional rhythms" since the pacemaker is not in the A-V node but in the A-V junction. However, these rhythms will be described in the classic manner for historical interest and understanding. The newer concepts follow.

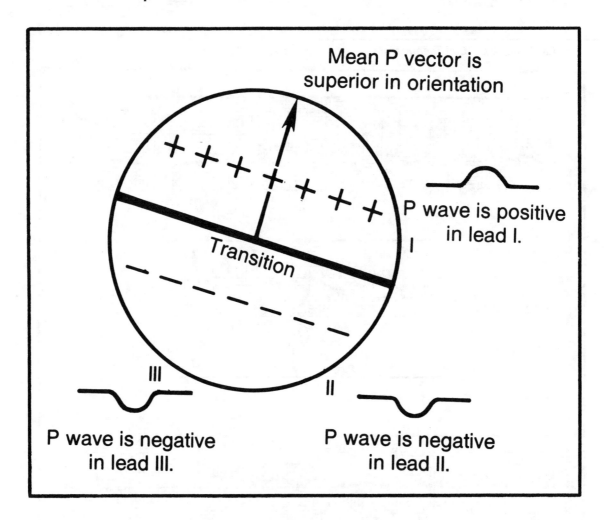

FIGURE 7-23. *Mean P vector in "A-V nodal rhythm."*

1. *Upper Nodal Rhythm*

In upper nodal rhythm the upper part of the A-V node initiates the impulse. Since it is closer to the atria (see below), the atria are first depolarized retrogradely, followed by the antegrade depolarization of the ventricles. The P wave precedes the QRS complex and the P-R interval is short (0.12 sec. or less).

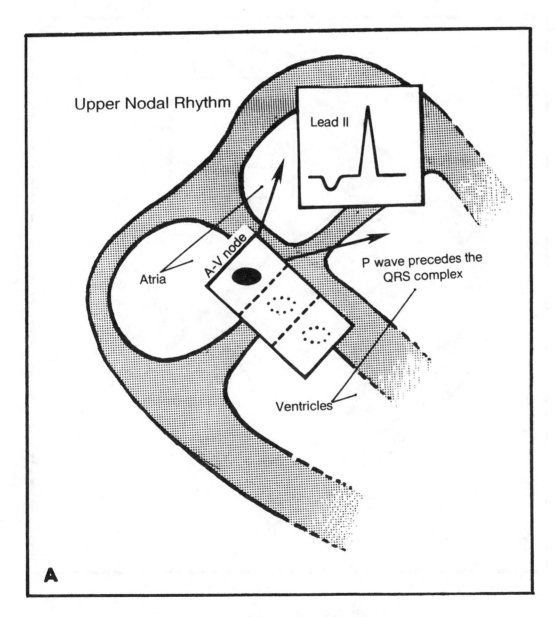

FIGURE 7-24A. Upper nodal rhythm.

2. *Middle Nodal Rhythm*

In middle nodal rhythm the atria and ventricles are depolarized at the same time, the atria in a retrograde and the ventricles in an antegrade manner. The P wave is not seen and is presumed to be within the QRS complex.

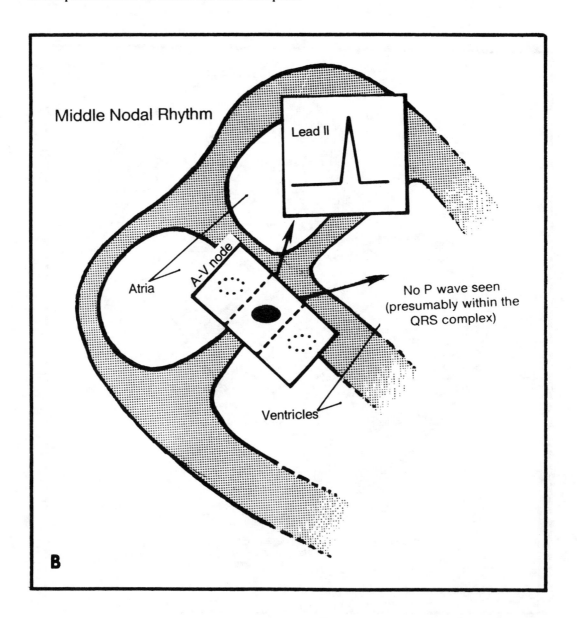

FIGURE 7-24B.   Middle nodal rhythm.

3. Lower Nodal Rhythm

In lower nodal rhythm the ventricles are depolarized antegradely, before the retrograde depolarization of the atria. The P wave follows the QRS complex. The relation of the retrograde P wave to the QRS complex depends not only on the *site* in the A-V node but also on the *speed* of antegrade and retrograde conduction. Examples of upper, middle, and lower nodal rhythms are seen in Figures 7-25, 7-26, and 7-27.

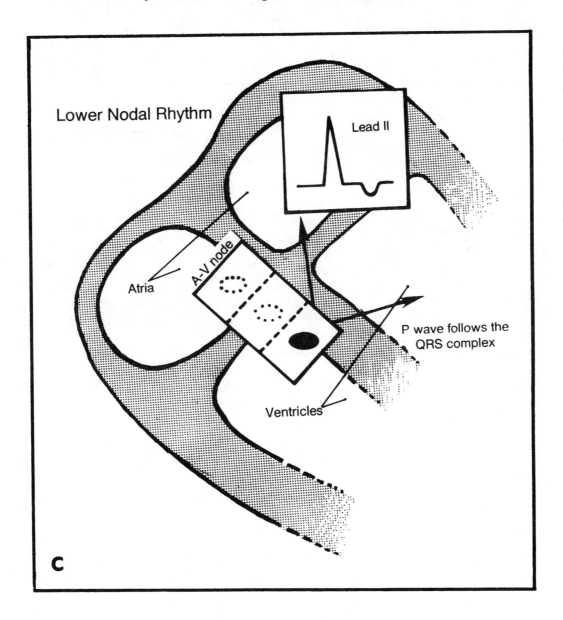

FIGURE 7-24C.   Lower nodal rhythm.

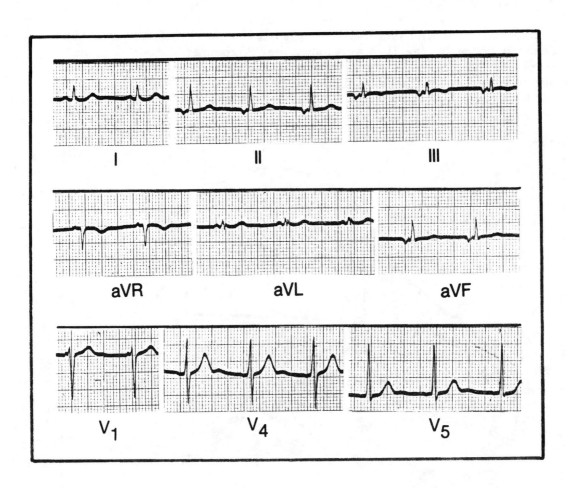

FIGURE 7-25.　Upper nodal rhythm. Describe the mean P vector. (Electrocardiogram reduced in size.)

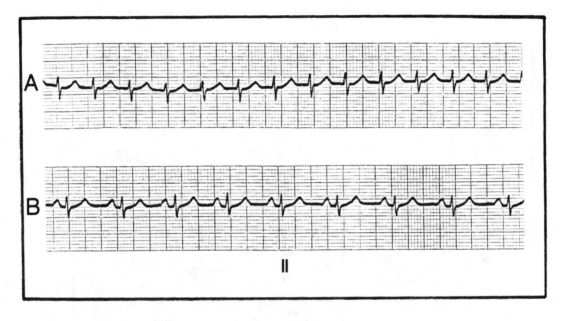

FIGURE 7-26A.   Middle nodal tachycardia. Where are the P waves? Are you sure? B, Restoration of sinus rhythm following the paroxysm. (Electrocardiogram reduced in size.)

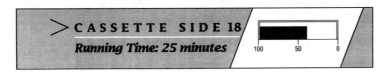

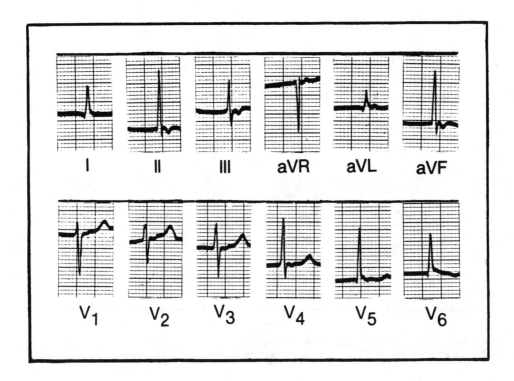

FIGURE 7-27. *Lower nodal rhythm. Locate the mean P vector. What is the relationship between the P wave and the QRS complex?*

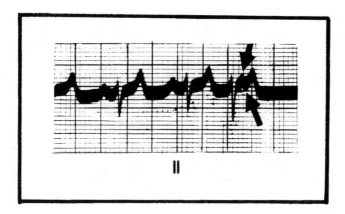

II

FIGURE 7-28.   A "lower nodal" premature beat is seen followed by a retrograde P wave (lower arrow). A more likely interpretation, since the strip is short and no esophageal or intra-atrial recordings are available, is that the premature beat is really a "middle nodal" premature beat followed by an upright "sinus" P wave (upper arrow), which is blocked because of the refractory state of the ventricular myocardium. (Electrocardiogram enlarged.)

4. His Bundle Studies

The classic upper, middle, and lower nodal rhythms have been explained for historical interest. We now know that the A-V node is not a pacemaker. The pacemaker is in the A-V junctional tissue; hence the term junctional rhythm. Bundle of His studies have contributed greatly to this understanding. The His bundle study is a technique where an electrode catheter is placed near the tricuspid valve via the femoral vein or an arm vein and recordings are made from the area of the His bundle. We see a sharp deflection, labeled H in Figure 7-29, between the atrial and ventricular deflections. The next two illustrations, Figures 7-30 and 7-31, are from His bundle studies.

His bundle recordings have terminated the "silence" of the P-R segment and have added an important tool to the understanding of arrhythmias.

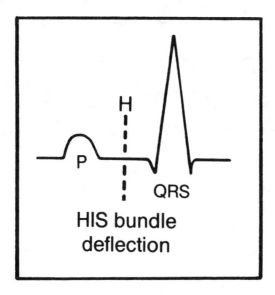

FIGURE 7-29.   Diagram showing location of His bundle deflection.

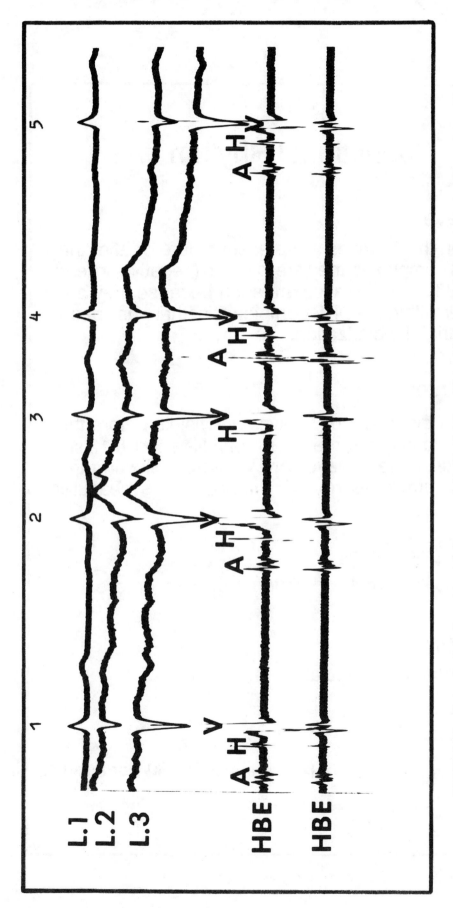

FIGURE 7-30. His bundle study. From above down are seen standard leads I, II, and III, in addition to recordings from within the heart. HBE is the His bundle electrogram; A, atrial deflection; H, His deflection; V, ventricular deflection. The five ventricular complexes are labeled 1, 2, 3, 4, and 5. Ventricular complexes (V 1, 2, 4, and 5) are preceded by an atrial deflection (A), lining up with the P wave on the clinical electrocardiogram, and a His deflection (H), representing normal A-V conduction. Complex number 3, on the other hand, might be called a "middle nodal" extra beat if we had only the clinical electrocardiogram at our disposal, since it is not preceded or followed by a P wave. The His bundle electrocardiogram shows us, however, that complex number 3 is preceded only by a His bundle (H) deflection—it is a His bundle or A-V junctional premature beat, and not a "middle nodal" beat. There is no "hidden" P wave within the QRS complex.

Junctional Rhythm

1. P Wave:

When the P waves are present before or after the QRS complexes, they are inverted (negative) in lead II . Often no P waves are seen because they are either within the QRS complexes or there has been no atrial depolarization.

2. P-R Interval:

When the inverted P waves are visible before the QRS complexes, the P-R interval is short, 0.12 sec. or less. If the P waves are within or following the QRS complexes, no P-R interval can be measured.

3. QRS Complex:

The QRS complex duration is 0.1 sec. or less.

4. Rhythm:

The rhythm is regular.

5. Rate:

The rate is constant between 40 and 60 per minute.

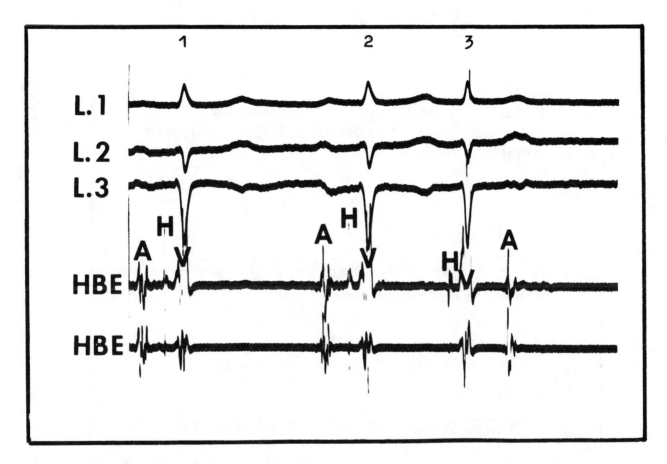

FIGURE 7-31.   *His bundle study. This recording is labeled in the same manner as Figure 7-30. Complexes 1 and 2 are normal, preceded by an atrial (A) deflection and a His bundle (H) deflection. Complex 3 is a premature contraction that might be labeled a "nodal" premature contraction on the clinical electrocardiogram. Why? As you can see on the His bundle electrogram (HBE), it is a His bundle or A-V junctional premature beat. This beat is then followed by a normal atrial deflection, which cannot conduct to the ventricles because the ventricular conduction system is in a refractory state caused by the premature contraction. Review Figure 7-28.*

On the basis of similar studies it has been determined that the classic upper, middle, and lower nodal rhythms should be called junctional rhythms since the pacemaker is not in the A-V node but in the A-V junctional tissue. Note how a technique came along which revolutionized time-honored concepts.

Review Figures 7-25, 7-26A, and 7-27 using the criteria for junctional rhythm presented on page 552 and refer to pages 601 to 603 for more illustrations.

>   Please refer to pages 601–603 for illustrations of junctional P waves, junctional rhythm, premature junctional contraction (PJC), and accelerated junctional rhythm.

Supraventricular Tachycardia

1. P Wave:

P waves, because of the rapid rate, cannot be clearly delineated to establish the diagnosis as atrial or junctional.

2. P-R Interval:

No P waves are seen; therefore, there is no measurable P-R interval.

3. QRS Complex:

The QRS complex duration is 0.1 sec. or less.

4. Rhythm:

The rhythm is regular.

5. Rate:

The rate is generally above 150 per minute.

An arrhythmia is not infrequently encountered where the ventricular rate is so rapid that P waves cannot be readily identified on the standard electrocardiogram. The rate appears fairly regular and the duration of the QRS complexes normal. In the absence of esophageal recordings or of more definitive laboratory studies, the diagnosis of atrial or junctional tachycardia cannot be clearly delineated. Such a tachycardia is frequently classified under the overall category of supraventricular tachycardia, the impulse originating above the ventricles. The normal QRS interval (0.1 sec. or less) identifies a supraventricular pacemaker.

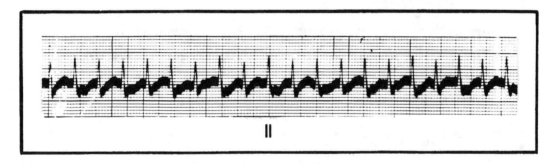

FIGURE 7-32. Supraventricular tachycardia. (Electrocardiogram reduced in size.)

Idioventricular Rhythm

1. P Wave:

    The P waves are not associated with the QRS complexes.

2. P-R Interval:

    Since there is no relationship between the P waves and the QRS complexes, there is no measurable P-R interval.

3. QRS Complex:

    The QRS complex duration is wide, greater than 0.1 sec., often greater than 0.12 sec. (three small boxes).

4. Rhythm:

    The ventricular rhythm is regular. The atrial rhythm will depend on the intrinsic atrial pacemaker.

5. Rate:

    The rate is that of the ventricular pacemaker, 20 to 40 per minute. The atria are often controlled by the S-A node.

C. Ventricles

Until now we have been studying arrhythmias where the impulse originates in the S-A node, atria, and A-V junction. These are supraventricular foci, with the pacemaker above the ventricles. Common to the supraventricular arrhythmias is a QRS complex that is of normal duration. The QRS complex duration is 0.1 sec. (two and a half small boxes) or less. Exceptions to this are described and illustrated on pages 608–610. In order to have a QRS complex duration of 0.1 sec. or less, the normal pathways of conduction, specialized for rapid conduction, are used. An impulse originating in the *ventricles* follows an abnormal pathway of conduction and cannot depolarize the ventricles within 0.1 sec. or less. In a ventricular rhythm the QRS complex is, therefore, abnormally wide, greater than 0.1 sec. and frequently greater than 0.12 sec. (three small boxes). The QRS complex is not only wide but also often bizarre in appearance. The T wave is generally opposite the QRS complex in orientation.

This section on ventricular rhythm disturbances includes: (1) idioventricular rhythm; (2) premature beats of the ventricle; (3) ventricular tachycardia; (4) ventricular flutter; and (5) ventricular fibrillation.

1. Idioventricular Rhythm

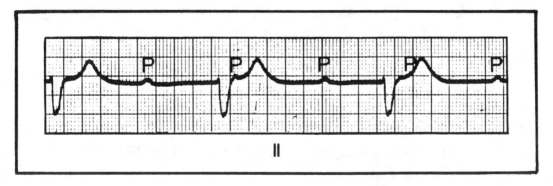

II

FIGURE 7-33. Idioventricular rhythm. When the dominant pacemaker is within the ventricles, because of drugs such as digitalis, or disease of the conduction system, the rate may be slow (20 to 40 beats per minute, which is the inherent rate of the ventricular pacemaker) and the rhythm is called idioventricular. The QRS complexes are wide (greater than 0.1 sec. and often greater than 0.12 sec.). In this figure the ventricular rate is 33 beats per minute and regular with an atrial rate of 62 beats per minute under control of the S-A node and not associated with the ventricles. With abnormal ventricular depolarization, the ventricular pacemaker is not as efficient as the supraventricular pacemakers. It is the lowest of the series of pacemakers and may become dominant when the higher pacemakers have failed. It may be an "escape" or "safety" rhythm and should not be suppressed since no other pacemaker may be available. "Accelerated" idioventricular rhythm (AIVR) is explained and illustrated on page 603.

> Accelerated idioventricular rhythm (AIVR) is explained and illustrated on page 603.

Premature Ventricular Contraction (PVC)

1. P Wave:

The premature ventricular deflection (QRS complex) is not preceded by a P wave.

2. P-R Interval:

There is no measurable P-R interval.

3. QRS Complex:

The QRS complex duration is at least 0.12 sec. The QRS complex is often bizarre in appearance compared with the normal QRS complexes.

4. Rhythm:

The regularity of the basic rhythm is disturbed by the PVC. It may be quite irregular when there are many PVCs.

5. Rate:

The rate depends on the basic rhythm and the number of PVCs present.

2. Premature Ventricular Contraction (PVC)

A premature ventricular contraction (PVC) is seen when an impulse is propagated from a ventricular focus before the next normal beat is due. The QRS is commonly widened and not preceded by a P wave. A "compensatory" pause usually follows. There may be retrograde activation of the atria following a premature ventricular contraction, or the normal sinus P waves may continue (as seen below). The sinus P waves following the premature ventricular contractions are blocked because of conduction system refractoriness.

In general, as stated in the introduction to this section, a normally narrow QRS complex is seen in supraventricular rhythms. An abnormally wide QRS complex may be seen in ventricular or supraventricular rhythms. After studying the wide QRS complex of the PVC, the ectopic beat of the ventricle (ventricular ectopy), it is important to study the causes of a wide QRS complex in a supraventricular rhythm. These will be described and illustrated on pages 608–610 as follows: bundle branch block, pre-excitation (W-P-W syndromes), and ventricular aberration or aberrancy, including the Ashman phenomenon.

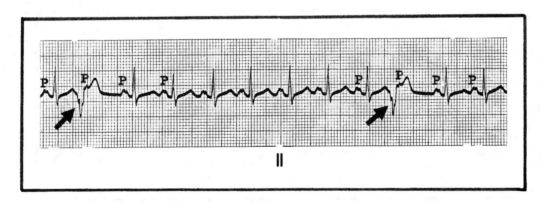

FIGURE 7-34.   *Premature ventricular contractions (arrows). (Electrocardiogram reduced in size.)*

> Compensatory pauses are illustrated on pages 604–606.

> Concealed conduction is defined and illustrated on page 607.

> The causes of a wide QRS complex with a supraventricular pacemaker, including the Ashman phenomenon,[7-7] are illustrated on pages 608–610.

Bigeminy or *coupling* describes the heart beating in groups of two, usually a normal beat followed by a premature ventricular contraction and separated from the next group by a compensatory pause. Beating in groups of three, such as two normal beats followed steadily by a premature ventricular contraction and separated by a compensatory pause, is known as *trigeminy*. The words bigeminy, trigeminy, etc., merely describe group beating; they do not tell you the components of the groups. As seen below, in bigeminy due to a premature ventricular contraction following a normal beat, the *coupling* interval is "fixed"—that is, there is an identical interval between each normal beat and each premature ventricular contraction. In this case, the true sinus rate is not known. The rate could be 35 or 70 beats per minute. If the latter is the case, the second, nonconducted p waves are completely buried within the ST-T complex. The PVCs shown here are *unifocal*, from one focus. Multifocal PVCs, couplets, salvos, fusion and parasystole are explained and illustrated on pages 611–614. The position of the PVC during ventricular repolarization is of importance. The "R-on-T" phenomenon is explained and illustrated on page 614.

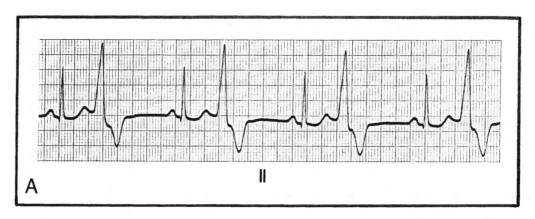

A   II

FIGURE 7-35A. *Bigeminy or coupling. (Electrocardiogram reduced in size.)*

> Multifocal PVCs, couplets, salvos, fusion, and parasystole are explained and illustrated on pages 611–614.

> The "R-on-T" phenomenon is explained and illustrated on page 614.

> The analysis of Figure 7-35A in the text and on the tape is the solution to Item 7 on the pretest.

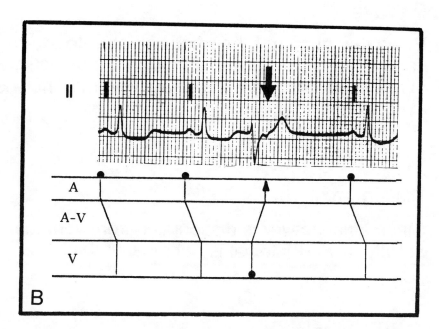

FIGURE 7-35B.   *Retrograde depolarization of the atria following a premature ventricular contraction. At times a premature ventricular contraction succeeds in penetrating the conducting system all the way to the atria, producing a retrograde P wave (arrow).*

Ventricular Tachycardia

1. **P Wave:**

   P waves may not be distinguishable during ventricular tachycardia, although atrial activity, dissociated from ventricular activity, may not be affected.

2. **P-R Interval:**

   Since atrial activity is dissociated from ventricular activity, a P-R interval is not measurable.

3. **QRS Complex:**

   The QRS complex duration is greater than 0.12 sec., and bizarre in appearance. The T wave may not be separated from the QRS complex.

4. **Rhythm:**

   The rhythm is regular or slightly irregular.

5. **Rate:**

   The ventricular rate is 150 to 250 per minute. Atrial activity is often not determinable.

3. Ventricular Tachycardia

The conduction system in the ventricles may propagate "runs" of premature contractions known as ventricular tachycardia. Once started, ventricular tachycardia may be sustained until terminated spontaneously, by medication, or by electrical cardioversion (Figure 7-36A), or it may be intermittent, with "runs" of premature ventricular contractions (Figure 7-36B). The QRS complexes are widened and the rate is usually from 150 to 250 per minute. The rhythm may be regular or slightly irregular. Ventricular tachycardia may be unifocal or multifocal ("polymorphic"). Refer to page 615 for explanation and illustration of "torsades de pointes."

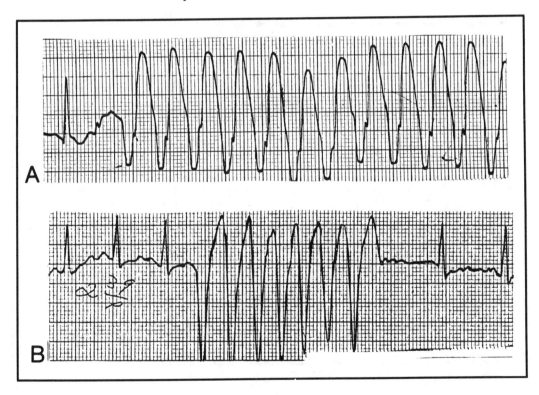

FIGURE 7-36.   Ventricular tachycardia.

> Explanation and illustration of "torsades de pointes" are found on page 615.

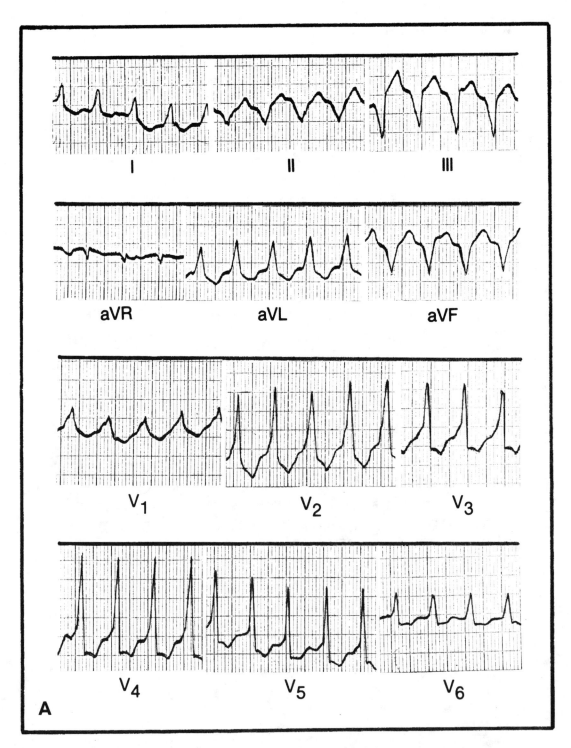

FIGURE 7-37A.   *Evaluation of this arrhythmia presents an interesting challenge. Review the analysis of the arrhythmia in Figure 7-21. Is this tachycardia, with a ventricular rate of 150 per minute, a ventricular tachycardia, or a supraventricular tachycardia with wide QRS complexes? Why? Make a decision before proceeding.*

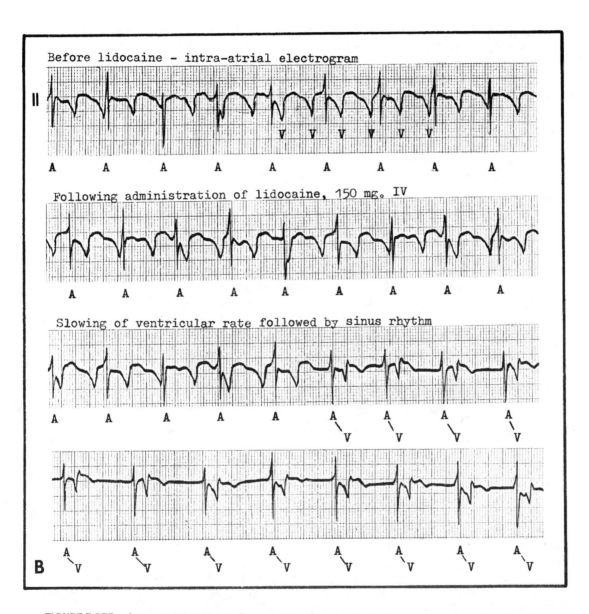

FIGURE 7-37B.   Intra-atrial electrogram. During ventricular tachycardia, the ventricles may activate the atria retrogradely. The atria, however, usually remain under sinus control and beat at the normal, slower rate and are dissociated from the ventricles. (Electrocardiogram reduced in size.)

Often it is important, in order to make the diagnosis of ventricular tachycardia, to evaluate the atrial activity. Atrial activity may or may not be obvious on the clinical electrocardiogram in the presence of a rapid ventricular rate. We may not even be dealing with a ventricular tachycardia, as we say earlier in this study with atrial flutter and left bundle branch block (Figure 7-21). All efforts to identify atrial activity on the clinical electrocardiogram may prove futile. Because of the importance of establishing the diagnosis, in terms of therapy, the cardiology laboratory may be of help. Figure 7-37A reveals a tachycardia with a ventricular rate of 150 per minute. Is this a ventricular tachycardia or a supraventricular tachycardia with wide QRS complexes? An electrode catheter was inserted into the right atrium and an intra-atrial electrogram recorded an atrial rate of 80 per minute. The demonstration of a slower atrial rate dissociated from the rapid ventricular rate facilitated the diagnosis of ventricular tachycardia and resulted in the initiation of proper therapy. The atrial deflections are marked by the letter A and the ventricular deflections by the letter V in Figure 7-37B. Note the slowing of the ventricular rate following the administration of lidocaine, with establishment of normal sinus rhythm seen in the third panel.

Another aid that may be obtained in the cardiology laboratory is the His bundle recording, as seen earlier in this chapter. If a His bundle deflection does not precede the QRS complex of the tachycardia, the origin of the impulses must be below the His bundle—for example, in the ventricle.

In the absence of a laboratory, esophageal recording can be of great value in locating the atrial deflections or P waves. When P waves are not obvious, and other differentiating features are obscured, it may help, in differentiating supraventricular tachycardia with wide QRS complexes (e.g., RBBB or LBBB) from ventricular tachycardia, to keep in mind that in *ventricular tachycardia,* the QRS complexes, when examined in all twelve leads, do not resemble classical bundle branch block of either type. In Figure 7-37A, lead V_1 suggests RBBB while other leads suggest LBBB.

Figure 7-21A is shown again on the next page. Compare the supraventricular tachycardia with a wide QRS complex with the ventricular tachycardia (Figure 7-37A).

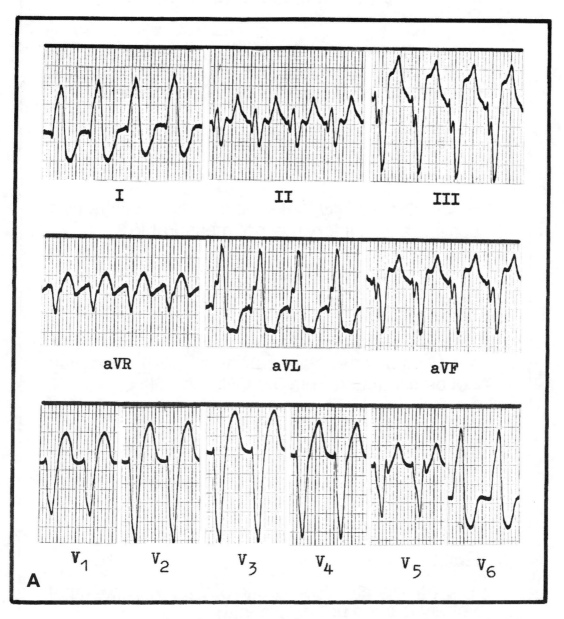

FIGURE 7-21A.   Supraventricular (atrial flutter with 2:1 A-V conduction), tachycardia with a wide QRS complex (due to LBBB). Compare with Figure 7-37A, ventricular tachycardia.

Ventricular Flutter

1. P Wave:

P waves may not be distinguishable during ventricular flutter, although atrial activity, dissociated from ventricular activity, may not be affected.

2. P-R Interval:

Since atrial activity is dissociated from ventricular activity, a P-R interval is not measurable.

3. QRS Complex:

The QRS complex duration is greater than 0.12 sec. and bizarre in appearance. The T wave may not be separated from the QRS complex.

4. Rhythm:

The rhythm is regular or slightly irregular.

5. Rate:

The ventricular rate is 250 to 350 per minute. Atrial activity is often not determinable.

4. Ventricular Flutter

In ventricular flutter undulating waves are seen rising and falling. This rhythm is often an intermediary stage between ventricular tachycardia and ventricular fibrillation. The rate is usually between 250 to 350 beats per minute. When the ventricular rate is at this level, the patient is acutely ill, and the pulse may be imperceptible. The differential diagnosis is ventricular flutter versus atrial flutter *in the presence of an aberrant pathway* (e.g., W-P-W). The normal A-V node cannot conduct 1:1 at this rate, and it is too fast for ventricular tachycardia (usually about 160 per minute).

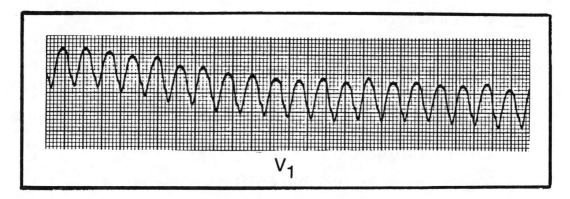

V_1

FIGURE 7-38.   *Ventricular flutter.*

Ventricular Fibrillation

1. P Wave:

   P waves are not identifiable.

2. P-R Interval:

   There is no measurable P-R interval.

3. QRS Complex:

   There are no identifiable QRS complexes.

4. Rhythm:

   The rhythm is chaotic, with multiple, disorganized contractions of the ventricles.

5. Rate:

   The rate cannot be determined accurately.

5. Ventricular Fibrillation

Ventricular fibrillation is characterized by very rapid, disorganized contractions of the ventricles, and represents cardiac arrest. It may be of sudden onset or may follow ventricular premature contractions and ventricular tachycardia as seen in Figure 7-39A. Chaotic action of the dying heart is seen in the bottom tracing in Figure 7-39A and in Figure 7-39B.

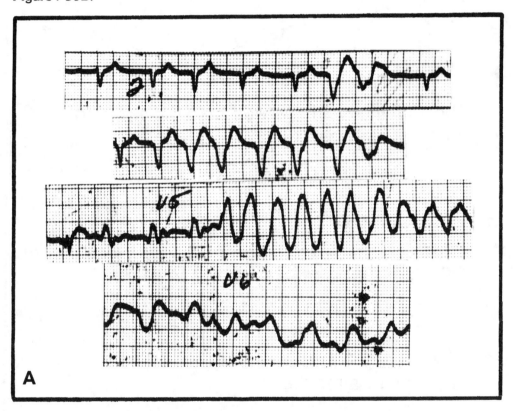

FIGURE 7-39A.   Ventricular fibrillation. (Electrocardiogram reduced in size.)

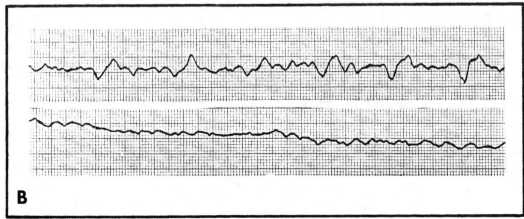

FIGURE 7-39B.   Chaotic action of the dying heart. (Electrocardiogram reduced in size.)

First Degree A-V Block

1. ## P Wave:

   The P waves are positive and uniform in leads I and II if the S-A node is the pacemaker. Every P wave is followed by a QRS complex.

2. ## P-R Interval:

   The P-R interval is greater than 0.2 sec. and constant from beat to beat.

3. ## QRS Complex:

   The QRS complex duration is 0.1 sec. or less. Every QRS complex is preceded by a P wave.

4. ## Rhythm:

   The rhythm is regular.

5. ## Rate:

   The rate is dependent on the basic rhythm. If the basic rhythm is sinus, the rate is constant between 60 and 100 per minute.

D. Atrioventricular (A-V) Conduction Disturbances

Atrioventricular conduction disturbances comprise: (1) first degree A-V block; (2) second degree A-V block; and (3) third degree, or complete A-V block.

1. First Degree A-V Block

First degree A-V block represents a delay in the transmission of impulses from the atria to the ventricles. A prolonged P-R interval (greater than 0.20 sec.) is seen on the electrocardiogram. The delay usually occurs in the A-V node but may occur elsewhere, e.g., the His-Purkinje system.

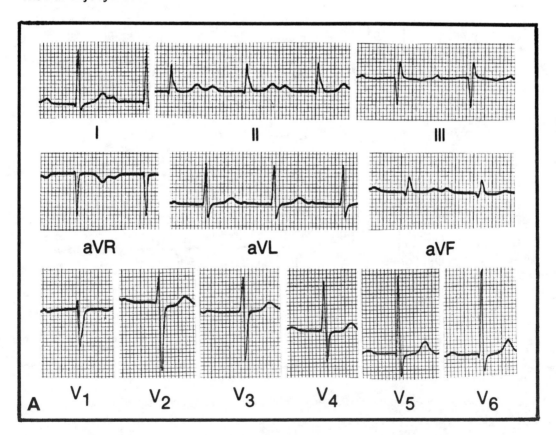

FIGURE 7-40A.   First degree A-V block in a patient with an old inferior myocardial infarction.

> The analysis of Figure 7-40A in the text and on the tape is the solution to Item 8 on the pretest.

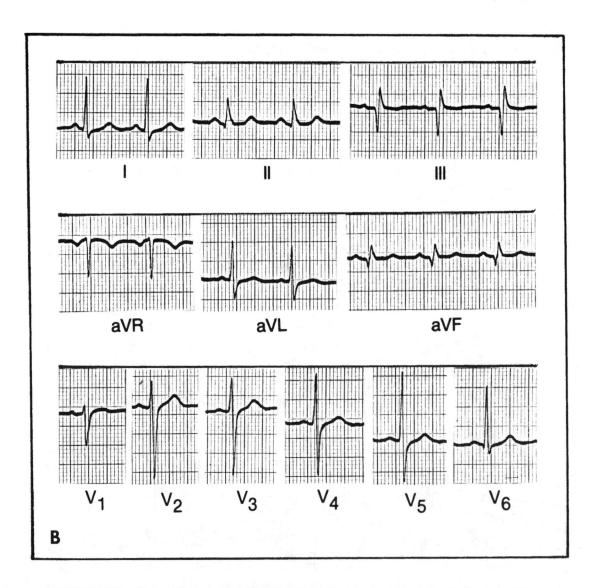

I   II   III

aVR   aVL   aVF

V_1 V_2 V_3 V_4 V_5 V_6

B

FIGURE 7-40B. Same patient as in Figure 7-40A following the infarct but prior to the development of first degree A-V block.

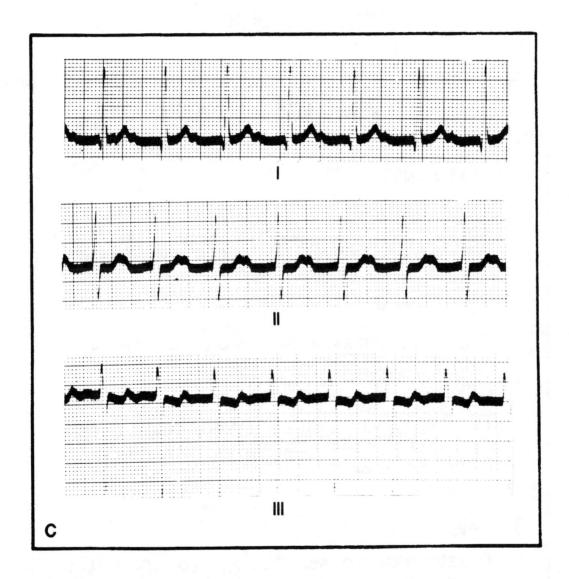

FIGURE 7-40C.   *First degree A-V block was recognized many years ago. This electrocardiogram will be seen again in the study of digitalis toxicity (Chapter 8).*

Second Degree A-V Block
(Mobitz I Block)

1. P Wave:

Not every P wave is followed by a QRS complex.

2. P-R Interval:

The P-R intervals become progressively longer until an atrial depolarization no longer initiates a ventricular response. The cycle is then resumed.

3. QRS Complex:

The QRS complex duration is 0.1 sec. or less.

4. Rhythm:

The rhythm is irregular with "group beating." As illustrated, there is a pause after each group of three ventricular beats.

5. Rate:

The atrial rate is constant between 60 and 100 per minute. The ventricular rate is slower due to the nonconducted beats.

2. Second Degree A-V Block

In second degree A-V block some atrial impulses do not reach the ventricles because of a conduction disturbance. The study will include Mobitz type I and Mobitz type II A-V block. Mobitz type I block has often been referred to as the "classic Wenckebach" block. Marriott has recommended that they simply be called type I and type II A-V block.[7,8]

Wenckebach described the phenomenon of progressive delay in conduction from the atria to the ventricles ending in a dropped beat. He later also described dropped beats when conduction time was *not* changed. Mobitz, years later, suggested that these forms of A-V block be called type I and type II.

In Mobitz type I or simply type I A-V block it is important to understand the Wenckebach phenomenon. Wenckebach conduction is characterized by progressive delay of conduction culminating in the failure of a single beat to conduct (single dropped beat). Wenckebach periods therefore have conduction ratios of (n + 1) : n. While Wenckebach conduction occurs commonly in the A-V node (i.e., A-V Wenckebach periods), the phenomenon may occur in any conducting tissue of the heart. In *typical* Wenckebach periods, the conduction times show progressive increase, but the intervals between the beats which are produced show progressive *decrease* prior to the drop. This occurs because the *increment*

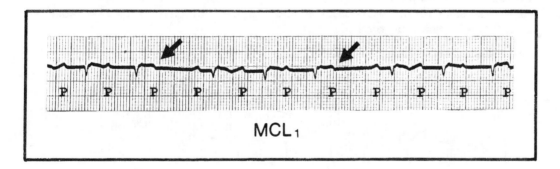

FIGURE 7-41.   *Mobitz type I A-V block. The P-R intervals become progressively longer until a P wave is not followed by a QRS complex. The cycle then starts again. The ratio in this electrocardiogram is 4:3, four P waves : three QRS complexes. The block in Mobitz type I A-V block has been shown to be above the bundle of His, in the A-V node (in contrast to Mobitz type II A-V block—Figure 7-42). (Electrocardiogram reduced in size.)*

> A ladder diagram of Mobitz type I A-V block is illustrated on page 616. Sinoatrial (S-A) Wenckebach periods are explained and illustrated on page 617.

> The analysis of Figure 7-41 in the text and on the tape is the solution to Item 9 on the pretest.

of delay of each beat over that of the previous beat progressively *decreases.* In typical Wenckebach periods, the pause containing the dropped beat is less than the sum of the two preceding interbeat intervals. In addition, the interval after the pause is longer than that preceding the pause (except in 3:2 Wenckebach periods, in which they are identical). In typical Wenckebach periods, those periods having the same conducting ratios (e.g., 5:4, 4:3, etc.) precisely replicate each other; that is, the length of each of the respective intervals, as well as that of the entire Wenckebach period, are identical. The entire Wenckebach period is measured from the first beat of the sequence to the beat terminating the long pause. In typical A-V Wenckebach periods, one can directly measure the underlying sinus rate, since it is equal to the (constant) P-wave rate. *Sinoatrial (S-A) Wenckebach periods* in contrast to A-V Wenckebach periods are explained and illustrated on page 617.

Another form of second degree A-V block is Mobitz type II or simply type II A-V block. It is far more serious than type I A-V block which is frequently short-lived. When the ventricles periodically do not respond to atrial stimuli, the P wave on the electrocardiogram is *not* followed by a QRS complex (arrows in Figure 7-42). The dropped beat occurs periodically with no change in the other P-R intervals. His bundle studies have shown the block to be below the His bundle, a warning of possible future development of complete A-V block. After studying type II A-V block, review Figure 7-8, which is "type II" S-A block. "Type I" S-A block is illustrated on page 617.

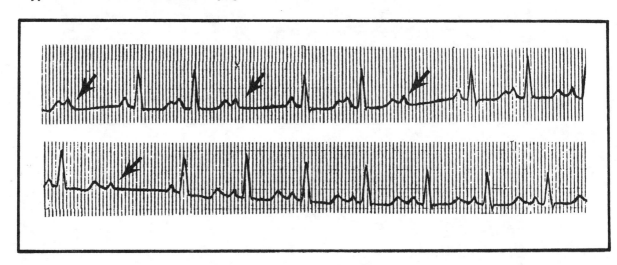

FIGURE 7-42. Mobitz II A-V block. Sporadic single dropped beats occur. The P-R intervals of the consecutively conducted beats are unchanging, indicating infranodal block.

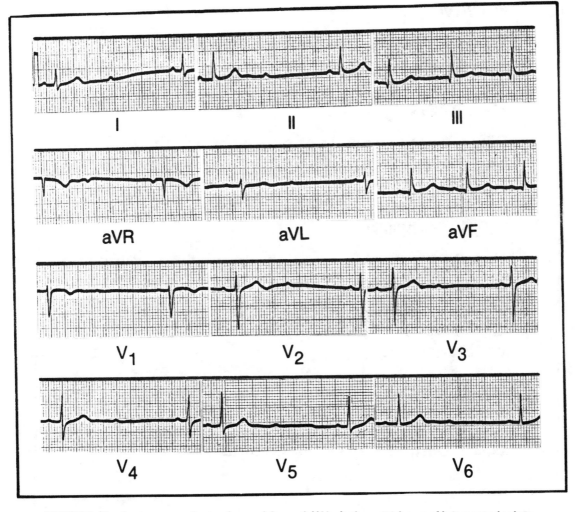

FIGURE 7-43. *In more severe forms of second degree A-V block, the ventricles are able to respond only to every second, third, fourth, or fifth beat. In this electrocardiogram, every other P wave (except in leads III and aVF) is not followed by a QRS complex. This is known as 2:1 A-V block (two atrial beats for every ventricular beat). (Electrocardiogram reduced in size.)*

> Examples of advanced (high grade) second degree A-V block are found on page 618.

Third Degree (Complete) A-V Block

1. **P Wave:**

   The P waves are not associated with the QRS complexes.

2. **P-R Interval:**

   Since there is no relationship between the P waves and the QRS complexes, there is no measurable P-R interval.

3. **QRS Complex:**

   The QRS complex duration, depending on the site of impulse formation, may be normal, with the pacemaker in the A-V junction, or quite wide and bizarre, with the pacemaker low in the ventricles.

4. **Rhythm:**

   The ventricular rhythm is regular. The atrial rhythm will depend on the intrinsic atrial pacemaker.

5. **Rate:**

   The atria are often controlled by the S-A node while the ventricles are controlled by either a junctional pacemaker with a normally narrow QRS complex or a ventricular pacemaker with a wide, bizarre QRS complex.

3. Third Degree (Complete) A-V Block

In *third degree,* or *complete A-V block,* there is no fixed relationship between the atria and the ventricles; they beat independently. On the electrocardiogram there is no constant relationship between the P waves and the QRS complexes. Depending on the site of impulse formation, the QRS complexes may be of normal duration and configuration, with the pacemaker in the A-V junction, or quite wide and bizarre, with the pacemaker low in the ventricles.

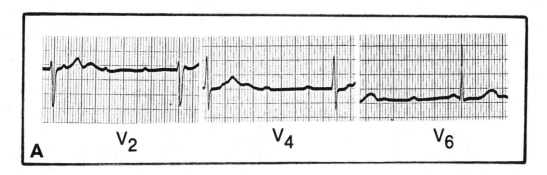

FIGURE 7-44A.   *Third degree (completed) A-V block. The atria and ventricles are beating independently, the atria under control of the S-A node are beating at a rate of 100 per minute and the ventricles, under control of the A-V junction, are beating at a rate of 33 per minute. The patient, who had a previous electrocardiogram with normal A-V conduction (Figure 7-44B), noted the sudden onset of the low heart rate; there was no accompanying chest pain and no evidence of myocardial infarction. What is the treatment of choice? (Electrocardiogram reduced in size.)*

> The analysis of Figure 7-44A in the text and on the tape is the solution to Item 10 on the pretest.

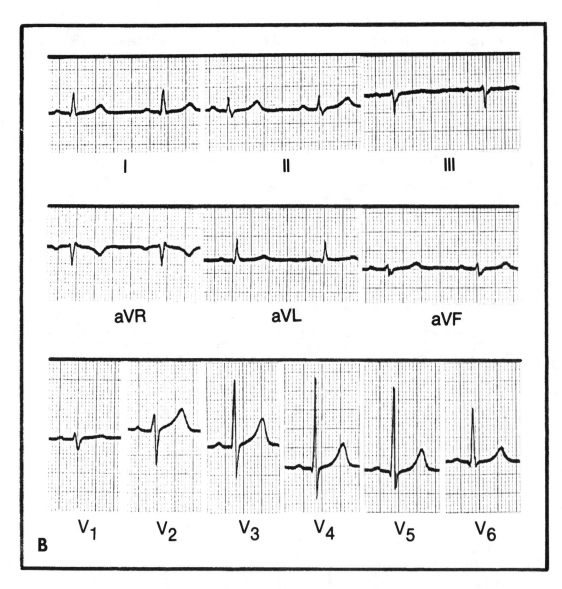

FIGURE 7-44B. Prior electrocardiogram of patient who presented with complete A-V block described in Figure 7-44A.

4. Pacemaker Therapy

Pacemaker therapy refers to electrical pacing of the ventricles and/or atria with an artificial pacemaker. A patient with complete A-V block, as seen in Figure 7-44A, may present with symptoms of cerebral insufficiency, such as dizziness or beclouded mentation, or may actually have lost consciousness because of the low rate and poor cardiac output, or to transient ventricular standstill or fibrillation. The present day treatment is electrical pacing to maintain a proper rate and good cardiac output.

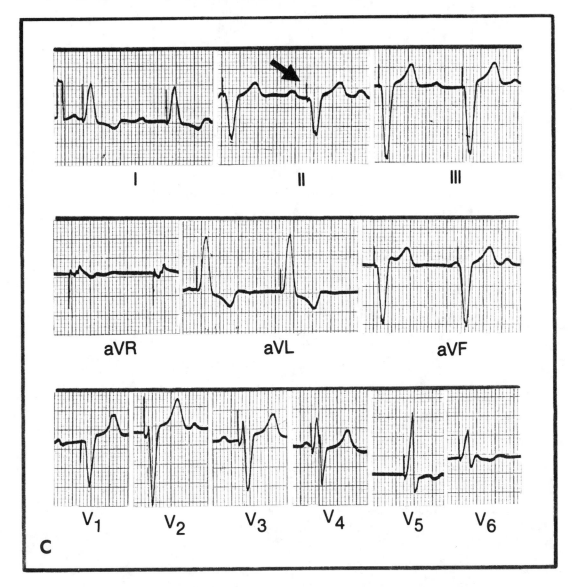

FIGURE 7-44C.   Following treatment with ventricular pacing; note the pacer impulse preceding each ventricular deflection, indicated by an arrow in lead II.

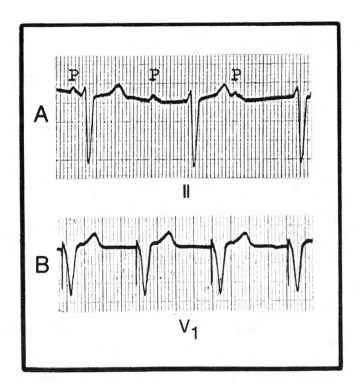

FIGURE 7-45.   Third degree A-V block. The atria and ventricles are beating independently (A), the atria at the usual sinus rate and the ventricles more slowly. This rhythm followed open heart surgery, and the patient was treated with permanent ventricular pacing (B).

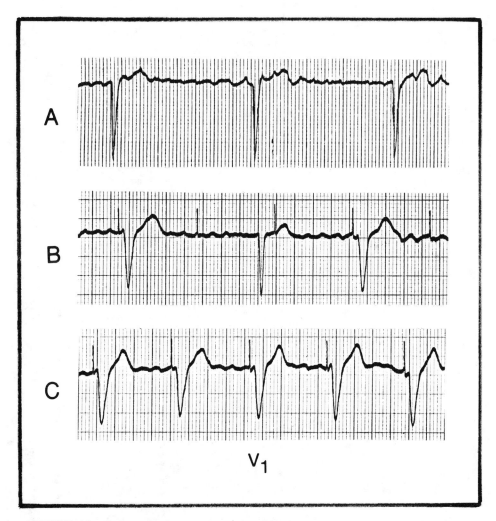

FIGURE 7-46. *Complete A-V block in a patient with coarse atrial fibrillation (flutter-fibrillation) (A). During adjustment of the pacemaker (B), the pacemaker impulse is producing a response only erratically; 1:1 pacing is accomplished in C.*

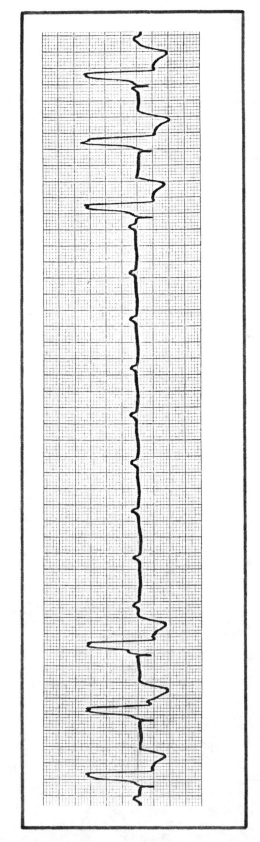

FIGURE 7-47. That pacemaker therapy has improved many lives is dramatically illustrated above. During adjustment of the pacemaker only atrial depolarization (P waves) is seen, with complete standstill of the ventricles. With resumption of electrical pacing (indicated by the pacemaker impulses), ventricular complexes follow. (Electrocardiogram reduced in size.)

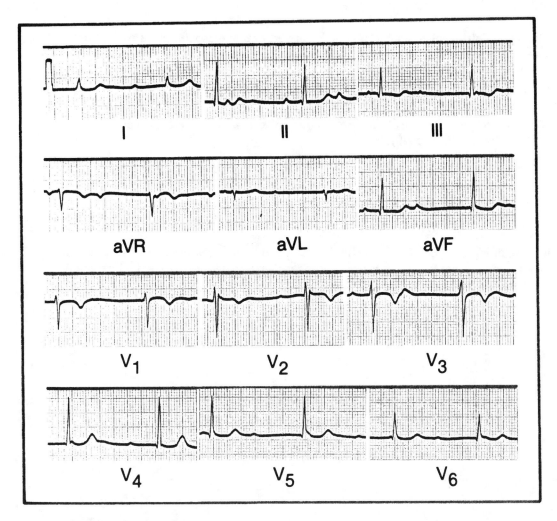

FIGURE 7-48.   Congenital third degree (complete) A-V block in a young, asymptomatic patient. How would you treat this patient? (Electrocardiogram reduced in size.)

We have been studying first, second, and third degree A-V block. Marriott has been stressing the importance of heart rate in the evaluation of patients with A-V block.[7,9] This patient with third degree A-V block (Figure 7-48) was asymptomatic with a heart rate of 46 while the patients with second degree A-V block, pages 579 and 618, with heart rates of 33 and 23, respectively, were symptomatic. The designation of third degree A-V block does not give a clear picture by itself. Once again compare this patient with a heart rate of 46 with the patient who had a heart rate of 14 beats per minute and syncope (page 619).

> The electrocardiogram of a patient who presented with a history of syncope and a heart rate of 14 beats per minute is seen on page 619.

The terms "atrioventricular block" and "atrioventricular dissociation" are often used interchangeably. *This is not correct.* You have just seen examples of third degree (complete) A-V block. A-V block is *not* synonymous with A-V dissociation. A-V dissociation merely means that the atria and ventricles are under separate control. A-V block is one category under A-V dissociation. Causes of A-V dissociation include:

1. Slowing or failure of the primary pacemaker (sinus), resulting in an escape rhythm (Figure 7-9).

2. Acceleration of the subsidiary pacemaker (see Figures 8-16 and 8-17, Chapter 8).

3. A-V block (complete) with slow idioventricular rhythm (Figures 7-44A, 7-45A, 7-46A, and 7-48).

4. Combination of numbers 1, 2, and 3.

In concluding our brief study of arrhythmias, the dynamic character of this subject must be stressed. Students should always be prepared to add new and revised information to their foundation of knowledge.

> Stop the tape and begin the post-test on the next page.

P O S T · T E S T

DIRECTIONS. Supply the information requested in each of the following.

1. List the criteria for "normal sinus rhythm."

2. In which group of people is "sinus arrhythmia" frequently found? Describe its characteristics.

3. Differentiate S-A block from sinus arrest.

4. Why is the Wolff-Parkinson-White (W-P-W) syndrome and the short P-R interval syndrome included in the study of arrhythmias?

5. In which group of patients is multifocal (chaotic) atrial tachycardia most frequently found?

6. What is the meaning of "bigeminy?" What are the components of bigeminy?

7. Describe atrial fibrillation as seen on the electrocardiogram.

8. Describe "upper, middle, and lower nodal" rhythms in the "classic" manner.

9. What is a His bundle study and what is its contribution?

10. The terms "atrioventricular block" and "atrioventricular dissociation" are often used interchangeably. Is this correct? If not, what is the difference?

> Check your responses on the following pages.

ANSWERS TO
POST-TEST

1. In normal sinus rhythm, the impulse starts in the S-A node and is propagated normally. The rate is regular, between 60 and 100 beats per minute. The P waves are constant and upright in at least leads I and aVF or I and II. Each P wave is followed by a QRS complex, and each QRS complex is preceded by a P wave. The P-R interval is from 0.12 to 0.2 sec. (3 to 5 small boxes), and constant from beat to beat. When the word "nodal" is used to describe a rhythm it refers to the A-V node and *not* to the S-A node; "nodal" is never an abbreviation for the S-A node. See Figure 7-2.

2. In sinus arrhythmia, the same characteristics as described under normal sinus rhythm apply except that there may be marked variation in rate that is often, but not always, associated with the respiratory cycles. It is commonly seen in the young. The P-R intervals are constant, but the R-R intervals are continually changing. See Figure 7-3.

3. In sinoatrial (S-A) block, the S-A node initiates the impulse but the *propagation* is blocked, so that the atria are not depolarized; hence there is no P wave. The pause is a multiple of the regular cycle length.

   Sinus arrest is a sudden failure of the S-A node to initiate an expected impulse; it is a failure of impulse *formation,* rather than a failure of impulse *propagation.* If no other pacemaker becomes dominant at this point, death follows quickly. When the S-A node fails to initiate an impulse, a lower pacemaker may become dominant. The beat that follows the "arrest" is then called an "escape" beat. If the pacemaker originating the escape beat remains the dominant one, the rhythm may then be called an escape rhythm. See Figures 7-8 and 7-9.

4. The W-P-W syndrome and the short P-R interval syndrome are associated with reentrant (reciprocating) tachycardias (see Figure 7-11A and B).

5. Multifocal (chaotic) atrial tachycardia is most frequently found in patients with chronic obstructive pulmonary disease with hypoxia. See Figure 7-22B.

6. Bigeminy refers to heart beats in groups of two. You must describe what you see since the word "bigeminy" does not tell you the component parts of each pair. See Figures 7-17 and 7-35A.

7. Disorganized, ineffective contractions of the atria (350 to 600 per minute) characterize atrial fibrillation. No P waves are seen, and the ventricular response is irregular, depending on how many of the 350 to 600 impulses are conducted to the ventricles. If the atrial rate is 500 per minute and the ventricular rate is 125 per minute, it means that one in every four atrial impulses is conducted, irregularly, to the ventricles. See Figure 7-22A.

8. The atrioventricular (A-V) node is a lower center of excitation and may become the dominant pacemaker when the S-A node is depressed. The A-V node may be the dominant pacemaker congenitally or may share dominance with the S-A node throughout life. The heart rate, with the A-V node as the pacemaker, is regular and from 40 to 60 beats per minute; however, the rate may be equivalent to the sinus rate or even quite rapid (A-V nodal tachycardia). The P waves are usually upright in lead I, but inverted in leads II and III (Figure 7-23), and may come before, during, or after the QRS complex.

    a. Upper nodal rhythm: The P wave precedes the QRS complex, with a P-R interval up to 0.12 sec.

    b. Middle nodal rhythm: The P wave is within the QRS complex.

    c. Lower nodal rhythm: The P wave follows the QRS complex.

9. The His bundle study is a technique whereby an electrode catheter is placed near the tricuspid valve via the femoral vein or an arm vein, and recordings are made from the area of the His bundle. The recordings reveal a sharp deflection, labeled H in Figure 7-29, between the atrial and ventricular deflections. His bundle recordings have terminated the "silence" of the P-R segment and have added an important tool to the understanding of arrhythmias. See also Figures 7-30 and 7-31.

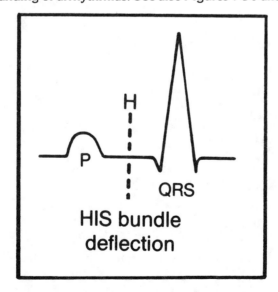

FIGURE 7-29. Diagram showing location of His bundle deflection.

10. The terms "atrioventricular block" and "atrioventricular dissociation" are often used interchangeably. *This is not correct.* A-V block is *not* synonymous with A-V dissociation. A-V dissociation merely means that the atria and ventricles are under separate control. A-V block is one category under A-V dissociation. Causes of A-V dissociation include:

    a. Slowing or failure of the primary pacemaker (sinus), resulting in an escape rhythm (Figure 7-9).

    b. Acceleration of the subsidiary pacemaker (see Figures 8-16 and 8-17, Chapter 8).

    c. A-V block (complete) with slow idioventricular rhythm (Figures 7-44A, 7-45A, 7-46A, and 7-48).

    d. Combination of numbers 1, 2, and 3.

NOTES AND
REFERENCES

From Page 493

The single leads commonly used for the constant monitoring of arrhythmias are leads II, MCL_1, and MCL_6. Lead II is a modified lead II since the positive and negative electrodes are not placed on the respective extremities, but on the chest as illustrated below. MCL_1 and MCL_6 are illustrated on the following page.

Lead II

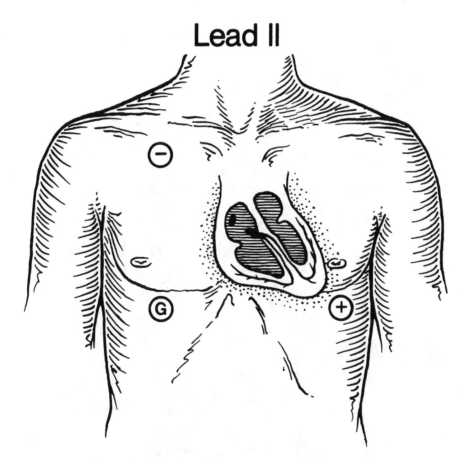

⊕ = Positive Electrode

⊖ = Negative Electrode

Ⓖ = Ground

From Page 493 (continued)

MCL_1 and MCL_6 are also modified leads, since the negative electrode is near the left shoulder and not on the left arm (in the "unmodified" CL lead the negative electrode is placed on the left arm and the positive on the chest as illustrated below).

> M = modified
> C = chest (positive electrode)
> L = left arm (negative electrode)

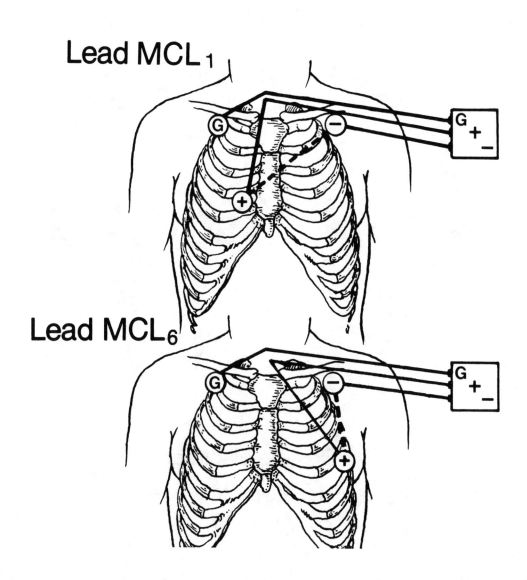

Lead MCL_1

Lead MCL_6

From Page 521:   Reentry

It is important to understand the concept of reentry in the study of arrhythmias since it is the mechanism of most supraventricular and many ventricular tachycardias. In order to have a reentrant (reciprocal) mechanism there must be two conduction pathways differing in refractoriness and conduction velocity.

In the schematic is represented a reentry circuit in the A-V node. A and B represent different stages in the same circuit. The circuit consists of a slow and a fast pathway with a final common pathway at either end. The slow pathway has slow antegrade (forward)

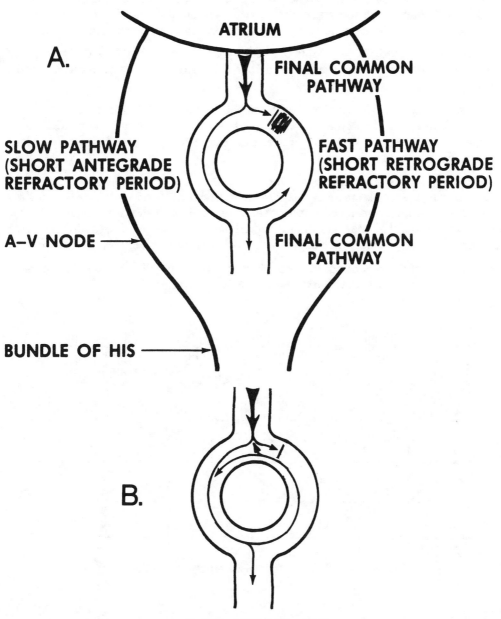

Model for A-V Nodal Reentry[7-3]

From Page 521 (continued)

conduction, but a relatively short antegrade refractory period. The fast pathway has more rapid antegrade conduction and a relatively short retrograde (backward) refractory period. Under certain conditions, an antegrade impulse may be blocked in the fast pathway while conducting slowly down the slow pathway. Given a critical degree of slowing, an impulse may arrive at the lower reaches of the A-V node via the slow pathway and find the fast pathway already recovered and able to conduct in the retrograde direction. The impulse then travels up the fast pathway to the upper reaches of the A-V node, from where it may (1) stimulate the atrium in retrograde fashion, and/or (2) find the slow pathway able to conduct in the antegrade direction, thus beginning another reentry loop, leading to a tachycardia. If one loop is made by the impulse, an extrasystole results.

The A-V node was used as an example of a reentry circuit. A reentry circuit may occur in other sites in the heart such as the Purkinje fiber sytem. Reentry involving the A-V node and bundle of Kent is illustrated below.

Tachycardias may result from reentry as described above or from a rapidly firing ectopic focus (increased automaticity). Ectopic beats are beats arising in any focus other than the S-A node. Automaticity is a property of pacemaking cells which form impulses spontaneously.

Some examples of reentrant (reciprocating) tachycardias are paroxysmal supraventricular tachycardia, ventricular tachycardia, pre-excitation (L-G-L and W-P-W) tachycardia and coupled premature beats. Examples of automatic tachycardias include atrial tachycardia with block and nonparoxysmal junctional tachycardia, both due to digitalis toxicity, ectopic atrial tachycardia, multifocal atrial tachycardia and idioventricular rhythm.

In the reentrant or reciprocating supraventricular tachycardia, illustrated below, a reentry loop became established within the A-V node, the common site.

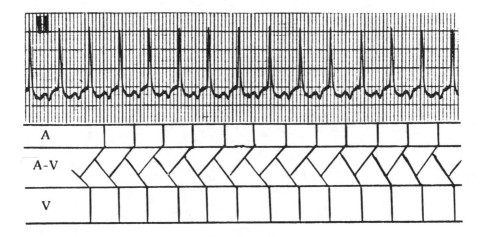

Reentrant (Reciprocating) Supraventricular Tachycardia

From Page 521 (continued)

The common reentrant circuit in W-P-W tachycardias involves antegrade conduction in the A-V node and retrograde conduction through the bundle of Kent, producing a normal narrow QRS complex. Much less common is antegrade conduction through the bundle of Kent with retrograde conduction through the A-V node, producing a wide, bizarre QRS complex.

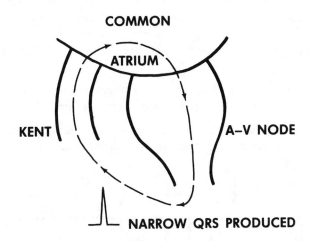

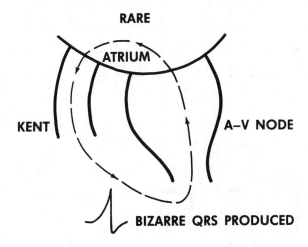

Reentry Involving the A-V Node and Bundle of Kent[7-3]

From Page 528:   Refractory Periods

In order to understand why a PAC is blocked (not conducted), it is important to know when the absolute and relative refractory periods of the ventricle occur. The process of depolarization reflects the flow of an electrical current to all cells along the pathway of conduction. The cells then return to their original resting state by the process of repolarization. Ventricular repolarization is complete at the end of the T wave, permitting a new impulse to start the process again. A new impulse, occurring before the peak of the T wave, finds the ventricular conduction system unable to accept it; this is the *absolute refractory period* (see Figure 7-16). Although the downslope of the T wave is still within the refractory period, an impulse may be conducted under certain circumstances; this is the *relative refractory period* (see Figure 7-15).

> *absolute refractory period*—the period after a stimulus when the conduction system cannot be stimulated no matter how great a stimulus is applied.

> *relative refractory period*—the period after a stimulus when partial repolarization of the conduction system has occurred and a greater than normal stimulus can stimulate a second response.

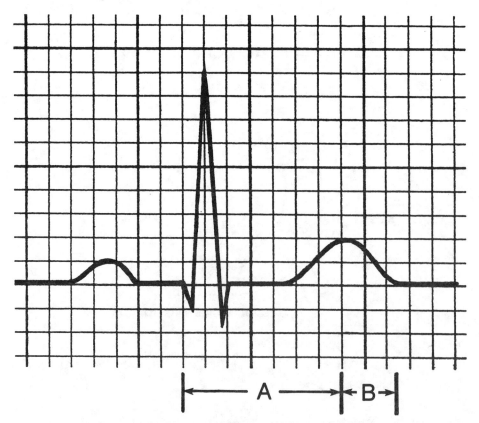

A. Absolute Refractory Period
B. Relative Refractory Period

From Page 553:
Junctional Rhythm P Waves

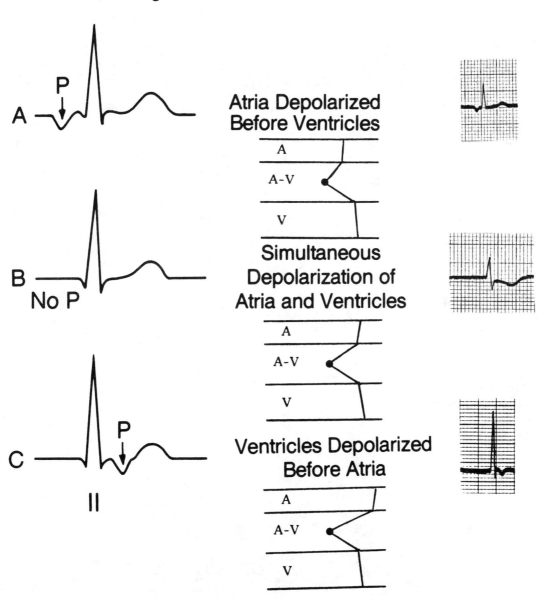

Atria Depolarized
Before Ventricles

Simultaneous
Depolarization of
Atria and Ventricles

Ventricles Depolarized
Before Atria

The position of the P wave depends on whether

1. The atria are depolarized *before* the ventricles. The P wave is inverted in lead II with a short (0.12 sec. or less) P-R interval (A).

2. The atria and ventricles are depolarized *simultaneously.* The P wave is then hidden within the QRS complex and is not visible on the electrocardiogram (B).

3. The atria are depolarized *after* the ventricles. The P wave is then inverted in lead II, following the QRS complex (C).

An additional possibility exists, as illustrated on the next page.

From Page 553 (continued):
Junctional Rhythm

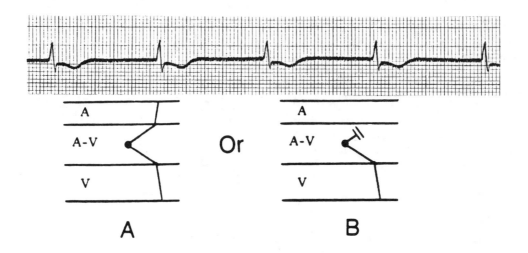

When no P waves are present in junctional rhythm, two possibilities exist. Either the atria and ventricles are depolarized simultaneously (A), or there is retrograde block and the atria are not depolarized (B).

From Page 553 (continued):
Premature Junctional
Contraction (PJC)

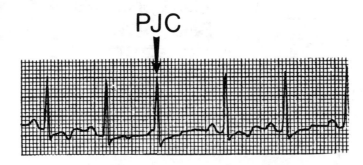

Premature junctional beats are seen when the A-V junction propagates an impulse before the next normal beat is due. In the illustration above, the PJC is seen shortly after the onset of the sinus P wave, interrupting the sinus rhythm.

From Page 553 (continued):
Accelerated Junctional Rhythm (AJR)

The normal junctional escape rate (inherent rate) is 40 to 60 beats per minute. In accelerated junctional rhythm (AJR) the rate exceeds 60 beats per minute (as seen below, at 88 beats per minute). The major causes of AJR are digitalis toxicity and myocardial infarction. Note the inverted (retrograde) P waves following the QRS complexes.

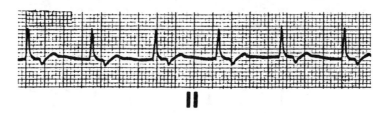

Accelerated Junctional Rhythm (AJR)

From Page 557:
Accelerated Idioventricular
Rhythm (AIVR)

Normally, the latent pacemakers of the ventricular Purkinje network have escape rates of 40 beats per minute or less. Under certain circumstances the escape rate of one of these pacemakers becomes enhanced to a rate between 60 and 130 beats per minute. Should the rate of the dominant supraventricular pacemaker fall below the rate of this accelerated lower pacemaker, it will discharge and control the ventricle for several beats but may last for minutes to hours. The morphology of the QRS complexes resembles that of PVCs; that is, at least 0.12 sec. in duration and not conforming to a classic bundle branch block pattern. It is usually observed in the setting of an acute myocardial infarction, although it occasionally appears on ambulatory monitor recordings. AIVR usually occurs in the presence of a relatively slow sinus rate (below 80 beats per minute). It may be regular or irregular, slightly accelerating ("warming up") or decelerating. It may terminate spontaneously, or when the sinus rate picks up and/or the P wave is able to conduct with resumption of the supraventricular rhythm. Fusion beats often occur. It rarely progresses to a serious tachycardia and should not be suppressed.

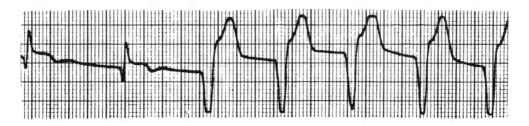

Accelerated Idioventricular Rhythm (AIVR)

From Page 559:
Compensatory Pause

1. Full Compensatory Pause

The PVC conducts retrogradely into the conducting system. The next sinus P wave finds the conducting system fully refractory, and is therefore not conducted. It is the *following* sinus beat that conducts normally. The R-R interval surrounding the PVC is therefore precisely equal to *two* sinus cycle lengths.

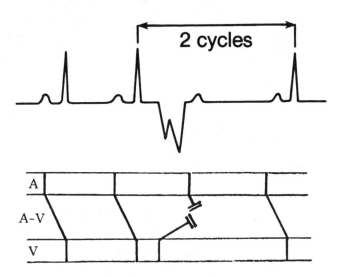

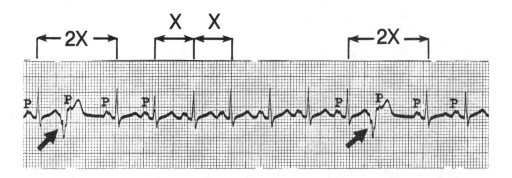

Full Compensatory Pause

From Page 559 (continued)

2. *Partial Compensatory Pause*

The PVC conducts retrogradely into the conducting system when the conducting system has *partially* recovered. This sinus P wave is therefore conducted, but with an *increased P-R interval,* so that the R-R interval surrounding the PVC is equal to *between* one and two sinus cycle lengths.

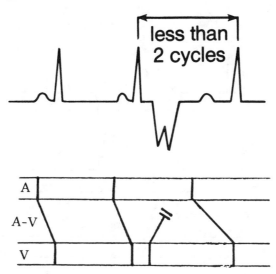

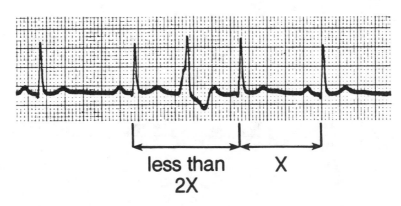

Partial Compensatory Pause

From Page 559 (continued)

3. *No Pause (Full Interpolation)*

The PVC barely penetrates the conducting system. The next sinus P wave encounters no conducting system delay, and thus conducts normally. The PVC therefore falls within precisely one sinus cycle R-R interval.

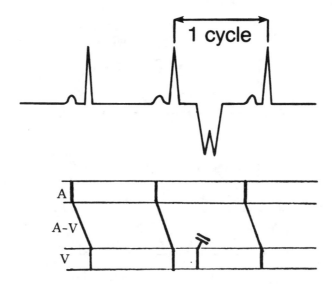

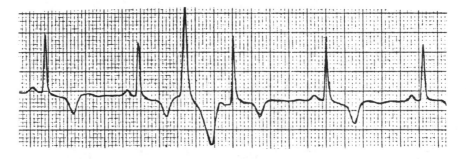

No Compensatory Pause (Full Interpolation)

From Page 559 (continued):
Concealed Conduction

Concealed conduction refers to an impulse, conducted within the conduction system, not visible (concealed) on the electrocardiogram, which influences the subsequent cycle. Using the example of the partial compensatory pause, note that the P-R interval of the fourth cycle is greater than the P-R intervals of cycles 1, 2 and 5. The PVC (4) penetrated the A-V junction sufficiently so that when the next sinus P wave came at the regular P-P interval, it encountered the A-V junction partially refractory resulting in delayed conduction in the A-V junction and prolonged P-R interval. The retrograde penetration of the A-V junction is an example of *concealed conduction* within the A-V junction (C on the ladder diagram) since it cannot be seen on the electrocardiogram but its effect is seen on the next cycle.

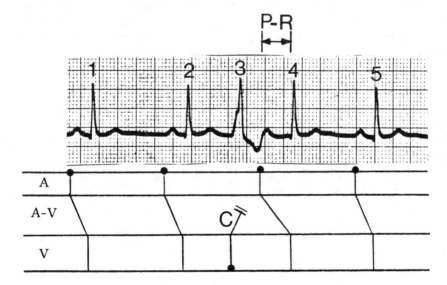

Concealed Conduction

From Page 559 (continued):
Wide QRS Complex with a
Supraventricular Pacemaker

1. *Bundle Branch Block*

Review of QRS Complex Width

a. A normally narrow (up to 0.1 sec.) QRS complex indicates a supraventricular rhythm (sinus, atrial, or junctional).

b. A ventricular rhythm has an abnormally wide QRS complex (usually 0.12 sec. or wider).

c. *An exception:* In the illustration below we have all the requirements of normal sinus rhythm except that the QRS complex is wide (greater than 0.1 sec.). The rhythm is supraventricular with a P wave before each QRS complex. Because there is an *intraventricular conduction disturbance,* in this case, *left bundle branch block (LBBB)* with delayed ventricular depolarization, there is a wide QRS complex.

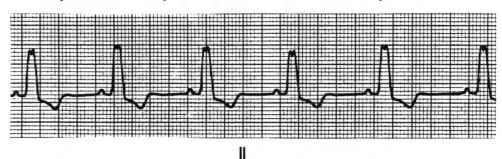

II

Wide QRS Complex with a Supraventricular Pacemaker

2. *Pre-excitation (Wolff-Parkinson-White or W-P-W Syndrome)*

Another example of a wide QRS complex with a supraventricular pacemaker is the W-P-W syndrome. As studied earlier, the W-P-W syndrome represents an anomalous pathway or bypass from the atria to the ventricles. The electrocardiographic characteristics include:

a. Short P-R interval (0.12 sec. or less).

b. Prolonged QRS interval (greater than 0.1 sec.).

c. Slurring of the upstroke by a *delta* wave (arrows).

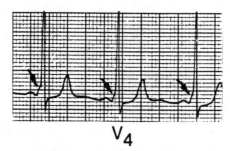

V₄

W-P-W Syndrome

From Page 559 (continued)

3. *Aberrancy or Ventricular Aberration*
   Including the Ashman Phenomenon

Aberrancy or aberrant ventricular conduction refers to abnormal ventricular depolarization following conduction of a supraventricular impulse. This occurs when a supraventricular impulse arrives while the ventricles are still partially refractory. In the example below, a premature supraventricular impulse found the right bundle branch refractory, hence the wide QRS complex of right bundle branch block (arrow) representing aberrant ventricular conduction. The wide QRS complex with the pattern of either RBBB or LBBB and preceding associated atrial activity indicates that the origin of the impulse is supraventricular.

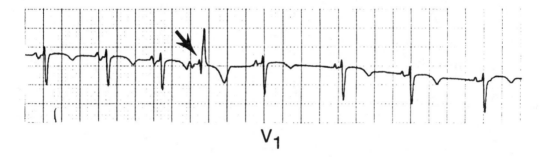

V_1

Ventricular Aberration

The refractory period of the conducting system adjusts to the heart rate, shortening with increasing heart rates (shorter cycles) and lengthening with lower heart rates (longer cycles). During the long cycle the refractory period lengthens and when a short cycle follows, the ventricular conducting system is still partially refractory leading to aberrant ventricular conduction. This was described by Gouaux and Ashman in patients with atrial fibrillation and is known as the Ashman phenomenon.[7-7] In the electrocardiogram below note the aberrancy in a patient with atrial fibrillation with long (A)-short (B) cycles. Single aberrant beats or the first aberrant beat of each multiple terminates a "long-short" sequence.

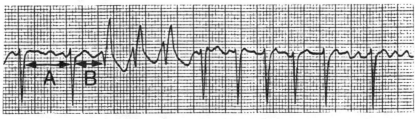

V_1

Ashman Phenomenon

From Page 559 (continued)

3. *Aberrancy or Ventricuar Aberration
    Including the Ashman Phenomenon
    (continued)*

In differentiating aberrant ventricular conduction from ventricular ectopy, atrial activity
and a RBBB or LBBB pattern point toward aberrancy. The availability of a baseline electrocardiogram with a bundle branch block pattern helps us, especially during a tachycardia, in determining the origin of the impulse. Below is the electrocardiogram of a patient
with a wide QRS tachycardia (A) whose baseline electrocardiogram revealed the same
LBBB pattern (B). The diagnosis of supraventricular tachycardia can be made with security. (See Figure 7-21A, B, and C for the complete evaluation of this patient.)

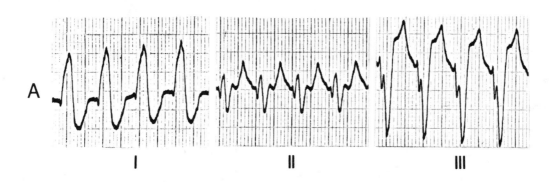

A

           I   II   III

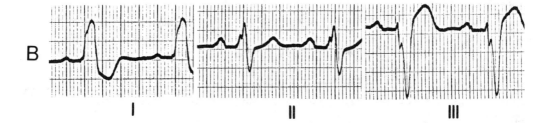

B

           I   II   III

From Page 560: Multifocal PVCs, Couplets, Salvos, Fusion, Parasystole, and the "R-on-T" Phenomenon

---

1. Multifocal PVCs

The three PVCs below originate in *two* foci. PVC 2 differs in configuration from PVCs 1 and 3. When PVCs originate in more than one focus, they are known as multifocal PVCs. The term "multiform" (or multiforme) has been recommended by some, since research has shown that PVCs of more than one configuration may originate in one focus.

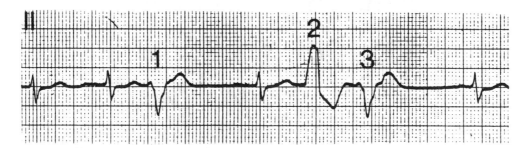

Multifocal PVCs

---

2. Couplets

A couplet refers to two closely coupled PVCs in a row. A couplet should not be confused with the term coupling, which refers to the relationship of the PVC to the previous normal beat, as seen in Figure 7-35A, page 560.

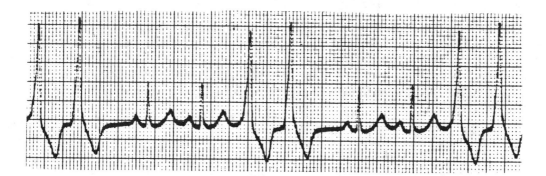

Couplets

_____

From Page 560 (continued)

_____

3. *Salvos*

A salvo is a run of three or more ventricular ectopic beats in a row. By definition, this is a burst of ventricular tachycardia.

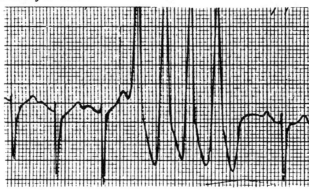

Salvos

_____

4. *Fusion*

A fusion beat occurs when more than one impulse conducts through the same myocardial area at approximately the same time, fusing into one beat. Fusion beats may occur in the ventricles or atria. The fusion beat (F below) is evident when the supraventricular impulse (in this case the sinus impulse) enters the ventricles at approximately the same time as an ectopic ventricular impulse fusing into one beat. Note that the P-R interval preceding the fusion beat is almost identical to the other P-R intervals. The underlying rhythm is sinus with 2:1 A-V block.

When the QRS complexes are wide, the presence of fusion beats favors ventricular ectopy rather than aberrant ventricular conduction. Fusion beats may be seen with PVCs, as in this electrocardiogram, during ventricular arrhythmias (accelerated idioventricular rhythm and ventricular tachycardia), ventricular pacing and ventricular parasystole. Atrial fusion may occur with simultaneous impulses from the S-A node and A-V junction depolarizing the atria.

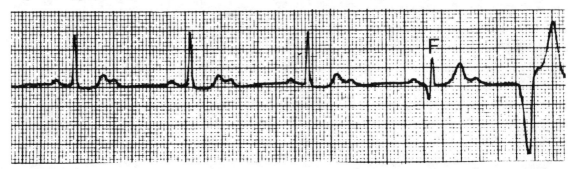

Fusion

From Page 560 (continued)

---

5. *Parasystole*

Under normal circumstances, the many latent pacemakers of the heart are continually penetrated and reset by the impulses arising in the S-A node. In this manner, they remain suppressed by the usually faster sinus. When a latent pacemaker acquires a protective shell of refractory tissue which prevents its penetration by the sinus, it may then reach threshold and discharge. Such a protected latent pacemaker is termed a parasystole, and may be located in the atria, junction, or ventricles. Upon firing, a parasystolic focus may find its impulse blocked either because the surrounding tissue has been rendered refractory by a sinus beat that it follows too closely, or because the immediately sur- rounding tissue is refractory because of intrinsic reasons.

On the electrocardiogram, a parasystole is recognized when a series of atrial, junctional, or ventricular extrasystoles are found to be related to each other, rather than either fixed- coupled to the dominant rhythm or randomly occurring. The interectopic intervals may be constant or varying. If varying, either the longer intervals are multiples of the shorter intervals, or all the intervals are multiples of some shorter interval not present. Fusion beats of the ectopic beats and normally conducted beats are common and must be counted when determining the interectopic intervals.

Ventricular parasystole is illustrated in this electrocardiogram. The diagnostic features are:

a. Non-fixed-coupling between the normally conducted beats and the PVCs.

b. Fusion (F) of a ventricular beat and a normally conducted beat.

c. Regular interectopic and a multiple of the basic interectopic interval.

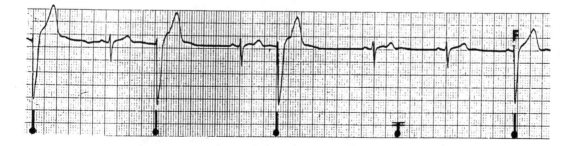

Ventricular Parasystole

From Page 560 (continued)

5. *Parasystole (continued)*

In junctional parasystole (below) nonfixed-coupled premature junctional contractions (PJCs) are present. All junctional cycles are multiples of a basic cycle.

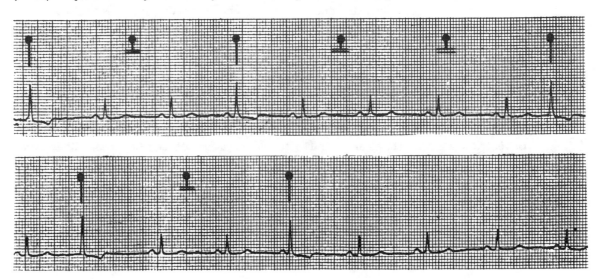

Junctional Parasystole

6. *"R-on-T" Phenomenon*

When a PVC occurs on or near the peak of the T wave of the previous beat, ventricular tachycardia, flutter, or fibrillation may be initiated. This is the vulnerable period or phase of ventricular repolarization. Here we see an "R-on-T" setting off a catastrophic arrhythmia.

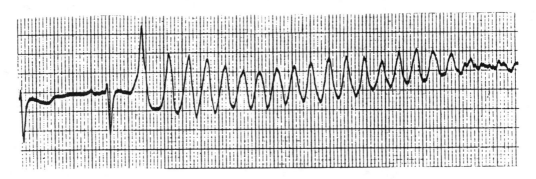

"R-on-T" Phenomenon

From Page 563:
"Torsades de pointes"

Ventricular tachycardia may be unifocal or multifocal ("polymorphic"); the form of the latter frequently involves a number of beats of one polarity in a given lead followed by beats of the opposite polarity. The two groups of beats may be separated from each other by beats of an intermediate form ("torsades de pointes"). "Torsades de pointes" means twistings of the points, describing the electrocardiographic appearance. Note, in the electrocardiographic tracings below, the upright and negative QRS complexes separated by transitional complexes. The usual causes are (1) type 1 antiarrhythmic drugs (toxicity or idiosyncratic reaction) and (2) the congenital Q-T prolongation syndrome. Prolonged Q-T intervals are often found in the supraventricular beats. Pacing the heart at a faster than the intrinsic sinus rate frequently suppresses the ventricular tachycardia (overdrive suppression).

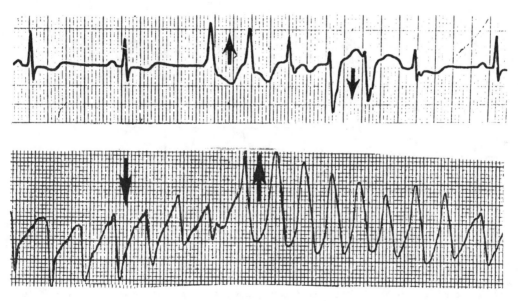

Torsades de Pointes

**From Page 577:   Mobitz Type I
or Simply Type I A-V Block**

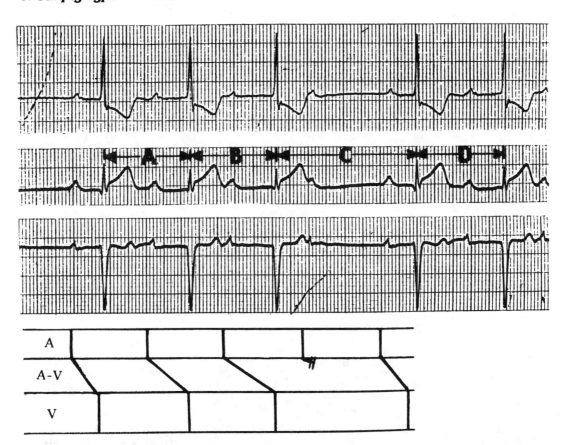

Sinus rhythm with A-V Wenckebach periods. A complete 4:3 A-V Wenckebach period is illustrated. The sinus rate is 70 beats per minute. A-V conduction time, represented by the P-R interval, progressively increases until one beat is finally dropped. This is a typical A-V Wenckebach period. The R-R intervals decrease as the P-R intervals increase (i.e., cycle A > cycle B). The length of the pause containing the dropped beat is less than that of the two previous cycles (i.e., C < A + B); it is also less than twice the length of the previous cycle (i.e., C < 2 × B). The length of the cycle following the pause is greater than that preceding (i.e., D > B). In a 3:2 A-V Wenckebach period they are equal. In this case there are 4 P waves producing 3 QRS complexes, hence, a 4:3 A-V Wenckebach period. The Wenckebach nature of the A-V conduction indicates that the site of block is in the A-V node.

From Page 577 (continued):
Sinoatrial (S-A) Wenckebach Periods

We have been studying Mobitz I A-V block with the site of block in the A-V node. The P-P intervals are stable while there is shortening of the R-R intervals and lengthening of the P-R intervals culminating in the failure of a single beat to conduct (single dropped beat). While Wenckebach conduction occurs commonly in the A-V node, the phenomenon may occur in other conducting tissue of the heart.

In *S-A Wenckebach periods* ("type I" S-A block) we see the progressive shortening of the *P-P intervals* until a *P wave* is dropped. The cycle including the dropped P wave is less than 2 times the shortest P-P cycle. The P-R intervals are stable.

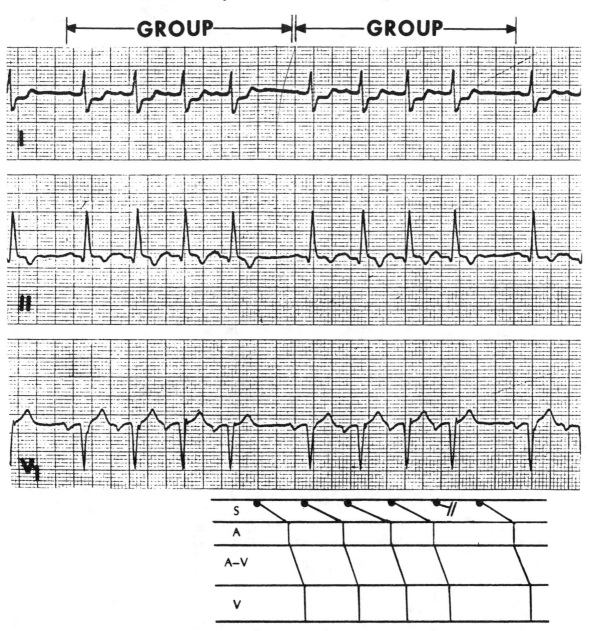

5:4 S-A Wenckebach periods. Group beating (brackets) of the QRS complexes follow group beating of the P waves; all P-R intervals are equal. The pause occurs when a P wave is dropped.

From Page 579: Advanced (High Grade) Second Degree A-V Block

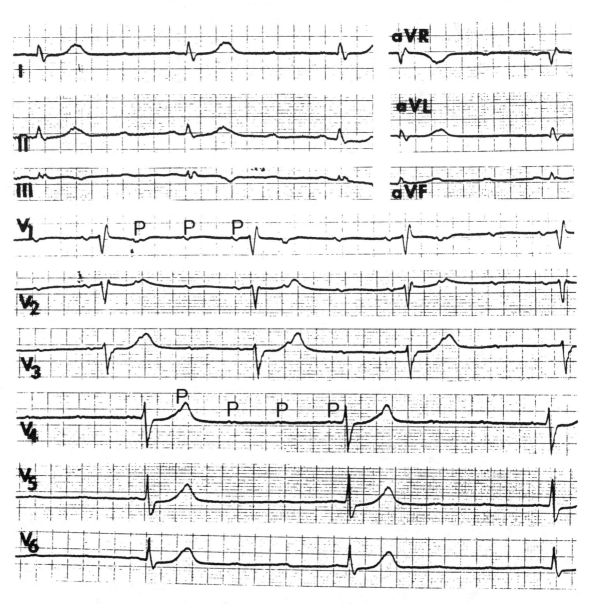

Advanced A-V block. Fixed 3:1 and 4:1 A-V block is present with right bundle branch block. During 4:1 block, the heart rate is 23 beats per minute. Note that every QRS complex is preceded by a P wave at a fixed interval.

From Page 587

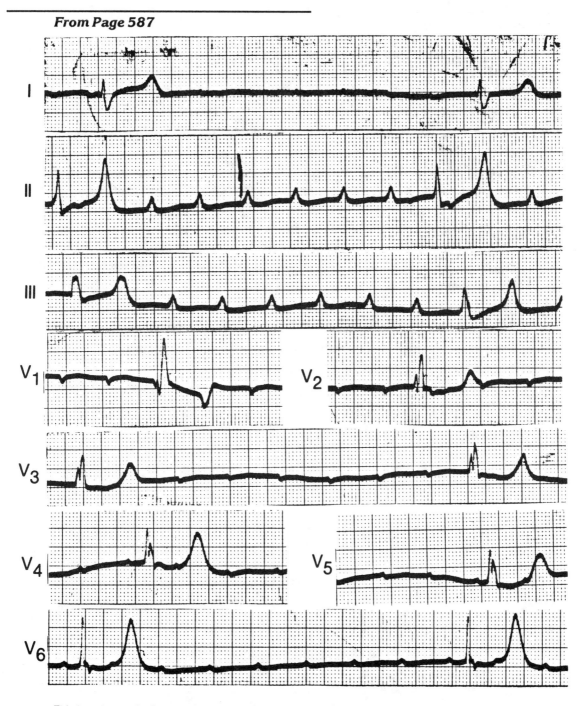

Elderly patient with a history of syncope and a heart rate of 14 beats per minute.

References

7-1. Scherlag, B.J., et al.: Catheter technique for recording His bundle activity in man. Circulation, *39*:13, 1969.

7-2. Fox, W., and Stein, E.: Cardiac Rhythm Disturbances: A Step-by-Step Approach. Philadelphia, Lea & Febiger, 1983.

7-3. Stein, E.: Interpretation of Arrhythmias: A Self-Study Program. Philadelphia, Lea & Febiger, 1988.

7-4. Borman, M.C., and Meek, W.J.: IV. Coronary sinus rhythm; rhythm subsequent to destruction by radon of the sino-auricular nodes in dogs. Arch. Intern. Med., *47:957*, 1931.

7-5. Scherf, D., and Gurbuzer, B.: Further studies on coronary sinus rhythm. Am. J. Cardiol., *1:*579, 1958.

7-6. Besoain-Santander, M., Pick, A., and Langendorf, R.: A-V conduction in auricular flutter. Circulation, *2:*604, 1950.

7-7. Gouaux, J.L., and Ashman, R.: Auricular fibrillation with aberration simulating ventricular paroxysmal tachycardia. Am. Heart J., *34:*366, 1947.

7-8. Marriott, H.J.L.: Practical Electrocardiography, 8th Ed. Baltimore, Williams & Wilkins, 1988, p. 363.

7-9. Marriott, H.J.L.: Practical Electrocardiography, 8th Ed. Baltimore, Williams & Wilkins, 1988, p. 382.

8

DIGITALIS

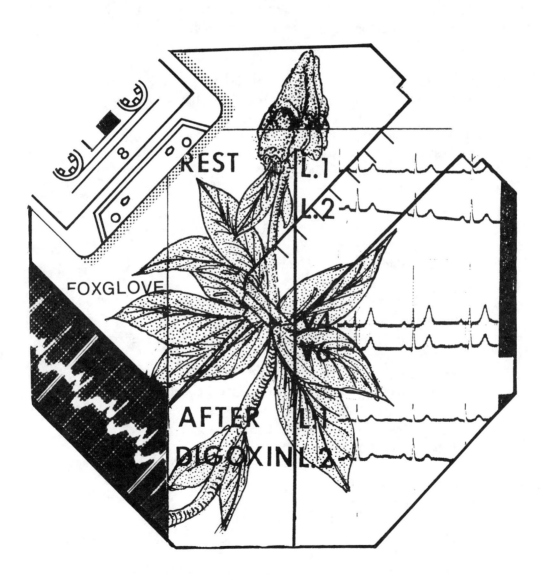

CHAPTER 8
CONTENTS

INTRODUCTION

In this chapter you will see some of the commonly seen electrocardiographic manifestations associated with digitalis *effects* and digitalis *toxicity*. Although this is not a course in pharmacology and therapeutics, some salient features concerning this potent medication will be emphasized. Digitalis can serve as the *prototype* for any medication in use today.

OBJECTIVES

Upon completion of this chapter, you should be able to:

1. Indicate that part of the electrocardiographic cycle in which the "effects" of digitalis are best seen.

2. Describe the "classic" electrocardiographic manifestations of digitalis.

3. State why a *positive* exercise test might not be reliable in a patient taking digitalis.

4. State how digitalis can slow the ventricular response in a patient with atrial fibrillation with a rapid ventricular response.

5. Recognize the electrocardiographic manifestations of digitalis "toxicity."

6. Indicate the predictability of "toxic" responses to digitalis.

7. State the circumstances under which atrial tachycardia *is* frequently due to digitalis "toxicity" and the circumstances under which it is generally *not* due to digitalis "toxicity."

8. State significance of "regularization" of heart rate in the presence of atrial fibrillation in a patient taking digitalis.

DIRECTIONS. This pretest consists of five electrocardiograms. Write a brief analysis of each in the space provided, taking care to include specific questions when indicated.

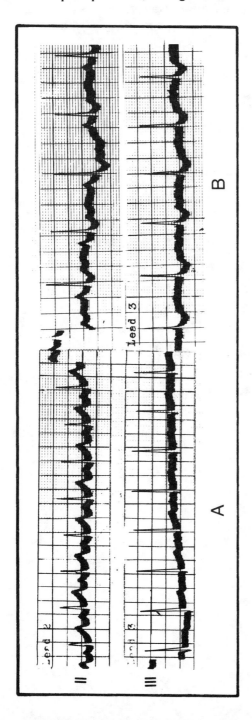

FIGURE 8-3.   Before (A) and after (B) "digitalization." Describe these changes.

1.   Analysis:

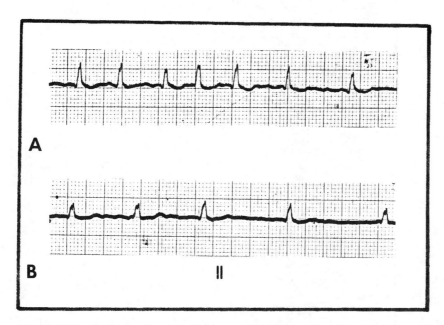

FIGURE 8-5.   A patient with electrocardiogram A was given additional digitalis. Describe the actions of digitalis leading to electrocardiogram B.

2. Analysis:

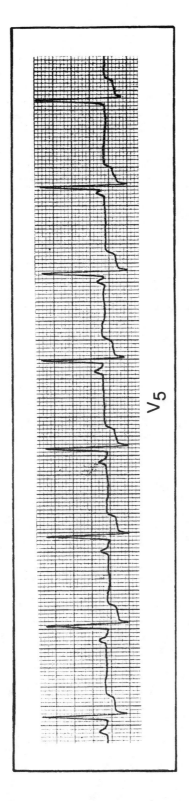

FIGURE 8-16. Patient taking digitalis.

V5

3.   Analysis:

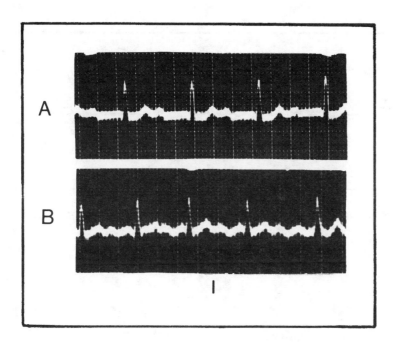

FIGURE 8-23.   Two rhythms in the same patient taking digitalis.

4. Analysis:

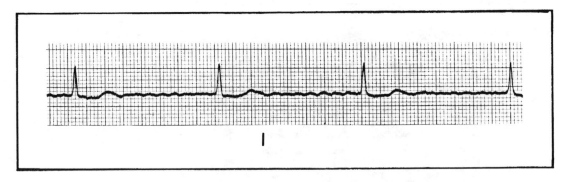

FIGURE 8-28.   Prior to receiving digitalis this patient's rhythm was atrial fibrillation with an irregularly irregular rate.

5.   Analysis:

> Solutions to the pretest are indicated in the chapter as well as on pages 661–662.

> When you have finished your analyses, start Cassette Side 19 and continue on the next page.

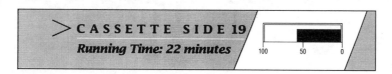

> CASSETTE SIDE 19
> *Running Time: 22 minutes*
> 100   50   0

ELECTROCARDIOGRAPHIC
MANIFESTATIONS OF DIGITALIS
EFFECTS AND DIGITALIS TOXICITY

As mentioned in the introduction to this chapter, although this is not a course in pharmacology and therapeutics, some salient features concerning this potent medication must be emphasized. It is a drug so often dispensed without much knowledge as to its effects and without recognition of specific evidence of toxicity. We occasionally hear of mistakes or drug accidents, such as reported in the *New York Times* years ago (Figure 8-1A). More recently, I received an urgent notice from a drug house advising of a dosage error on a digitalis preparation (Figure 8-1B). A physician who is familiar with the preparation and its dosage should recognize the typographic error immediately. The danger, however, arises when a physician who is unfamiliar with a preparation uses it according to the accompanying literature.

In patient populations, there is a spectrum response to an "average digitalizing" dose of digitalis preparation. Each patient's treatment must be individualized and "tailored." Even the "average" dosage schedules represent a spectrum. At one end of the spectrum a certain number of patients will be digitalis toxic, while at the other end a certain number will be underdigitalized (Figure 8-1C).

Because of the extent of the tragedy cited in Figure 8-1A, this example received worldwide attention, but it is not a rare nor isolated incident. Digitalis must not be used without thorough familiarity with its actions, its effect on the myocardium and on the periphery, its relationship to calcium and potassium metabolism and renal function, specific indications, preparations, dosage, absorption, excretion, interaction with concomitant medication, side effects, and toxic manifestations. If you are not familiar with this information, even for the purpose of this course in electrocardiography, stop here and study the subject in one of the many good standard textbooks.

Digitalis can serve as the prototype for any medication in use today. A physician must never affix his signature to a prescription or hand out samples without knowledge of the information listed above. How many times has the practicing cardiologist seen a patient in consultation who had been given digitalis and told to take the pills until the onset of

THE NEW YORK TIMES

20 BELGIANS DEAD AFTER DRUG ERROR

Clerk Sent Wrong Substance to Clinic for Elderly

By CLYDE H. FARNSWORTH
Special to The New York Times

BRUSSELS, Jan. 7—An error made by a Brussels pharmaceutical house has resulted in the death of at least 20 elderly persons taking cancer treatment at a Belgian clinic.

It is one of the worst drug tragedies yet brought to public attention in Belgium and promises to stir new controversy in medicine. Belgium has had two doctor strikes in less than three years.

The drug house was identified in a brief announcement of the tragedy as the Arthur Gailly Clinic of Charleroi, an institution run by a Socialist insurance body.

An inexperienced stock clerk in the Brussels company substituted the drug Digitaline, a heart stimulant, for benzoate of estradiol, a hormone used in the treatment of cancer of the prostate.

The error was compounded, the clinic said, by the failure of pharmacists, both in the company and in the drug dispensary in the clinic, to take requisite control measures.

The clinic ordered 50 grams of the hormone in March, 1965, and instead of 50 grams of Digitaline.

The hormone can be admisistered in three daily doses of 10 milligrams each, while the maximum dosage for Digitaline is three milligrams daily.

After several of the patients died, doctors concluded that there was something wrong with the drug and asked the company to verify what it had delivered.

The company was unable to identify it. Last April a sample was sent to the drug control bureau of the Belgian Phammaceutical Association, which in a report last month said only that the product was not the hormone.

In the end a company pharmacist identified it as the heart drug. The long, involved process of identification came to a close with a letter from the company to the clinic saying that since digitaline is less expensive than the hormone, the clinic was being given a credit.

Of the 50 grams that the clinic received 23 grams were dispensed to patients. No one is sure how many patients died from the dosage.

There was public anger and bitterness. It was asked why it took so long to make the identification and bring the matter to public notice.

The law makes drug companies responsible for what they sell, but some of the blame is almost certain to fall on the clinic, especially since it is of the type that is already under heavy criticism from doctors.

The Socialist clinics pay their doctors a flat salary and have a reputation for mass production treatment in which individual patients get short shrift.

The doctors' organizations believe the standards would rise if the doctors were paid according to the scale and kind of work they do.

A

FIGURE 8-1A.   *From the* New York Times, *January 8, 1967. Reprinted by permission of the New York Times Company.*

nausea without a baseline electrocardiogram having been taken? Whether using digitalis to treat congestive heart failure or an arrhythmia, always keep the end points of the spectrum response in mind, relative to a given patient. Patients' responses may be quite variable and unpredictable, and careful follow-up is essential. How many times has the practicing cardiologist seen a patient who was given a digitalizing dose of digitalis preparation for congestive heart failure, instructed about maintenance dosage, and told to come back 1 month later? A sense of exhilaration is often prevalent in digitalized patients who feel better after having been in congestive heart failure. They remember

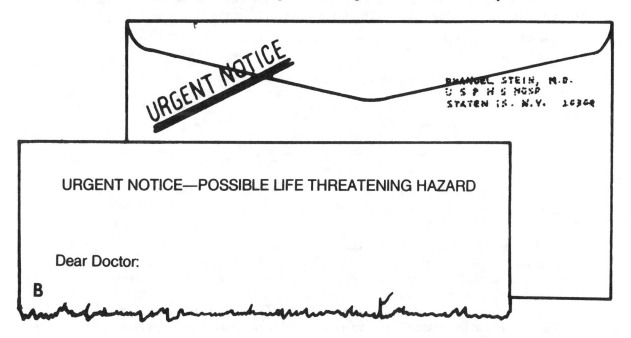

FIGURE 8-1B.   *Notification of a typographical dosage error in the literature accompanying a digitalis preparation.*

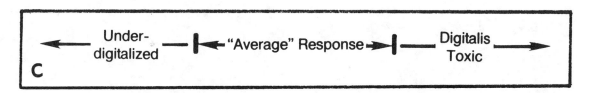

FIGURE 8-1C.   *Response to an "average digitalizing" dose of a digitalis preparation.*

the dramatic response to the digitalizing dose, and when they are not feeling well, even though it may be due to overdosage, they will take more tablets of digitalis, returning to the physician severely ill with digitalis toxicity. If this stage is missed, the next may be a complete halt of heart action—death caused by a "lifesaving" medicine. Patient instruction and understanding of the drug's actions are as vital as careful and frequent patient follow-up.

Perspectives must be kept in mind. However universal digitalis may be, it is used to treat certain signs and symptoms. What is presently needed is a way to prevent or remove the "cause" of the signs and symptoms. This is the subject of intensive investigation today.

William Withering, in the eighteenth century, noted the beneficial effcts of the foxglove plant on "dropsy." He wrote:

> The Foxglove's leaves, with caution given,
> Another proof of favouring Heav'n
>   Will happily display;
> The rapid pulse it can abate;
> The hectic flush can moderate
> And, blest by Him whose will is fate,
> May give a lengthen'd day.[8-1]

Withering studied digitalis, the product of the foxglove plant and observed that "it has a power over the motion of the heart to a degree yet unobserved in any other medicine, and this power may be converted to salutary ends."[8-2]

Some of the electrocardiograms in this chapter have already been seen in previous chapters; the study of digitalis effects, and especially digitalis toxicity, is a study of repolarization alterations, conduction disturbances and arrhythmias.[8-3] This chapter will serve as both a review and a reminder that digitalis, a most common medicine in cardiology today, may be both a blessing and a curse—a blessing for its "salutary" action on the heart and a curse in that it is so common a cause of devastating arrhythmias and drug toxicity.

A. Electrocardiographic Manifestations of Digitalis Effects

1. Digitalis Effects on Ventricular Repolarization (S-T Segment and T Wave)

Digitalis is commonly used to treat congestive heart failure as well as arrhythmias such as atrial fibrillation, atrial flutter, and atrial tachycardia (when these arrhythmias are not caused by digitalis).

The electrocardiogram may be helpful in following patients taking digitalis. Electrocardiographically, digitalis effects are seen in the ventricular repolarization phase affecting the S-T segment and the T wave. The whole repolarization phase may be accelerated, hence a shorter Q-T interval. The "classic" alterations of digitalis are described as a "fist-like" depression of the S-T segment (as if you were placing your fist in the S-T segment

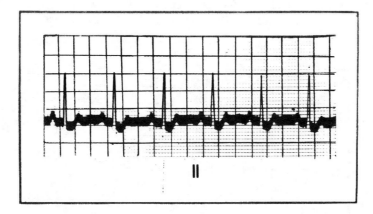

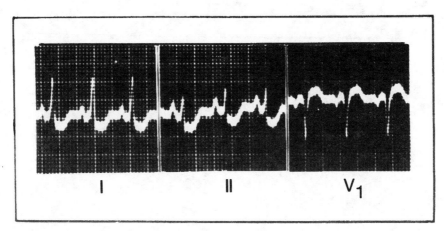

FIGURE 8-2. "Classic" alterations of the S-T segment caused by digitalis in two patients. (Electrocardiograms reduced in size.)

and depressing it), as "paintbrush" inscription (as if you were painting the S-T segment with gradual widening of the paintbrush as you approach the S-T segment from the downslope of the R wave), or as "scooping" of the S-T segment. The elevation of the S-T segment in lead V_1 (Figure 8-2) represents the same phenomenon as the S-T segment depression in leads I and II. With a good imagination you should have no difficulty with these descriptions. Figure 8-3 compares the electrocardiograms before and after digitalis administration.

As seen earlier, in our study of the S-T segment and T wave (Chapter 4), the repolarization phase of the ventricles is the energy consuming phase, the active phase, as compared with depolarization, and is therefore, more labile and more prone to alterations. It is best to study the repolarization phase as a unit, including both the S-T segment and the T wave, rather than trying to ascribe one set of the rules to the S-T segment and another set to the T wave. Although early repolarization changes affecting the S-T segment are considered a classic sign of digitalis effect, late repolarization changes affecting the T wave may be seen even as the first, and often as the only, effect. This is well illustrated in our studies with digitalis. Review Figures 4-13 to 4-17 in Chapter 4.

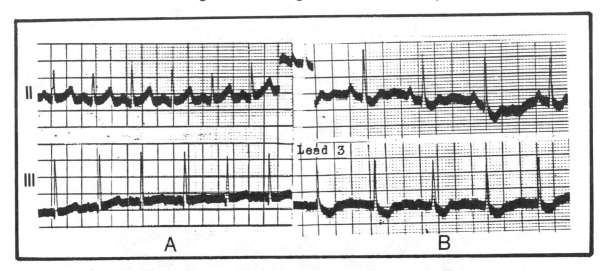

FIGURE 8-3.   Before (A) and after (B) "digitalization." In (B) the "classic" alterations of the ventricular repolarization phase are seen. Note the "fist-like" depression ("paintbrush" inscription or "scooping") of the S-T segment. Note also that the T wave is not as tall in (B) as in (A). In this patient the entire phase of repolarization (both the S-T segment and the T wave) is affected. (Electrocardiogram reduced in size.)

> The analysis of Figure 8-3 on this page, on the tape, and on page 661 is the solution to Item 1 on the pretest.

Review of Figures 4-13 through 4-16 in Chapter 4 reveals that in a significant number of patients it was not possible to predict which part, or whether the entire phase (both the S-T segment and the T wave), of repolarization would be affected. In a given patient digitalis effects may be seen in the T wave, S-T segment, both, or neither. This again stresses the need to follow each patient very closely without relying on "predictable" changes. Because of the increased lability of the repolarization phase in patients taking digitalis, a positive exercise test might not be reliable in these patients.

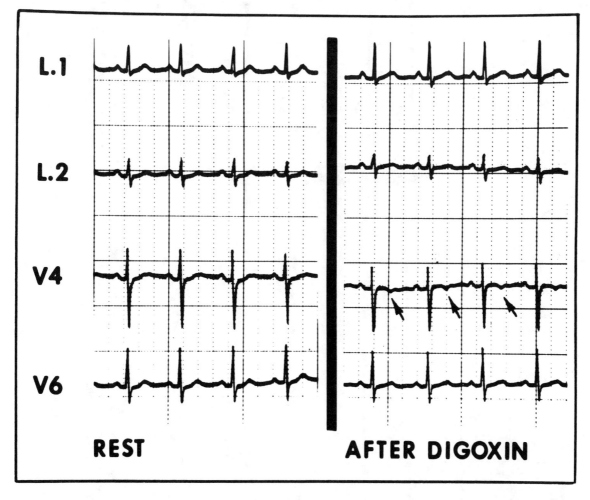

FIGURE 4-13.   *Repolarization changes due to a digitalis preparation (digoxin). In spite of the "classic" changes ascribed to digitalis on the early part of repolarization (S-T segment), note the effect of a subdigitalizing dose of digoxin on late repolarization (T wave). (Electrocardiogram reduced in size.)*

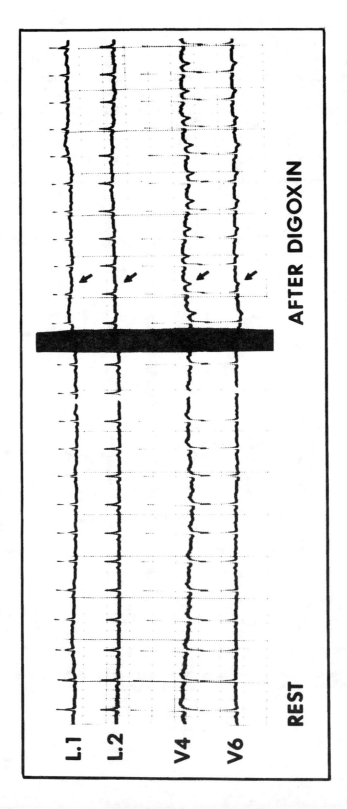

FIGURE 4-14.   Repolarization changes due to digitalis. A dramatic effect is seen in late repolarization (T wave) due to a small dose of the digitalis preparation digoxin. There was no other intervention here; the thick black line in the center is where the recording machine was stopped for one hour following the administration of digoxin. It cannot, therefore, be said dogmatically that digitalis affects only the early part of repolarization; the effect on the T waves may be much more marked than the effect on the S-T segments. Repolarization should be dealt with as a unit; the S-T segments and T waves should not be categorically separated. Digitalis may affect one, the other, or both. (Electrocardiogram reduced in size.)

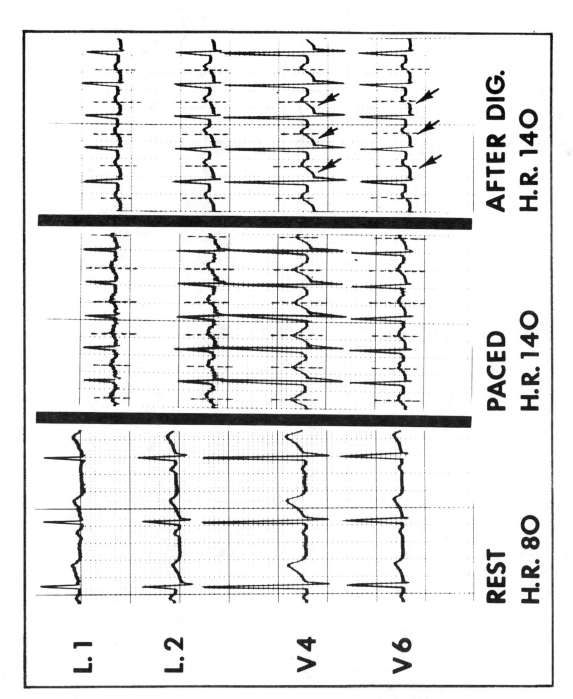

FIGURE 4-15.   Repolarization changes due to digitalis. The arrows point to the effects of digitalis on the S-T segments at a given paced heart rate, compared with the same paced heart rate without digitalis. (Electrocardiogram reduced in size.)

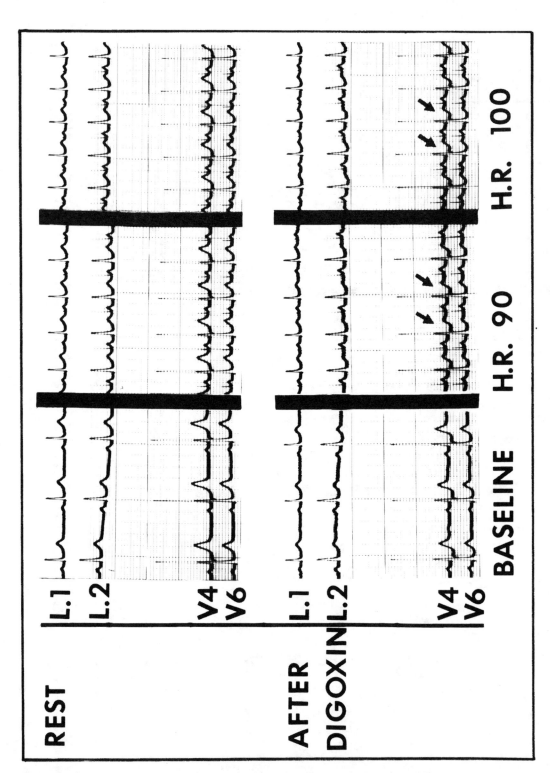

FIGURE 4-16. *Digitalis effects on repolarization. Compare the effects on each of the paired heart rates, baseline, 90 per minute, and 100 per minute. (Electrocardiogram reduced in size.)*

2. Digitalis Effects on Atrioventricular Conduction

The question has frequently arisen as to whether prolongation of the P-R interval represents digitalis effect or digitalis toxicity. In our studies of effect of digitalis on atrioventricular conduction no significant differences were noted in the P-R interval at rest. As the rate of the heart was increased by atrial pacing, however, atrioventricular conduction time was prolonged as an effect of digitalis, resulting in a significant prolongation of the P-R interval. His bundle studies confirmed that the increase was within the interval from the atrial deflection to the His bundle deflection (A-H interval). Clinically, an increase in the baseline P-R interval, or advancement to higher degrees of A-V block, as seen in Figures 8-4A and B, has been associated with toxic manifestations of digitalis. Although the subject of digitalis toxicity will be studied in a later section of this chapter, it is introduced here to emphasize the importance of close and careful patient follow-up.

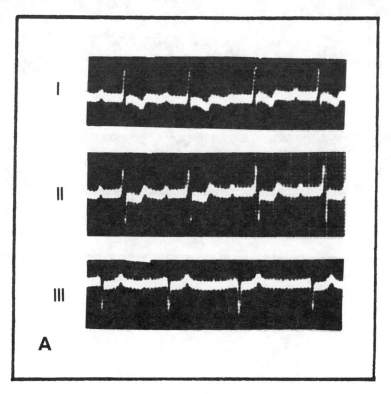

FIGURE 8-4A.   First degree A-V block. Digitalis toxicity is represented in progressive atrioventricular block.

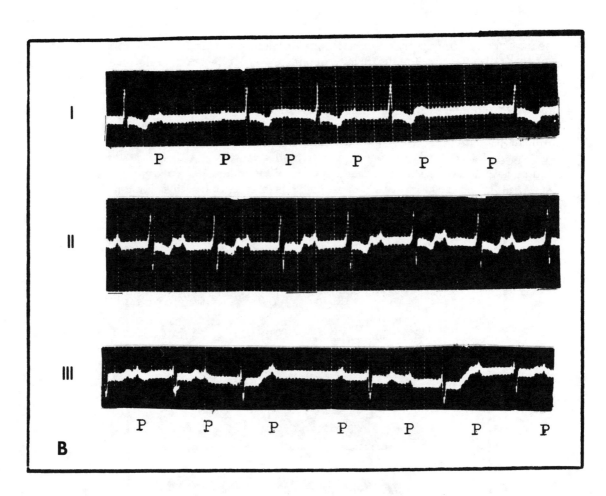

FIGURE 8-4B.   Progression of A-V block due to digitalis toxicity.

3. *Digitalis effects on an Arrhythmia*
   (Atrial Fibrillation with a Rapid
   Ventricular Response)

Figure 8-5A and B illustrates an effect of digitalis on atrial fibrillation with a rapid ventricular response. The patient was a 35-year-old man with mitral valve disease who presented with atrial fibrillation and a ventricular rate of approximately 125 beats per minute on an inadequate dose of digitalis. With proper adjustment of the dose the ventricular rate fell to approximately 75 beats per minute.

Atrial fibrillation with a rapid ventricular response is an excellent arrhythmia for the study of digitalis effects on heart rate. In normal sinus rhythm digitalis does not have much effect on the ventricular rate per se. In atrial fibrillation, most of the atrial impulses are blocked in the A-V conduction system. However, if there are 500 atrial impulses per minute and 1 impulse of every 4 reaches the ventricles, irregularly, the average ventricular rate would be 125 beats per minute. Digitalis acts on the A-V conduction system,

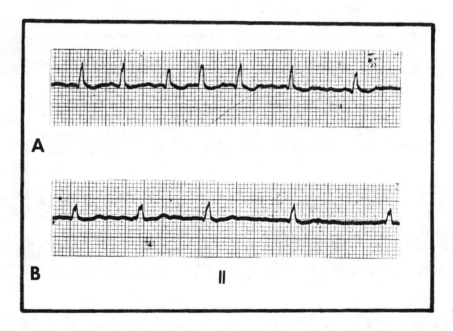

FIGURE 8-5.   Digitalis effects on atrial fibrillation with rapid ventricular response; A, baseline; B, following increase in digitalis dosage.

> The analysis of Figure 8-5 on this page, on the tape, and on page 661 is the solution to Item 2 on the pretest.

allowing fewer impulses to go through, effectively slowing the ventricular rate. In atrial fibrillation (longstanding) the aim with digitalis therapy is not to convert to sinus rhythm, but to slow the ventricular rate.

In spite of the good response with digitalis, the physician must use caution in treating a patient with this arrhythmia. Patients respond in different ways to overdosage of digitalis. As more and more digitalis is given, for instance to a patient with baseline atrial fibrillation or flutter-fibrillation, that patient may show no irritability of the heart whatever, no premature contractions and no tachycardia. The ventricular rate may, however, decrease from 125 to 85 to 75 to 60 to 50 to 40 and so on down to the point where the heart stops (Figure 8-6). Responses may not be predictable. This example of digitalis toxicity is introduced at this point to caution physicians treating patients with atrial fibrillation (Figure 8-6). Careful follow-up is essential.

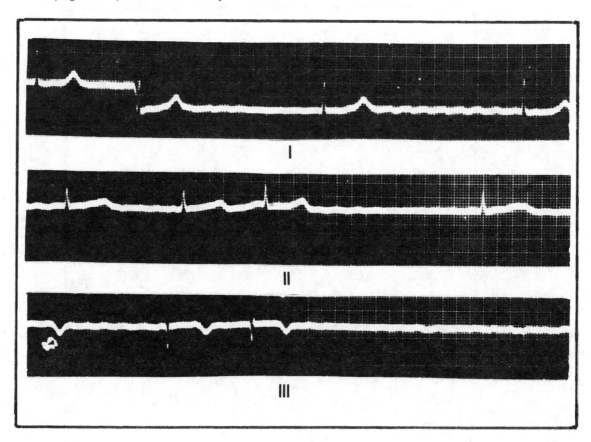

FIGURE 8-6.   Digitalis toxicity. (Electrocardiogram reduced in size.)

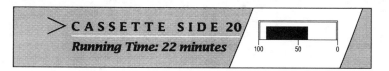

> CASSETTE SIDE 20
>
> *Running Time: 22 minutes*
>
> 100   50   0

B. Electrocardiographic Manifestations of Digitalis Toxicity

The prevalence of digitalis toxicity must be continually emphasized and both the physician and the patient must be ever watchful—all the more so because toxic manifestations do not necessarily mean that the dose has been changed. The response may be altered by changes in absorption caused by gastrointestinal upset, by electrolyte imbalance due to diuretics, and so forth. Remember also that toxicity may be manifest before any therapeutic effects of digitalis are seen.

In a course in electrocardiography major emphasis must be placed on the electrocardiographic manifestations of digitalis, and it has often been stated that a study of digitalis includes a study of all of electrocardiography. A knowledge of digitalis, however, in all its facets, is vital; this has been emphasized. It is not possible to accurately predict which sign or signs of digitalis toxicity a given patient may develop. All the more care is necessary since, not infrequently, a patient may "feel better" while in digitalis toxicity. This has been seen many times, especially when a rapid heart rate is effectively reduced by alternate premature beats of the ventricle, or by alternate sinoatrial block. More than a cursory "How do you feel?" and quick pulse check are necessary in following a patient taking digitalis. Knowledge of the subject must be combined with knowledge of, and interest in, the patient.

1. Depressed Sinoatrial (S-A) Pacemaker Leading to:

a.   *Atrial Fibrillation.* When the sinoatrial pacemaker is depressed by digitalis and sinus rhythm is no longer dominant, another rhythm must supervene for the patient to

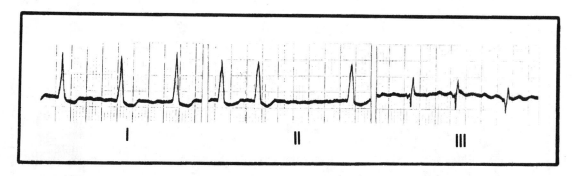

FIGURE 8-7.   *Atrial fibrillation in a patient with suppression of the S-A node due to digitalis. (Electrocardiogram reduced in size.)*

continue living. A most important rule to remember is that an arrhythmia or conduction disturbance developing in a patient on digitalis should be considered as resulting from digitalis.

Atrial fibrillation may replace sinus rhythm when the atria become disorganized upon suppression of the S-A node (Figure 8-7). Note the electrocardiographic signs of digitalis effects. It is important to know the patient and to have baseline electrocardiograms available. The onset of atrial fibrillation in a patient with normal sinus rhythm may be paroxysmal and not necessarily related to the administration of digitalis, since it is an uncommon manifestation of digitalis toxicity.

b.   *Atrial Flutter.* Atrial flutter is a rare arrhythmia in a patient with digitalis toxicity.[84] It must be considered, however, lest the patient receive more digitalis in an attempt to "break" the flutter. The onset of atrial flutter with a slow ventricular rate (less than 90 beats per minute) and varying A-V block (Figure 8-8), should arouse suspicion in a digitalized patient. Figure 8-9 is an example of atrial flutter with 2:1 A-V conduction, which is usually *not* due to digitalis toxicity.

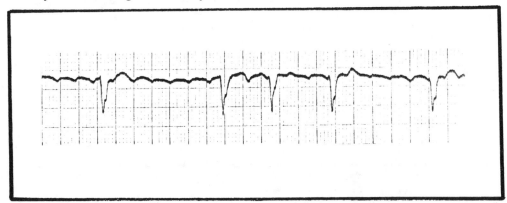

FIGURE 8-8.   *Atrial flutter with varying A-V block.*

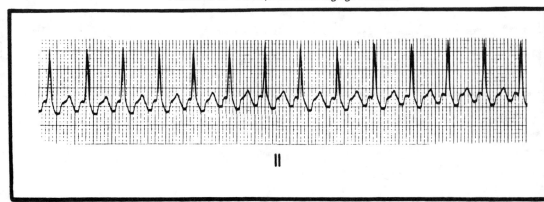

FIGURE 8-9.   *Atrial flutter with 2:1 A-V conduction.*

c. *Atrial Tachycardia.* Atrial tachycardia with atrioventricular block is a common arrhythmia in digitalis toxicity. In fact, atrial tachycardia with atrioventricular block represents digitalis toxicity until proven otherwise (Figure 8-10).

Atrial tachycardia with 1:1 atrioventricular conduction (no A-V block) is usually *not* due to digitalis toxicity (Figure 8-11). An esophageal lead recording may help establish the diagnosis since P waves are not obvious. Digitalis was used to terminate the tachycardia.

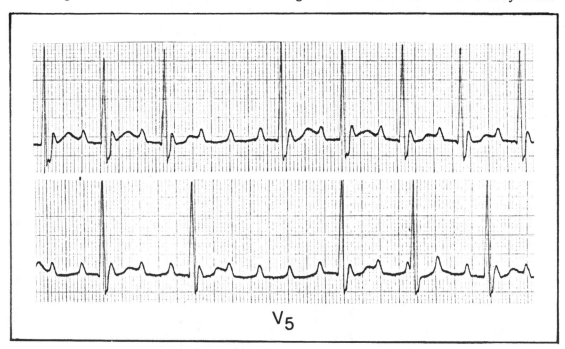

V_5

FIGURE 8-10.   *Atrial tachycardia with varying A-V block.*

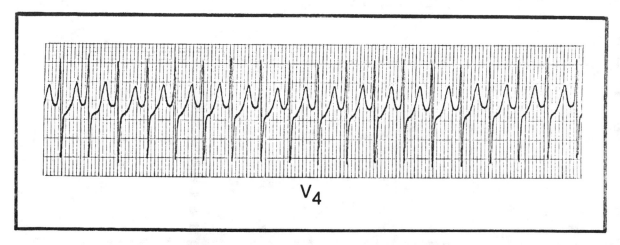

V_4

FIGURE 8-11.   *Atrial tachycardia with 1:1 A-V conduction (no A-V block).*

The paroxysmal tachycardia with 1:1 atrioventricular conduction heralded by premature atrial contractions seen in Figure 8-12 is also unlikely to be due to digitalis toxicity. Digitalis was used to treat the arrhythmia.

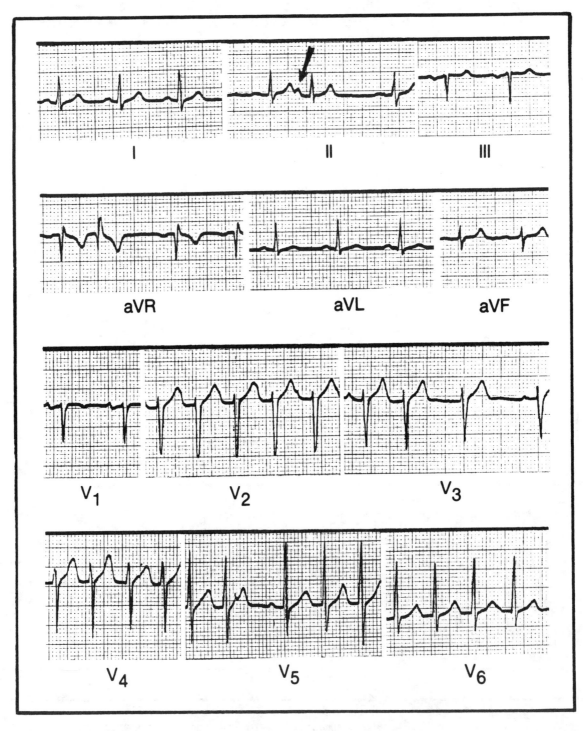

FIGURE 8-12.   Premature beats of the atria and paroxysms of atrial tachycardia.

d. *Sinoatrial (S-A) Block (Type II).* The sinoatrial node initiates an impulse but the propagation is blocked, so the atria are not depolarized and hence, there is no P wave. The pause is a multiple of the regular cycle length. The block, represented by the letter B in Figure 8-13 is seen where the P wave should normally be. This may be an exceedingly dangerous arrhythmia in that every other beat may be blocked as seen in the upper tracing of Figure 8-13, with a resulting low rate. The physician may consider the patient well digitalized with a regular rhythm, instead of digitalis toxic. The next stage may be sinus arrest, with no other pacemaker taking over, and death of the patient.

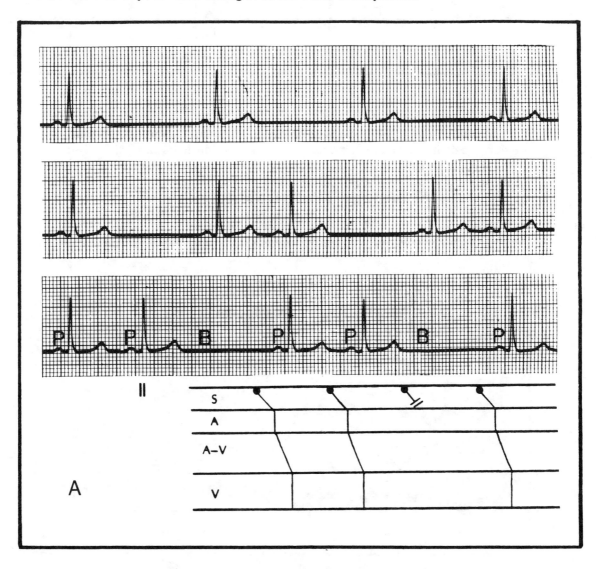

FIGURE 8-13.   Sinoatrial (S-A) block ("type II.") "Type I" S-A block is explained and illustrated on page 617. It may also be seen in digitalis toxicity, especially when the atrial rate is slow.

e. *Sinus Arrest.* Sinus arrest is a sudden failure of the sinoatrial node to initiate an expected impulse (Figure 8-14); it is a failure of impulse formation, rather than a failure of impulse propagation. If no other pacemaker becomes dominant at this point, death quickly follows.

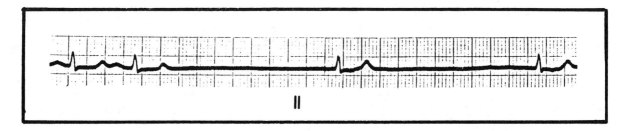

FIGURE 8-14.   *Sinus arrest with junctional escape rhythm.*

f. *Coronary Sinus Rhythm (Ectopic Atrial Rhythm).* Always beware of a change in rhythm in a digitalized patient; it may be an ominous sign. In Figure 8-15B we see the onset of coronary sinus rhythm without a significant change in heart rate. If the physician checks the pulse rate for 15 sec. and sends the patient on his way, this ectopic rhythm is missed, possibly forfeiting the only chance to detect digitalis toxicity.

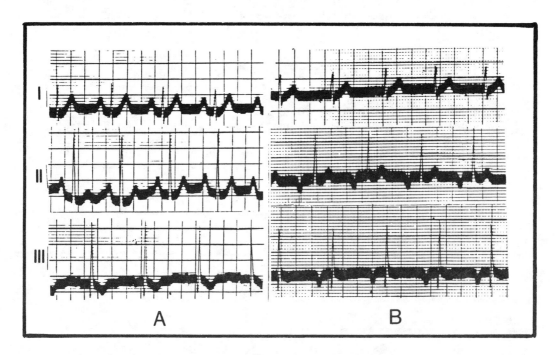

FIGURE 8-15.   *Onset of coronary sinus rhythm (B) in a patient taking digitalis; there is no significant change in heart rate. (Electrocardiogram reduced in size.)*

2. Junctional Rhythm

Atrioventricular dissociation due to acceleration of the junctional pacemaker is frequently seen in digitalis toxicity. In Figure 8-16 we see the acceleration of the junctional pacemaker resulting in A-V dissociation in digitalis toxicity. The P waves "merge" with the QRS complexes. The junctional rhythm, although the rate is under 70 per minute, is really a junctional tachycardia because the junctional pacemaker is faster than its maximum inherent rate of 60 per minute.

Figure 8-17 is from a patient with more advanced digitalis toxicity. The rate of the junctional pacemaker is between 95 and 100 per minute, and the atrial rate, under sinus control, is between 80 and 90 per minute.

Review the "nodal" rhythms in Chapter 7 (pages 542–553). Although we use the term "junctional" rhythm you should be familiar with the terminology of "upper, middle, and lower nodal" rhythms. What are some of the newer thoughts regarding the origin and propagation of these rhythms?

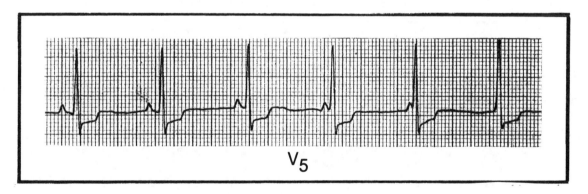

V_5

FIGURE 8-16. Acceleration of junctional pacemaker resulting in A-V dissociation in digitalis toxicity. The P waves "merge" with the QRS complexes.

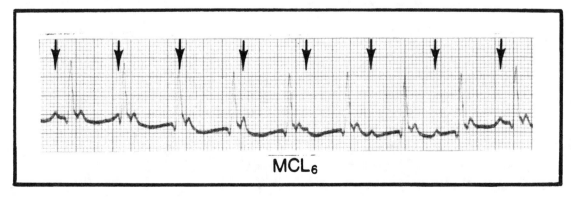

MCL_6

FIGURE 8-17. Acceleration of junctional pacemaker with A-V dissociation in a digitalis toxic patient. The arrows point to the slower sinus P waves "marching through" the QRS complexes.

> The analysis of Figure 8-16 on this page, on the tape, and on page 661 is the solution to Item 3 on the pretest.

Another arrhythmia associated with digitalis toxicity is "bidirectional tachycardia," illustrated in Figure 8-18. This rhythm appears as a regular tachycardia with wide QRS complexes of alternating polarity in some of the leads, and is associated with severe digitalis toxicity. Marriott pointed out that bidirectional tachycardia is a descriptive term with various possible mechanisms.[8-5] There have been numerous studies on the subject of bidirectional tachycardia.[8-6–8-9]

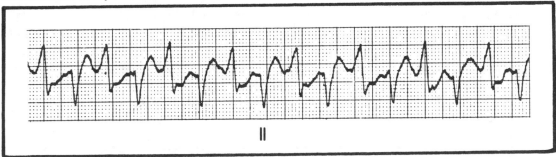

FIGURE 8-18.   Bidirectional tachycardia. (Electrocardiogram reduced in size.)

3.   *Increased Ventricular Irritability or
     Automaticity Leading to:*

a.   *Premature Beats of the Ventricle.* Premature beats of the ventricle are common in digitalis toxicity. When they originate in more than one focus, they are said to be multifocal (often called multiform or multiforme, see page 611), as seen in Figure 8-19. Note the different contours of the premature ventricular contractions. The multifocal origin of these beats is ominous, revealing an irritable heart. The next stages may be ventricular tachycardia, ventricular fibrillation and death.

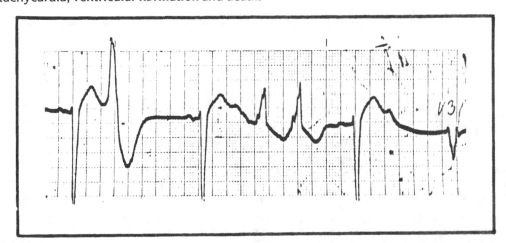

FIGURE 8-19.   Multifocal (multiform or multiforme) premature ventricular contractions. In patients with chronic heart disease and premature ventricular contractions, it may be extremely difficult to decide whether the premature ventricular contractions are secondary to the intrinsic heart disease or to the digitalis. This is also true of the high degree of atrioventricular block discussed at the end of this chapter. You must know your patient. (Electrocardiogram reduced in size.)

b.   *Group Beating (Bigeminy) Due to Alternate Premature Beats of the Ventricle.* When the premature beats of the ventricle are of the same contour in any given lead they are said to be unifocal, from one ventricular focus. Figure 8-20 is from a patient with digitalis toxicity and is an example of bigeminy due to alternate premature beats of the ventricle. Note the fixed interval between the normal beat and the premature beat.

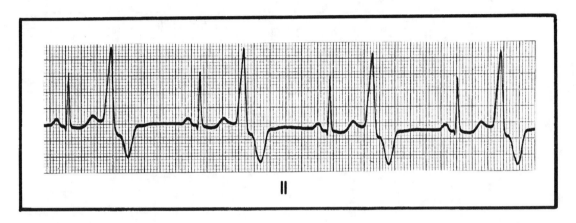

FIGURE 8-20.   *Bigeminy in a digitalis toxic patient. (Electrocardiogram reduced in size.)*

c.   *Ventricular Tachycardia, Flutter, and Fibrillation.* Of great concern is the occurrence of ventricular tachycardia, flutter, and fibrillation associated with digitalis toxicity. Ventricular flutter is not often seen since it tends to be short-lived, deteriorating into ventricular fibrillation, often within seconds. Review the illustrations of ventricular tachycardia, flutter, and fibrillation (pages 562-571), the compensatory pause (pages 604-606), couplets (page 611), salvos (page 612), the R-on-T phenomenon (page 614), and torsades de pointes (page 615).

That physicians, like the rest of mankind, do not learn from history is well illustrated by the electrocardiographic tracings in Figure 8-21. On July 6 the patient arrived, digitalis toxic, with low effective heart rate and alternate premature beats of the ventricle (bigeminy). Digitalis was discontinued and the rate gradually increased until July 11, when digitalis treatment was restarted. On August 2 the patient was back to where he was on July 6. Although this sequence of events occurred decades ago, it is being repeated to this very day.

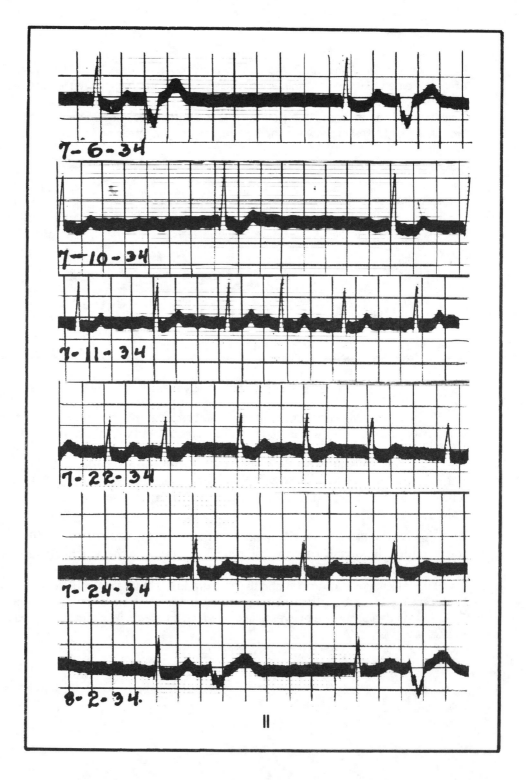

FIGURE 8-21. Patient with atrial fibrillation and digitalis toxicity. (Electrocardiogram enlarged.)

4. *Atrioventricular (A-V) Conduction*
   Disturbances Leading to:

a. *Marked First Degree A-V Block.* As seen earlier (review discussion of digitalis effects on A-V conduction, also Figure 8-4A and B), clinically, an increase in the baseline P-R interval, or advancement to higher degrees of A-V block, has been associated with toxic manifestations of digitalis. This stage should not be missed (Figure 8-22), since it is a step along the path to disaster. An electrocardiographic rhythm tracing, at the very least, should be taken since the pulse rate may not change.

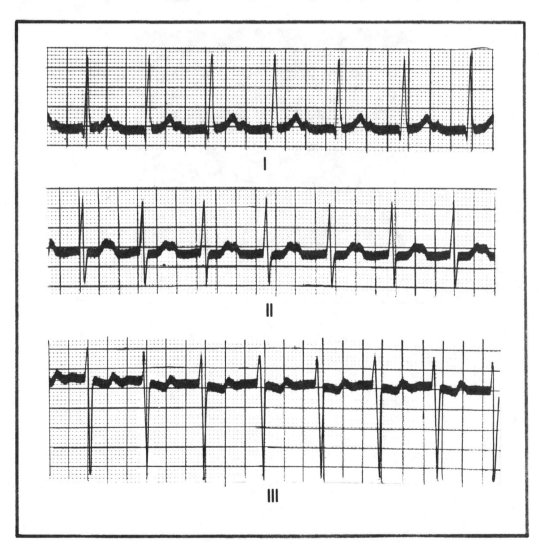

FIGURE 8-22. *Marked first degree A-V block. (Electrocardiogram enlarged.)*

A patient may present with various rhythms during stages of digitalis toxicity. Figure 8-23A and B is from a digitalis toxic patient who had both first degree atrioventricular block and atrial flutter at different times. You must know your patient and have serial electrocardiograms to be sure that the atrial flutter is not merely a coincidental paroxysmal arrhythmia.

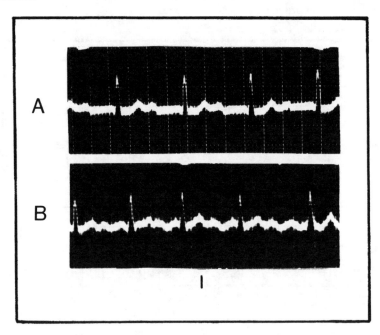

FIGURE 8-23.   First degree A-V block (A) and atrial flutter (B) may be manifestations of digitalis toxicity. (Electrocardiogram enlarged.)

> The analysis of Figure 8-23 on this page, on the tape, and on page 662 is the solution to Item 4 on the pretest.

b. *Second Degree A-V Block.* A form of second degree A-V block is what is known as a Mobitz I block or simply type I A-V block. The rhythm is sinus rhythm with A-V Wenckebach periods. Ventricular beats are "dropped" in a cyclic manner. The P-R interval is less prolonged at first but becomes progressively longer until an atrial contraction no longer initiates a ventricular response. The cycle is then resumed. In Figure 8-24 the first P-R interval is shorter than the second and the third P wave does not conduct (first arrow). The fourth P wave starts the cycle again. The seventh P wave does not conduct (second arrow) and the cycle begins again with the eighth P wave. The block in Wenckebach periods has been shown to be above the bundle of His (by the use of His bundle recordings), in the A-V node. Note that before the "dropped" ventricular beat, as the P-R intervals are progressively prolonged, the R-R intervals shorten.

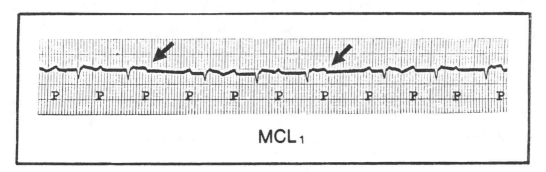

FIGURE 8-24.   Mobitz I (Wenckebach) block. (Electrocardiogram reduced in size).

Figure 8-25 is another example of second degree A-V block. Here only every second P wave conducts through to the ventricle. The ventricular rate is one half the atrial rate.

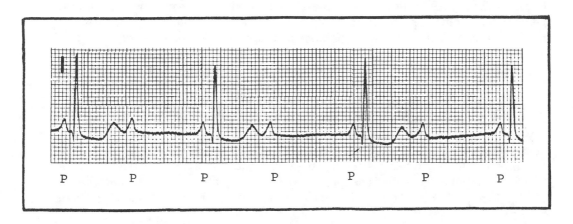

FIGURE 8-25.   Second degree A-V block. The various grades of second degree A-V block are recognized by the frequency and characteristics of blocked atrial conduction. Seen above are two atrial deflections for every ventricular deflection, or 2:1 A-V block. Three and four P waves for every QRS complex are classified as 3:1 and 4:1 A-V block, respectively.

c.   *Third Degree (Complete) A-V Block.* In third degree (complete) A-V block there is no constant relationship between the atria and the usually much slower ventricles. In Figure 8-26 the atria are beating at a rate of approximately 65 per minute and the ventricles at approximately 29 per minute.

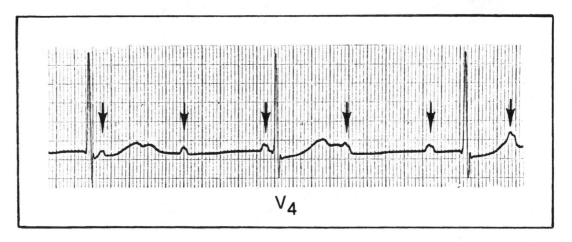

FIGURE 8-26.   Third degree (complete) A-V block. The arrows point to the P waves, which are not related to the QRS complexes.

Figure 8-27 is an example of complete A-V block in a patient with atrial fibrillation.[8-10] The ventricular rate is low, with no clear evidence of atrial activity. The atrial activity is fine fibrillation, with no impulses entering the ventricular conduction system from the atria.

Figures 8-27 to 8-29 illustrate a principle of great importance. When the QRS complexes become regular in the presence of atrial fibrillation in a patient on digitalis, it usually means that complete atrioventricular block has supervened. When the ventricular rate is very low (40 per minute in Figure 8-27 and 37 per minute in Figure 8-28), the physician and the patient would generally become suspicious that all is not well. However, when a junctional rhythm becomes dominant and the regular rate is not very slow (Figure 8-29), the patient may actually feel well in the presence of digitalis toxicity. If the physician examines the patient with a quick pulse check and congratulates himself on the regular rhythm, he may be sending his patient home to disaster. This stage, which already represents significant digitalis toxicity, is tragically common and too often missed. The important principle to remember is that if a patient on digitalis with known atrial fibrillation develops a regular rhythm, it is dangerous to assume, whatever the rate, that the new rhythm is sinus rhythm. At the very least, en electrocardiographic rhythm strip should be inspected.

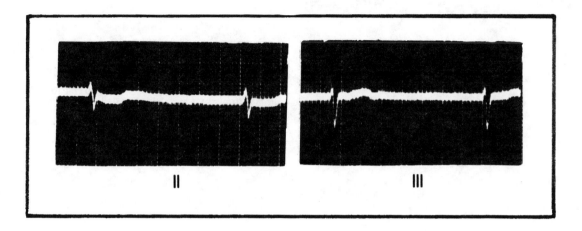

FIGURE 8-27.　Complete A-V block in a patient with atrial fibrillation. (Electrocardiogram enlarged.)

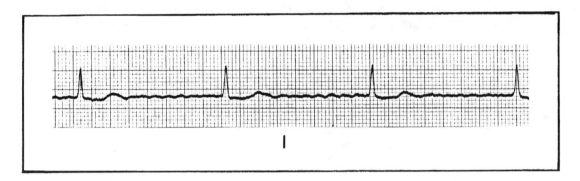

FIGURE 8-28.　Complete A-V block in a patient with atrial fibrillation.

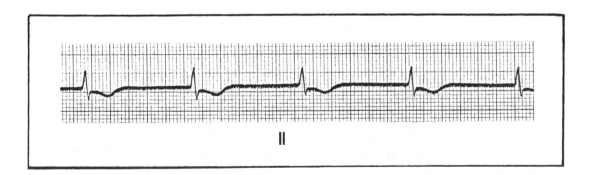

FIGURE 8-29.　Complete A-V block in a patient whose baseline rhythm was atrial fibrillation with an irregular ventricular response.

> The analysis of Figure 8-28 on this page, on the tape, and on page 662 is the solution to Item 5 on the pretest.

> Stop the tape and begin the post-test on the next page.

P O S T - T E S T

DIRECTIONS. Supply the information requested in each of the following.

1. Why might a positive exercise test not be reliable in a patient taking digitalis?

2. Does the prolongation of the P-R interval in a patient taking digitalis represent digitalis "effects" or digitalis "toxicity?"

3. How predictable are the "toxic" responses to digitalis?

4. When is atrial tachycardia frequently due to digitalis "toxicity," and when is it generally *not* due to digitalis "toxicity?"

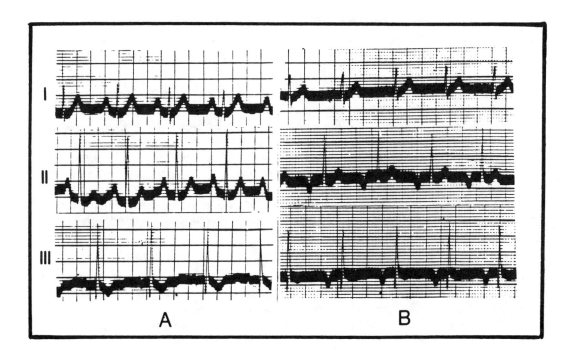

FIGURE 8-15.

5. What electrocardiographic changes have occurred between A and B in a patient taking digitalis? Why are they significant?

> Check your responses on the following pages.

ANSWERS TO
POST-TEST

1. In evaluating exercise tests the ventricular repolarization phase (S-T segment and T wave) is of the utmost importance. Because of the effect of digitalis on this phase and its increased lability, a positive exercise test might not be reliable in these patients.

2. The question has frequently arisen whether prolongation of the P-R interval represents digitalis *effect* or digitalis *toxicity*. In our studies of effect of digitalis on atrioventricular conduction no significant differences were noted in the P-R interval at rest. As the rate of the heart was increased by atrial pacing, however, atrioventricular conduction time was prolonged as an effect of digitalis, resulting in a significant prolongation of the P-R interval. His bundle studies confirmed that the increase was within the interval from the atrial deflection to the His bundle deflection (A-H interval). Clinically, an increase in the baseline P-R interval, or advancement to higher degrees of A-V block, as seen in Figure 8-4A and B, has been associated with *toxic* manifestations of digitalis.

3. The prevalence of digitalis toxicity must be continually emphasized, and both the physician and the patient must be ever watchful—all the more so because toxic manifestations do not necessarily mean that the dose has been changed. The response may be altered by changes in absorption caused by gastrointestinal upset, by electrolyte imbalance due to diuretics, and so forth. Remember also that toxicity may be manifested before any therapeutic effects of digitalis are seen.

   It is not possible to predict accurately which sign or signs of digitalis toxicity a given patient may develop. All the more care is necessary since, not infrequently, a patient may "feel better" while in digitalis toxicity. This has been seen many times, especially when a rapid heart rate is effectively reduced by alternate beats of the ventricle or by alternate sinoatrial block. More than a cursory "How do you feel?" and quick pulse check are necessary in following a patient taking digitalis.

4. Atrial tachycardia *with* atrioventricular block is a common arrhythmia in digitalis toxicity. In fact, atrial tachycardia with atrioventricular block represents digitalis toxicity until proven otherwise (Figure 8-10).

   Atrial tachycardia with 1:1 atrioventricular conduction (no A-V block) is usually *not* due to digitalis toxicity (Figure 8-11). An esophageal lead recording may help establish the diagnosis since P waves are not obvious. Digitalis was used to terminate the tachycardia.

   The paroxysmal tachycardia with 1:1 atrioventricular conduction heralded by premature atrial contractions seen in Figure 8-12 is also unlikely to be due to digitalis toxicity. Digitalis was used to treat the arrhythmia.

5. The rhythm is sinus in A and coronary sinus rhythm (ectopic atrial rhythm) in B. Always beware of a change in rhythm in a digitalized patient; it may be an ominous sign. In Figure 8-15B we see the onset of coronary sinus rhythm without a significant change in heart rate. If the physician checks the pulse rate for 15 seconds and sends the patient on his way, this ectopic rhythm is missed, possibly forfeiting the only chance to detect digitalis toxicity.

ANSWERS TO PRETEST

1. The electrocardiogram may be helpful in following patients taking digitalis. Electro-cardiographically, digitalis effects are mainly seen in the ventricular repolarization phase affecting the S-T segment and the T wave. The "classic" alterations of digitalis are described as a "fist-like" depression of the S-T segment (as if you were placing your fist in the S-T segment and depressing it), as "paintbrush" inscription (as if you were painting the S-T segment with gradual widening of the paintbrush as you approach the S-T segment from the downslope of the R wave), or as "scooping" of the S-T segment. These "classic" changes are well illustrated in Figure 8-3B. Note also that the T wave is less prominent in B.

2. Figure 8-5A and B illustrates an effect of digitalis on atrial fibrillation with a rapid ventricular response. The patient was a 35-year-old man with mitral valve disease who presented with atrial fibrillation and a ventricular rate of approximately 125 beats per minute on an inadequate dose of digitalis. With proper adjustment of the dose the ventricular rate fell to approximately 75 beats per minute.

   Atrial fibrillation with a rapid ventricular response is an excellent arrhythmia for the study of digitalis effects on heart rate. In normal sinus rhythm digitalis does not have much effect on the ventricular rate per se. In atrial fibrillation, most of the atrial impulses are blocked in the A-V conduction system. However, if there are 500 atrial impulses per minute and 1 impulse of every 4 reaches the ventricles, irregularly, the average ventricular rate would be 125 beats per minute. Digitalis acts on the A-V conduction system, allowing fewer impulses to go through, effectively slowing the ventricular rate. In atrial fibrillation (longstanding) the aim with digitalis therapy is not to convert to sinus rhythm, but to slow the ventricular rate.

3. Atrioventricular dissociation due to acceleration of the junctional pacemaker is frequently seen in digitalis toxicity. In Figure 8-16 we see the acceleration of the junctional pacemaker resulting in A-V dissociation in digitalis toxicity. The P waves "merge" with the QRS complexes.

   Review the "nodal" rhythms in Chapter 7. Although we use the term "junctional" rhythm you should be familiar with the terminology of "upper, middle, and lower nodal" rhythms.

4. A patient may present with various rhythms during stages of digitalis toxicity. Figure 8-23A and B is from a digitalis toxic patient who had both first degree atrioventricular block and atrial flutter at different times. You must know your patient and have serial electrocardiograms to be sure that the atrial flutter is not merely a coincidental paroxysmal arrhythmia.

5. When the QRS complexes become regular in the presence of atrial fibrillation in a patient on digitalis, it usually means that complete atrioventricular block has supervened. The patient may actually feel well in the presence of digitalis toxicity. If the physician examines the patient with a quick pulse check and congratulates himself on the regular rhythm, he may be sending his patient home to disaster. This stage, which already represents significant digitalis toxicity, is tragically common and too often missed. The important principle to remember is that if a patient on digitalis with known atrial fibrillation develops a regular rhythm, it is dangerous to assume, whatever the rate, that the new rhythm is sinus rhythm. At the very least, an electrocardiographic rhythm tracing should be inspected.

REFERENCES

8-1. Goodman, L.S., and Gilman, A.: The Pharmacological Basis of Therapeutics, 2nd Ed. New York, Macmillan, 1956, p. 702.

8-2. Goodman, L.S., and Gilman, A.: The Pharmacological Basis of Therapeutics, 2nd Ed. New York, Macmillan, 1956, p. 669.

8-3. Castellanos, A., et al.: Digitalis-indiced arrhythmias: recognition and therapy. Cardiovasc. Clin., *1:*107, 1969.

8-4. Delman, A.J. and Stein, E.: Atrial flutter secondary to digitalis toxicity—report of three cases and review of the literature. Circulation *29:*593, 1964.

8-5. Marriott, H.J.L.: Practical Electrocardiography, 8th Ed. Baltimore, Williams & Wilkins, 1988, p. 485.

8-6. Rosenbaum, M.B., et al.: The mechanism of bidirectional tachycardia. Am. Heart J., *78:*4, 1969.

8-7. Cohen, S.I., et al.: Infra-His origin of bidirectional tachycardia. Circulation, *47:*1260, 1973.

8-8. Morris, S.N., and Zipes, D.P.: His bundle electrocardiography during bidirectional tachycardia. Circulation, *48:*32, 1973.

8-9. Gavrilescu, S., and Luca, C.: His bundle electrogram during bidirectional tachycardia. Br. Heart J., *37:*1198, 1975.

8-10. Kastor, J.A.: Digitalis intoxication in patients with atrial fibrillation. Circulation, *47:*888, 1973.

E P I L O G U E

We have now come to the end of our course. I want to express my thanks to all of you. I have done the best as I saw it to present a clear picture of a frequently misunderstood subject. My aim was clarity of presentation to facilitate understanding, to break through the quagmire of technical terminology, to present the concepts with a few basic rules.

I have had much satisfaction in the excellent grasp of the material among the people who were with us throughout the course. Within the framework of the time, the scope, the group, and the subject, I have tried, to the best of my ability and experience, to shed some light.

It is my hope that you will be stimulated to continue reading electrocardiograms and remain ever ready to add new information to your foundation of knowledge. For your continued self-assessment, a course post-test is provided. The answers are on page 693.

COURSE POST-TEST

DIRECTIONS (Items 1–25): Each of the numbered questions or incomplete statements in the course post-test is followed by answers or by completions of the statement. Select the *ONE* lettered answer or completion that is *BEST* in each case.

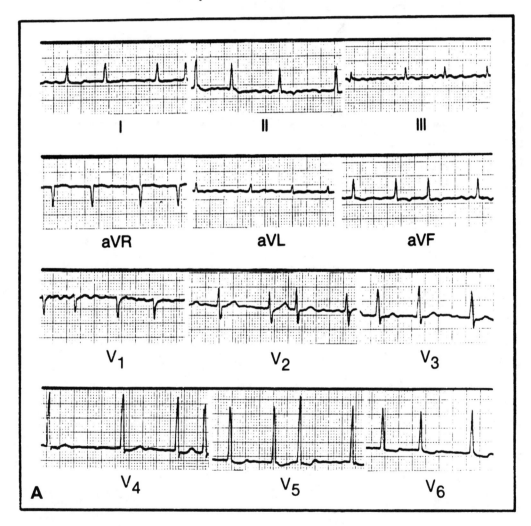

1. This rhythm is:

   A. Atrial standstill
   B. Junctional
   C. Multifocal atrial tachycardia
   D. Atrial fibrillation
   E. Normal sinus rhythm

> Refer to pages 692 and 693 for answers to the course post-test including references.

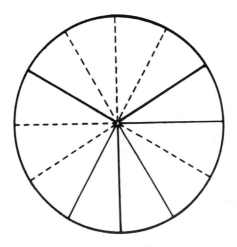

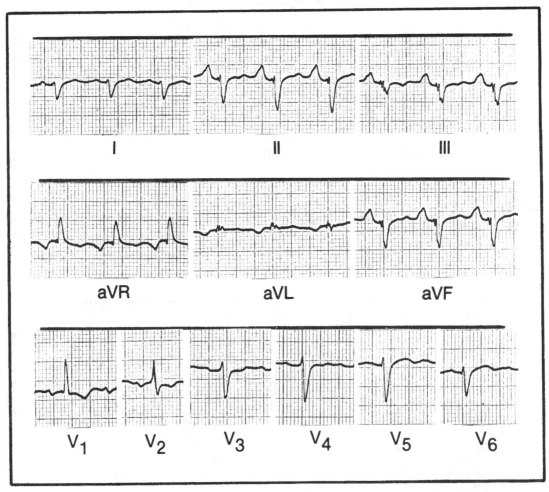

2. The mean electrical axis (mean QRS vector or "axis") is at:

A. −120°
B. −45°
C. 0°
D. 45°
E. 120°

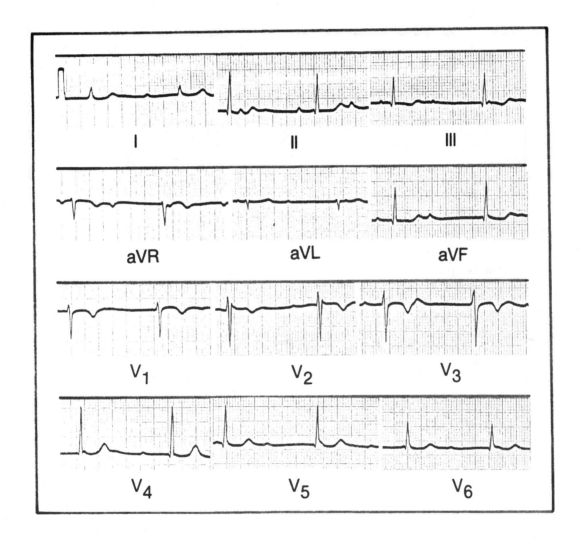

3. This young, asymptomatic patient has:

   A. A normal electrocardiogram
   B. First degree atrioventricular block
   C. Third degree (complete) atrioventricular block
   D. Sinus bradycardia
   E. Atrial tachycardia

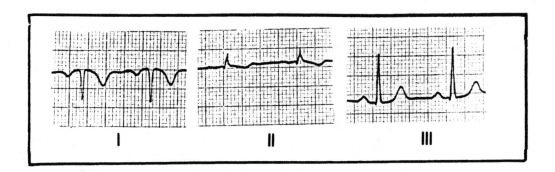

4. The most common cause of this entity is:

   A. Dextrocardia
   B. Sinus arrest
   C. Inferior myocardial infarction
   D. Apical myocardial infarction
   E. Technical error

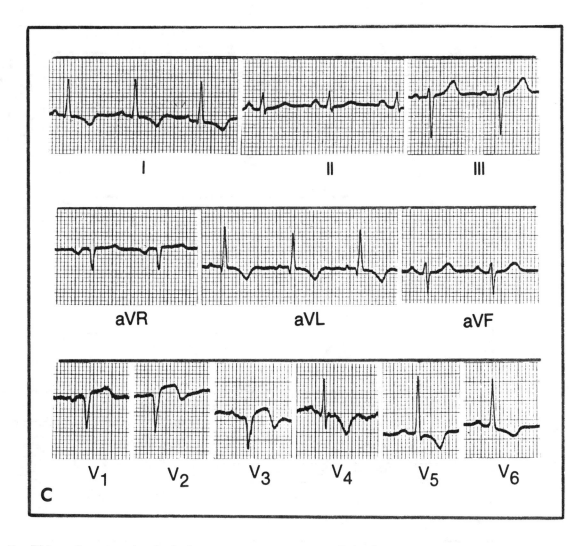

5. This patient sustained a (an) _____ myocardial infarction.

    A. Anterolateral (or lateral)
    B. Diaphragmatic (or inferior)
    C. Apical
    D. Anterior (or anteroseptal)
    E. True posterior

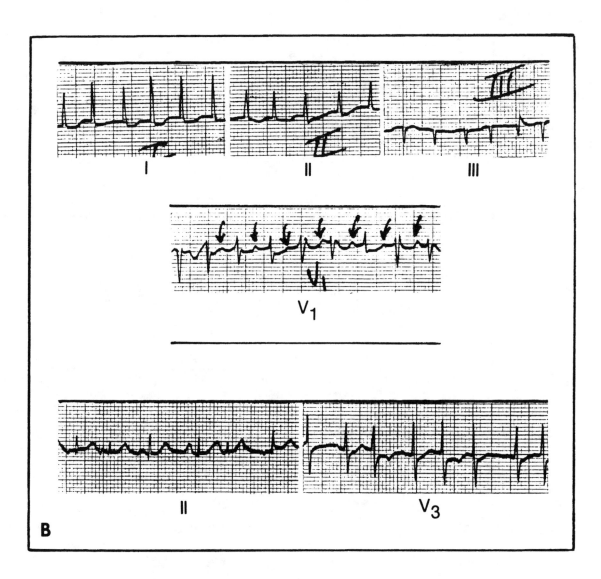

6. This patient has:

   A. Normal sinus rhythm
   B. Junctional rhythm
   C. Atrial standstill
   D. Multifocal atrial tachycardia
   E. Atrial fibrillation

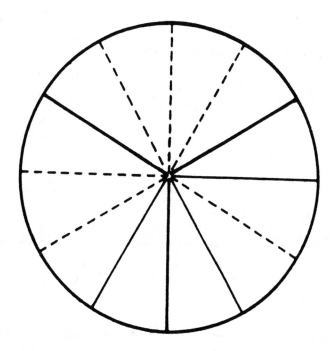

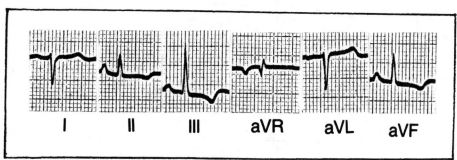

7. The angle formed by the QRS and T waves (QRS-T angle) is:

    A.   0°

    B.   60°

    C.   90°

    D. 120°

    E. 180°

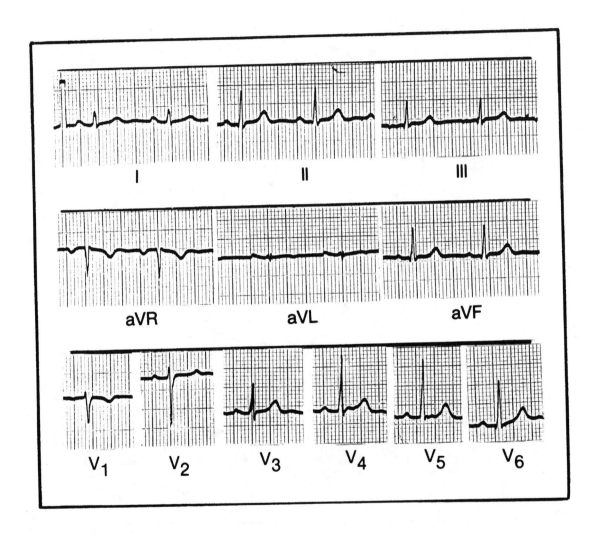

8. Analysis of this electrocardiogram reveals:

   A. Normal sinus rhythm
   B. Junctional rhythm
   C. First degree atrioventricular block
   D. The Wolff-Parkinson-White (W-P-W) syndrome
   E. Reversed arm leads

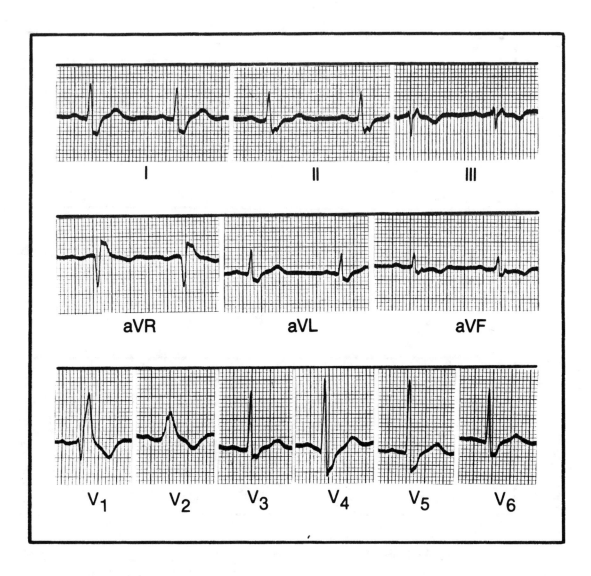

9. Analysis of this electrocardiogram reveals:

    A. Left ventricular hypertrophy
    B. Right ventricular hypertrophy
    C. Left bundle branch block
    D. Right bundle branch block
    E. Sinus tachycardia

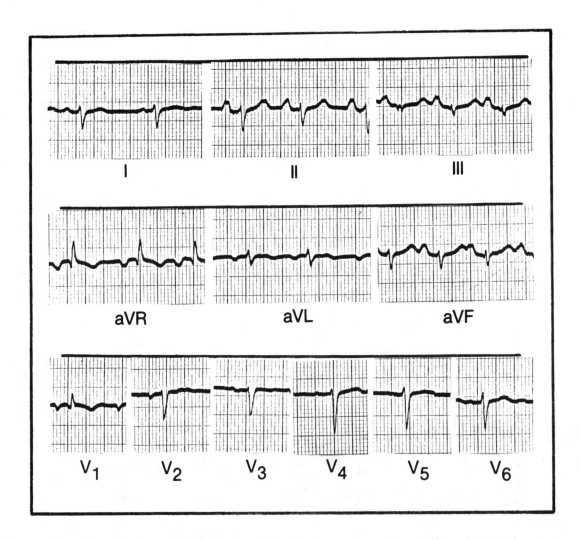

10. This electrocardiogram is from a patient with:

   A. Left ventricular hypertrophy
   B. Chronic lung disease
   C. An anterior (or anteroseptal) myocardial infarction
   D. A normal heart
   E. A diaphragmatic (or inferior) myocardial infarction

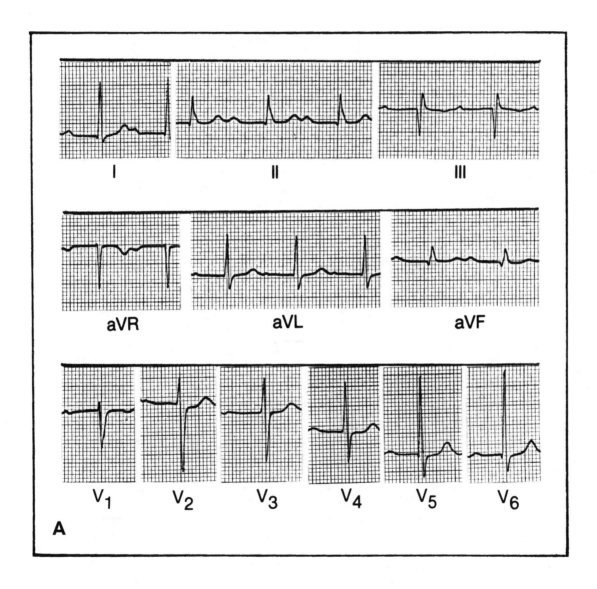

A

11. This patient was found to have:

    A. First degree atrioventricular block
    B. Third degree (complete) atrioventricular block
    C. Sinus tachycardia
    D. Right axis deviation
    E. Junctional rhythm

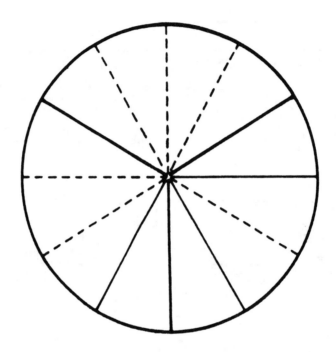

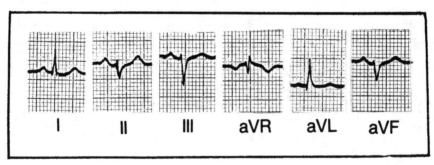

12. The mean electrical axis (mean QRS vector or "axis") is at:

    A. −60°
    B. 0°
    C. 60°
    D. 90°
    E. 120°

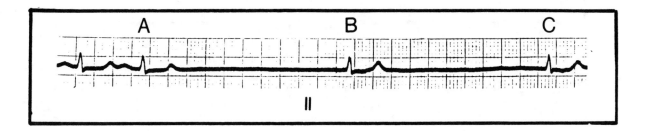

II

13. The pauses between A and B and between B and C are due to:

    A. Sinus bradycardia
    B. Sinus arrest
    C. Sinus arrhythmia
    D. Sinoatrial block
    E. Atrial fibrillation

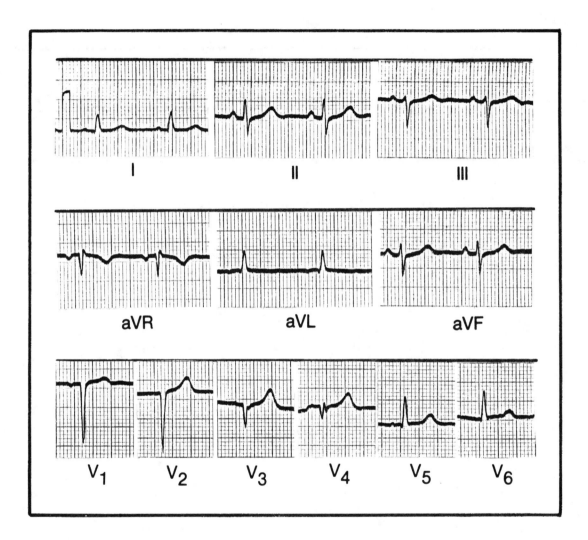

I   II   III

aVR   aVL   aVF

V₁   V₂   V₃   V₄   V₅   V₆

14. This patient sustained a (an) _____ myocardial infarction.

    A. Anterolateral (or lateral)
    B. Diaphragmatic (or inferior)
    C. Apical
    D. Anterior (or anteroseptal)
    E. True posterior

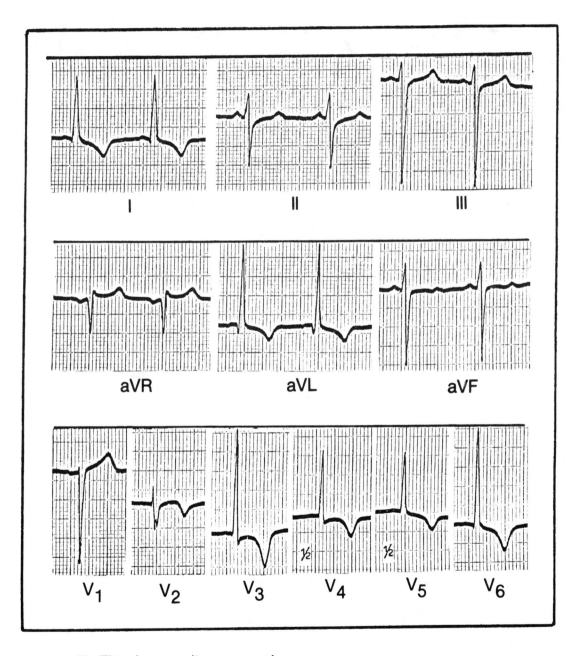

15. This electrocardiogram reveals:

    A. Right ventricular hypertrophy
    B. Left bundle branch block
    C. Junctional rhythm
    D. Right axis deviation
    E. Left ventricular hypertrophy

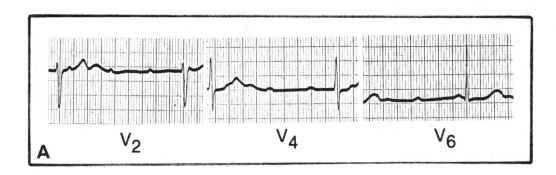

A   V₂   V₄   V₆

16. This electrocardiogram is from a patient with:

    A. Sinus bradycardia
    B. Sinus arrest
    C. Normal sinus rhythm
    D. First degree atrioventricular block
    E. Third degree (complete) atrioventricular block

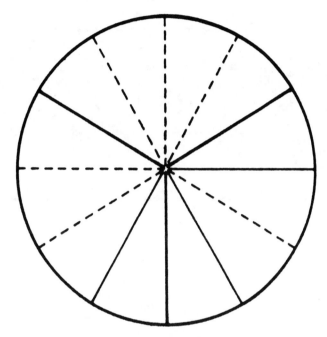

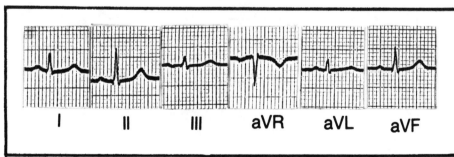

17. The mean electrical axis (mean QRS vector or "axis") is at:

    A. −45°
    B. −5°
    C. 45°
    D. 95°
    E. 120°

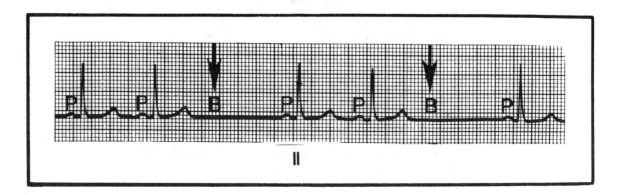

18. The pauses (arrows) are due to:

    A. Sinus bradycardia
    B. Sinus arrest
    C. Sinoatrial block
    D. Venricular fibrillation
    E. Atrial fibrillation

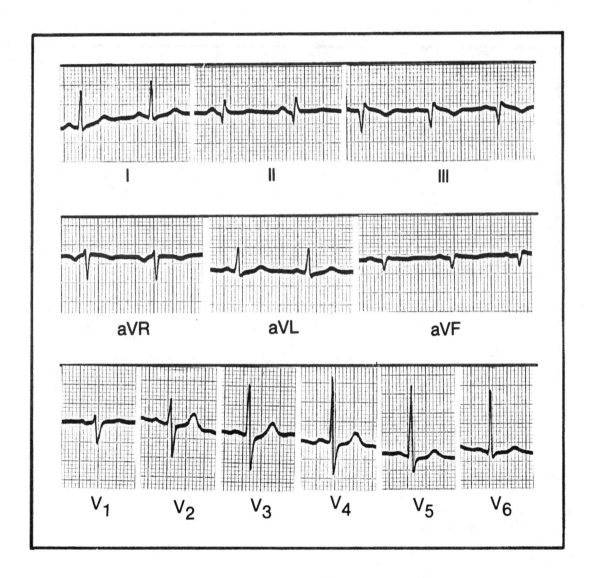

19. This patient sustained a (an) _____ myocardial infarction.

    A. Anterolateral (or lateral)
    B. Diaphragmatic (or inferior)
    C. Apical
    D. Anterior (or anteroseptal)
    E. True posterior

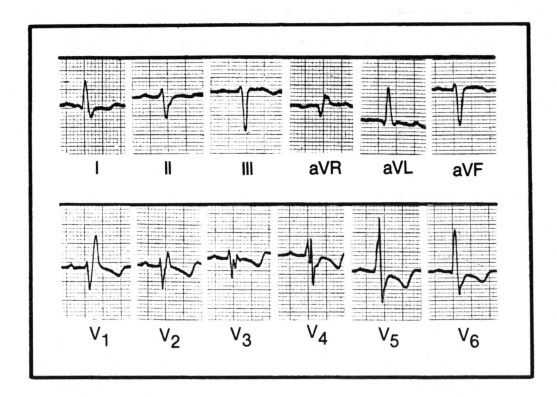

20. Evidence of _____ is present.

    A. Left bundle branch block
    B. Right axis deviation
    C. Bifascicular block
    D. Normal mean electrical axis
    E. Third degree (complete) atrioventricular block

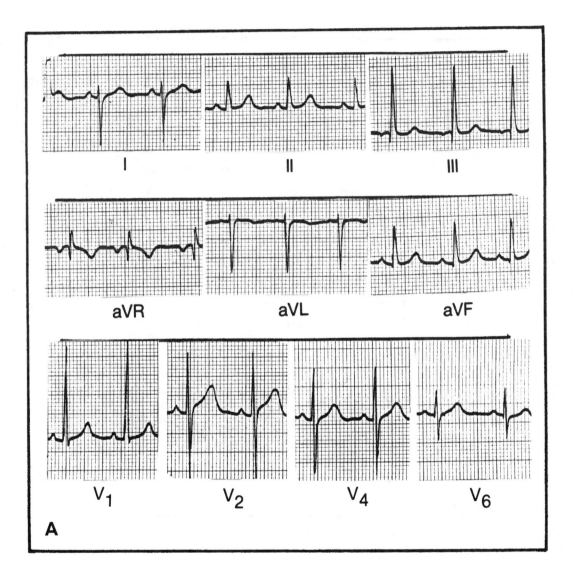

A

21. A child with this electrocardiogram was found to have:

    A. Right ventricular hypertrophy
    B. Left ventricular hypertrophy
    C. Bifascicular block
    D. Right bundle branch block
    E. Left axis deviation

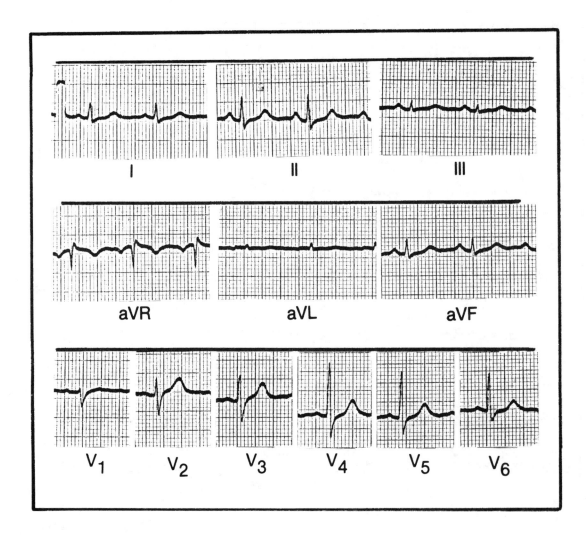

22. Analysis of this electrocardiogram reveals:

   A. Junctional rhythm
   B. Sinus bradycardia
   C. Normal sinus rhythm
   D. Atrial tachycardia
   E. Left ventricular hypertrophy

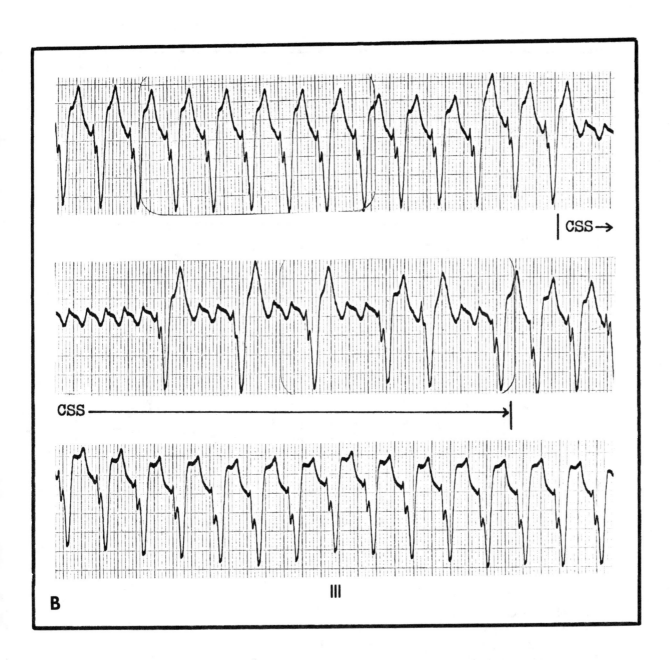

23. Carotid sinus stimulation (CSS) revealed the basic rhythm to be:

    A. Atrial flutter
    B. Normal sinus rhythm
    C. Sinus tachycardia
    D. Sinus arrhythmia
    E. Ventricular tachycardia

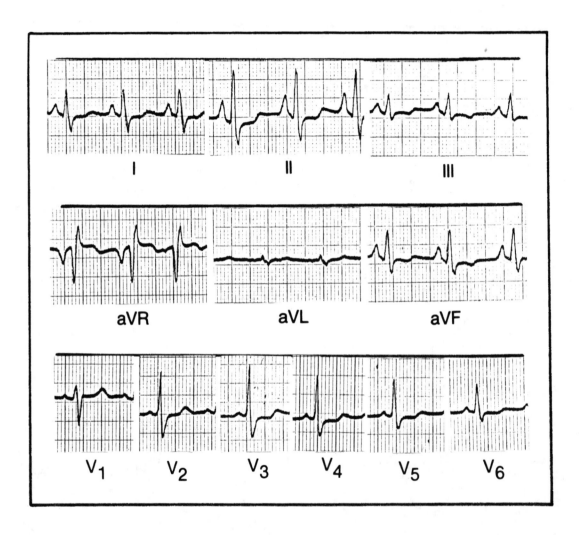

24. Evidence of _____ is present.

    A. Left bundle branch block
    B. Left atrial enlargement
    C. Right atrial enlargement
    D. Left axis deviation
    E. Right axis deviation

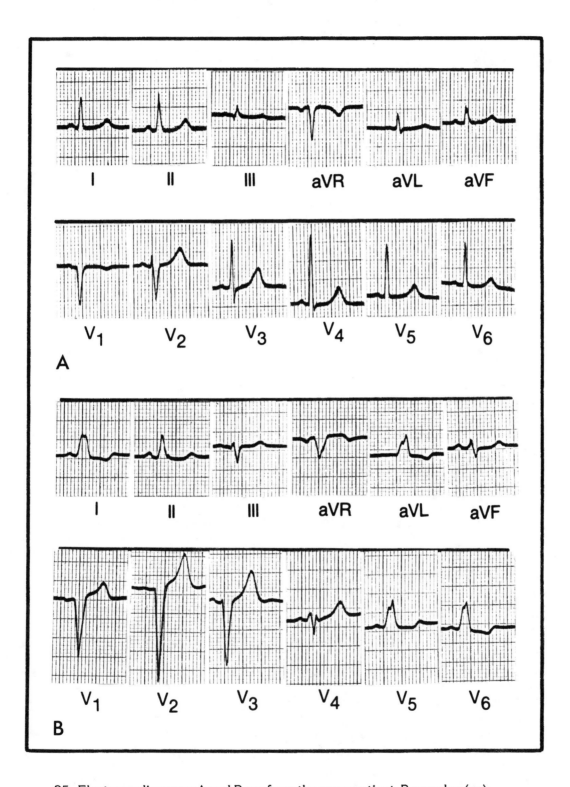

25. Electrocardiograms A and B are from the same patient. B reveals a (an):

    A. Inferior (diaphragmatic) myocardial infarction
    B. Apical myocardial infarction
    C. Lateral myocardial infarction
    D. Left bundle branch block
    E. Anterior myocardial infarction

ELECTROCARDIOGRAPHIC INTERPRETATION: ANSWERS TO COURSE POST-TEST

All referenced pages and figures are in your text/workbook *Electrocardiographic Interpretation.*

1. D.   Atrial fibrillation. Figure 7-22A, page 587.

2. A.   –120°. Figures 1-73 to 1-75, pages 94-95.

3. C.   Third degree (complete) atrioventricular block. Figure 7-48, page 587.

4. E.   Technical error. Figure 1-46A, page 69.

5. D.   Anterior (or anteroseptal). Figure 5-14A to D, pages 344-347.

6. D.   Multifocal atrial tachycardia. Figure 7-22B, page 541.

7. E.   180°. Figure 1-39, page 60.

8. A.   Normal sinus rhythm. Figure 1-77, page 100.

9. D.   Right bundle branch block. Figure 6-4, page 420.

10. B.   Chronic lung disease. Figure 2-21, page 173.

11. A.   First degree atrioventricular block. Figure 7-40A, page 573.

12. A.   –60°. Figure 1-32, page 49.

13. B.   Sinus arrest. Figure 7-9, page 519.

14. D.   Anterior (or anteroseptal). Figure 5-45, page 392.

15. E.   Left ventricular hypertrophy. Figure 3-4, page 211.

16. E.   Third degree (complete) atrioventricular block. Figure 7-44A, page 581.

17. C.   45°. Figure 1-42, page 63.

18. C.   Sinoatrial block. Figure 7-8, page 517.

19. B.   Diaphragmatic (or inferior). Figure 5-32, page 373.

20. C.   Bifascicular block. Figure 6-30, page 453.

21. A.   Right ventricular hypertrophy. Figure 2-7A, page 150.

22. C.   Normal sinus rhythm. Figure 1-80, page 103.

23. A.   Atrial flutter. Figures 7-21A to C, pages 535-537.

24. C.   Right atrial enlargement. Figure 2-16, page 162.

25. D.   Left bundle branch block. Figure 6-14, page 432.

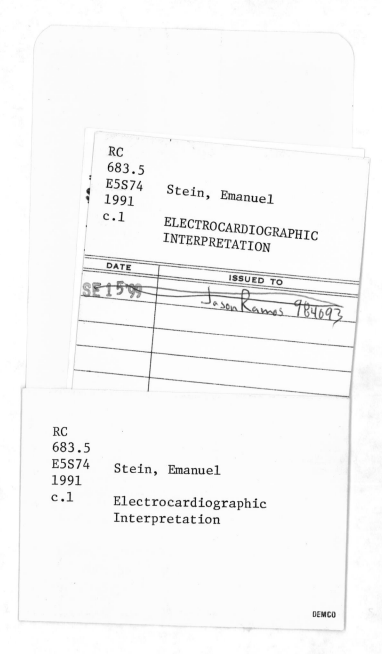